New Trends in the Treatment of Sarcoma

Editors

ANDREA S. PORPIGLIA
JEFFREY M. FARMA

SURGICAL CLINICS
OF NORTH AMERICA

www.surgical.theclinics.com

Consulting Editor
RONALD F. MARTIN

October 2016 • Volume 96 • Number 5

ELSEVIER

1600 John F. Kennedy Boulevard ● Suite 1800 ● Philadelphia, Pennsylvania, 19103-2899

http://www.surgical.theclinics.com

SURGICAL CLINICS OF NORTH AMERICA Volume 96, Number 5
October 2016 ISSN 0039–6109, ISBN-13: 978-0-323-46337-9

Editor: John Vassallo, j.vassallo@elsevier.com

Developmental Editor: Colleen Viola

Surgical Clinics of North America (ISSN 0039–6109) is published bimonthly by Elsevier Inc., 360 Park Avenue South, New York, NY 10010-1710. Months of publication are February, April, June, August, October, and December. Business and Editorial Offices: 1600 John F. Kennedy Blvd., Suite 1800, Philadelphia, PA 19103-2899. Periodicals postage paid at New York, NY and additional mailing offices. Subscription prices are $375.00 per year for US individuals, $707.00 per year for US institutions, $100.00 per year for US students and residents, $455.00 per year for Canadian individuals, $895.00 per year for Canadian institutions, $510.00 for international individuals, $895.00 per year for international institutions and $250.00 per year for Canadian and foreign students/residents. To receive student/resident rate, orders must be accompanied by name of affiliated institution, date of term, and the *signature* of program/residency coordinator on institution letterhead. Orders will be billed at individual rate until proof of status is received. Foreign air speed delivery is included in all *Clinics* subscription prices. All prices are subject to change without notice. POSTMASTER: Send address changes to *Surgical Clinics*, Elsevier Health Sciences Division, Subscription Customer Service, 3251 Riverport Lane, Maryland Heights, MO 63043. **Customer Service (orders, claims, online, change of address): Telephone: 1-800-654-2452 (U.S. and Canada); 314-447-8871 (outside U.S. and Canada). Fax: 314-447-8029. E-mail: journalscustomerservice-usa@elsevier.com (for print support); journalsonline support-usa@elsevier.com (for online support)**.

Reprints. For copies of 100 or more, of articles in this publication, please contact the Commercial Reprints Department, Elsevier Inc., 360 Park Avenue South, New York, New York 10010-1710. Tel. 212-633-3874, Fax: 212-633-3820, E-mail: reprints@elsevier.com.

The *Surgical Clinics of North America* is also published in Spanish by McGraw-Hill Interamericana Editores S.A., P.O. Box 5-237 06500 Mexico D.F. Mexico; and in Portuguese by Interlivros Edicoes Ltda., Rua Comandante Coelho 1085, CEP 21250, Rio de Janeiro, Brazil; and in Greek by Paschalidis Medical Publications, Athens Greece.

The *Surgical Clinics of North America* is covered in *MEDLINE/PubMed (Index Medicus)*, *EMBASE/Excerpta Medica*, *Current Contents/Clinical Medicine*, *Current Contents/Life Sciences*, *Science Citation Index*, and *ISI/BIOMED*.

Contributors

CONSULTING EDITOR

RONALD F. MARTIN, MD, FACS
Colonel (ret.), United States Army Reserve York Hospital, York, Maine

EDITORS

ANDREA S. PORPIGLIA, MD, MS
Surgical Oncologist, Department of Surgery, Crozer Keystone Health Network, Drexel Hill, Pennsylvania

JEFFREY M. FARMA, MD, FACS
Associate Professor, Department of Surgical Oncology, Fox Chase Cancer Center, Philadelphia, Pennsylvania

AUTHORS

JOHN A. ABRAHAM, MD, FACS
Associate Professor of Orthopedic Surgery and Radiation Oncology and Director of Sarcoma and Bone Tumor Center, Sidney Kimmel Cancer Center at Thomas Jefferson University Hospital; Chief, Orthopedic Oncology, Rothman Institute; Consultant Orthopedic Oncology Surgeon, Fox Chase Cancer Center, Philadelphia, Pennsylvania

ATRAYEE BASU-MALLICK, MD
Clinical Assistant Professor of Medical Oncology, Sarcoma and Bone Tumor Center, Sidney Kimmel Cancer Center at Thomas Jefferson University Hospital, Philadelphia, Pennsylvania

MARILYN M. BUI, MD, PhD
Department of Anatomic Pathology, H. Lee Moffitt Cancer Center & Research Institute; Department of Pathology and Cell Biology, University of South Florida Morsani College of Medicine, Tampa, Florida

JAMIE T. CARACCIOLO, MD, MBA
Associate Member and Section Head, Musculoskeletal Imaging, Department of Diagnostic Imaging, Moffitt Cancer Center; Associate Professor, Departments of Radiology and Orthopedics/Sports Medicine, University of South Florida Morsani College of Medicine, Tampa, Florida

AIMEE M. CRAGO, MD, PhD, FACS
Assistant Attending Surgeon, Sarcoma Disease Management Team, Department of Surgery, Memorial Sloan Kettering Cancer Center; Department of Surgery, Weill Cornell Medical College, New York, New York

JEREMIAH L. DENEVE, DO, FACS
Department of Surgery; Assistant Professor of Surgery, Division of Surgical Oncology, University of Tennessee Health Science Center, Memphis, Tennessee

MARK FAIRWEATHER, MD
Department of Surgery, Brigham and Women's Hospital, Boston, Massachusetts

JEFFREY M. FARMA, MD, FACS
Associate Professor, Department of Surgical Oncology, Fox Chase Cancer Center, Philadelphia, Pennsylvania

ISRAEL FERNANDEZ-PINEDA, MD
Assistant Member, Department of Surgery, St Jude Children's Research Hospital, Memphis, Tennessee

THOMAS J. GALLOWAY, MD
Department of Radiation Oncology, Fox Chase Cancer Center, Philadelphia, Pennsylvania

JULIE GIBBS, MD
Department of Pathology and Cell Biology, University of South Florida Morsani College of Medicine, Tampa, Florida

RICARDO J. GONZALEZ, MD, FACS
Chair, Sarcoma Department, H. Lee Moffitt Cancer Center, Tampa, Florida

ANKUSH GOSAIN, MD, PhD
Associate Professor, Department of Surgery, University of Tennessee Health Science Center, Memphis, Tennessee

VALERIE P. GRIGNOL, MD
Division of Surgical Oncology, Fellow, Department of Surgery, The Ohio State University, Columbus, Ohio

WHITNEY M. GUERRERO, MD
Department of Surgery, University of Tennessee Health Science Center, Memphis, Tennessee

CHRISTINA J. GUTOWSKI, MD
Chief Resident, Orthopedic Surgery, Thomas Jefferson University Hospital, Philadelphia, Pennsylvania

EVITA HENDERSON-JACKSON, MD
Department of Anatomic Pathology, H. Lee Moffitt Cancer Center & Research Institute; Department of Pathology and Cell Biology, University of South Florida Morsani College of Medicine, Tampa, Florida

JOHN HARRISON HOWARD, MD
Division of Surgical Oncology, Assistant Professor, Department of Surgery, The Ohio State University, Columbus, Ohio

CARY HSU, MD
Assistant Professor, Department of Surgery, Baylor College of Medicine, Houston, Texas

JANE Y.C. HUI, MD, MSc, FRCSC
Assistant Professor, Division of Surgical Oncology, Department of Surgery, University of Minnesota, Minneapolis, Minnesota

STEVEN C. KATZ, MD, FACS
Department of Surgery, Roger Williams Medical Center, Providence, Rhode Island;
Department of Surgery, Boston University School of Medicine, Boston, Massachusetts

EMILY Z. KEUNG, MD
Department of Surgery, Brigham and Women's Hospital, Boston, Massachusetts

BROOKE K. LEACHMAN, MD
Department of Radiation Oncology, Fox Chase Cancer Center, Philadelphia, Pennsylvania

ANN Y. LEE, MD
Fellow, Complex Surgical Oncology, Sarcoma Disease Management Team, Department of Surgery, Memorial Sloan Kettering Cancer Center, New York, New York

G. DOUGLAS LETSON, MD
Professor, Departments of Radiology, Orthopedics/Sports Medicine, University of South Florida Morsani College of Medicine; Executive Vice President, Physician-in-Chief, Moffitt Cancer Center; Professor, Department of Surgery, University of South Florida Morsani College of Medicine, Tampa, Florida

SUSAN A. McCLOSKEY, MD
Assistant Clinical Professor, Department of Radiation Oncology, University of California, Los Angeles, Los Angeles, California

SUJANA MOVVA, MD
Associate professor, Department of Hematology/Oncology, Fox Chase Cancer Center, Philadelphia, Pennsylvania

JOHN E. MULLINAX, MD
Instructor, Sarcoma Department, H. Lee Moffitt Cancer Center, Tampa, Florida

PARVIN F. PEDDI, MD
Assistant Clinical Professor, Division of Hematology & Oncology, Department of Medicine, University of California, Los Angeles, Los Angeles, California

RAPHAEL POLLOCK, MD, PhD
Division of Surgical Oncology, Professor, Department of Surgery, The Ohio State University, Columbus, Ohio

ANDREA S. PORPIGLIA, MD, MS
Surgical Oncologist, Department of Surgery, Crozer Keystone Health Network, Drexel Hill, Pennsylvania

CHANDRAJIT P. RAUT, MD, MSc
Department of Surgery, Brigham and Women's Hospital; Center for Sarcoma and Bone Oncology, Dana-Farber Cancer Institute, Boston, Massachusetts

SANJAY S. REDDY, MD
Assistant Professor, Fox Chase Cancer Center, Philadelphia, Pennsylvania

JEFFREY REHA, MD, FACS
Department of Surgery, Roger Williams Medical Center, Providence, Rhode Island

JENNIFER Y. SHENG, MD
Fellow, Department of Oncology, Sidney Kimmel Comprehensive Cancer Center, Johns Hopkins University School of Medicine, Baltimore, Maryland

MARGARET VON MEHREN, MD
Professor of Medical Oncology, Director, Sarcoma Oncology, Associate Director of Clinical Research, Fox Chase Cancer Center, Philadelphia, Pennsylvania

REGAN F. WILLIAMS, MD
Assistant Professor, Department of Surgery, University of Tennessee Health Science Center, Memphis, Tennessee

Contents

> Sarcomas are rare malignancies of mesenchymal origin and are broadly divided into soft tissue sarcomas and bone sarcomas. The etiology of these tumors is largely unknown, and most sarcomas are sporadic. A small subset of sarcomas is associated with certain genetic syndromes and environmental factors. Ionizing radiation is the strongest environmental factor linked to sarcoma development.

> Soft tissue and bone tumors are a heterogeneous group of tumors most often classified according to the type of tissue they most closely histologically resemble. Although sarcomas are rare, greater than 100 histologic subtypes of benign and malignant soft tissue and bone tumors are currently recognized. In this article, the authors review the current pathologic definitions, the classification and grading systems, supportive ancillary techniques, and the prognostic implications for some of the more common soft tissue and bone tumors.

> Diagnostic imaging plays an important role in evaluation and treatment planning of patients with musculoskeletal tumors. This article discusses various imaging modalities available in the work-up, staging, and surveillance of patients with primary bone and soft tissue neoplasms. A systematic approach to initial evaluation of newly suspected bone lesions and soft tissue masses is presented. Reviewed are relevant imaging features of musculoskeletal neoplasms that help predict tumor biology and risk of malignancy and findings that define internal tumor composition and allow for accurate preoperative histopathologic diagnosis before intervention. Finally, the role of diagnostic imaging in tumor staging, evaluation of response to neoadjuvant therapy, and postoperative surveillance is discussed.

Dermatofibrosarcoma protuberans (DFSP) is a rare superficial soft tissue sarcoma. Its rarity precludes large prospective studies. Clinical diagnosis requires an high index of suspicion. Effective management requires an appreciation of tumor biology and the nature of the characteristic infiltrative growth pattern. DFSP tends to recur locally, with a low risk of dissemination. Aggressive surgical resection with widely negative margins is essential to management. Radiotherapy may be indicated in special circumstances. Understanding the molecular pathogenesis has resulted in use of tyrosine kinase inhibitor therapy for patients with locally advanced disease or in metastatic disease. DFSP patients require long-term follow-up.

Breast sarcomas are exceptionally rare mesenchymal neoplasms composed of many histologic subtypes. Therapy is guided by principles established in the management of extremity sarcomas. The anatomic site does influence treatment decisions, particularly the surgical management. Surgery should be undertaken with the aim of achieving a widely negative margin. Selected patients can be managed with breast-conserving surgery. Breast reconstruction is increasingly being undertaken for selected patients. Radiation therapy and chemotherapy are used selectively for large, high-grade sarcomas for which there is significant concern for local and distant recurrence.

Gastrointestinal stromal tumors had the reputation for poor outcomes because of their lack of response to nonsurgical interventions. The discovery of gain-of-function mutations involving receptor tyrosine kinase growth factor receptors altered the biological understanding and management. Beginning in 2000, management of these tumors has changed dramatically because of the availability of tyrosine kinase inhibitors. The role of surgery continues to be refined. This article reviews how surgery and systemic therapy are being used, incorporating definitions of risk. Decisions on how to treat a patient is based on the risk of progression, pathologic characteristics, and tumor location.

Treatment of bone sarcoma requires careful planning and involvement of an experienced multidisciplinary team. Significant advancements in systemic therapy, radiation, and surgery in recent years have contributed to improved functional and survival outcomes for patients with these difficult tumors, and emerging technologies hold promise for further advancement.

Pediatric sarcomas are a heterogeneous group of tumors accounting for approximately 10% of childhood solid tumors. Treatment is focused on multimodality therapy, which has improved the prognosis over the past two decades. Current regimens focus on decreasing treatment for low-risk patients to decrease the long-term side effects while maximizing therapy for patients with metastatic disease to improve survival. Pediatric sarcomas can be divided into soft tissue sarcomas and osseous tumors. Soft tissue sarcomas are further delineated into rhabdomyosarcomas, which affect young children and nonrhabdomyosarcomas, which are most common in adolescents. The most common bone sarcomas are osteosarcomas and Ewing's sarcoma.

Although there is no consensus regarding the optimal sequencing of external beam radiotherapy and surgery for extremity soft tissue sarcoma, radiation therapy delivered before or after limb-sparing surgery significantly improves local control, particularly for high-grade tumors. Large database analyses suggest that improved local control may translate into an overall survival benefit. Best practices require ample communication between the radiation and surgical teams to ensure appropriate tissues are targeted, unnecessary radiation is avoided, and patients are afforded the best opportunity for cure while maintaining function. Modern experiences with intensity-modulated radiotherapy/image-guided radiation therapy suggest toxicity is reduced through field size reduction and precise targeting, improving the therapeutic ratio.

Soft tissue sarcomas are rare tumors that present with distant metastasis in up to 10% of patients. Survival has improved significantly because of advancements in histologic classification and improved management approaches. Older agents such as doxorubicin, ifosfamide, gemcitabine, and paclitaxel continue to demonstrate objective response rates from 18% to 25%. Newer agents such as trabectedin, eribulin, aldoxorubicin, and olaratumab have demonstrated improvements in progression-free survival, overall survival, or toxicity profiles. Future studies on treatment of advanced soft tissue sarcoma will continue to concentrate on reducing toxicity, personalization of therapy, and targeting novel pathways.

The management of recurrent soft tissue sarcoma is a challenging problem for clinicians and has a significant physical, mental, emotional, and oncologic impact for the patient. Despite excellent limb-preservation therapies, approximately one-quarter of patients may eventually develop recurrence of disease. How to most appropriately manage these patients is a matter of debate. Several treatment options exist, including surgical resection, irradiation, systemic chemotherapy, amputation, and regional therapies. This article highlights the management of recurrent extremity soft tissue sarcoma.

Emily Z. Keung, Mark Fairweather, and Chandrajit P. Raut

Sarcomas are rare cancers of mesenchymal cell origin that include many histologic subtypes and molecularly distinct entities. For primary resectable sarcoma, surgery is the mainstay of treatment. Despite treatment, approximately 50% of patients with soft tissue sarcoma are diagnosed with or develop distant metastases, significantly affecting their survival. Although systemic therapy with conventional chemotherapy remains the primary treatment modality for those with metastatic sarcoma, increased survival has been achieved in select patients who receive multimodality therapy, including surgery, for their metastatic disease. This article provides an overview of the literature on surgical management of pulmonary and hepatic sarcoma metastases.

SURGICAL CLINICS
OF NORTH AMERICA

FORTHCOMING ISSUES

December 2016
Pancreatic Cancer and Periampullary
Neoplasms
Jeffrey M. Hardacre, *Editor*

February 2017
Emergency Pediatric Surgery
Todd A. Ponsky and Aaron P. Garrison,
Editors

April 2017
Gastric Neoplasms
Douglas S. Tyler and Kelly Olino, *Editors*

RECENT ISSUES

August 2016
Metabolic and Bariatric Surgery
Adrian G. Dan, *Editor*

June 2016
Practical Urology for the General Surgeon
Lisa T. Beaule and Moritz H. Hansen,
Editors

April 2016
Technical Aspects of Oncologic Hepatic
Surgery
Clifford S. Cho, *Editor*

February 2016
Development of a Surgeon: Medical School
through Retirement
Ronald F. Martin and Paul J. Schenarts,
Editors

ISSUE OF RELATED INTEREST

Surgical Oncology Clinics, October 2016 (Vol. 25, Issue 4)
Contemporary Management and Controversies of Sarcoma
Chandrajit P. Raut, *Editor*
Available at: www.surgonc.theclinics.com

THE CLINICS ARE AVAILABLE ONLINE!
Access your subscription at:
www.theclinics.com

Foreword

Sarcoma

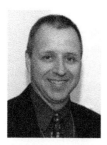

Ronald F. Martin, MD, FACS
Consulting Editor

One of the recurrent themes in the *Surgical Clinics of North America* is what "belongs" to General Surgery and what "belongs" to subspecialty care. Of course, the answer to that is not black and white under the best of circumstances. Some aspects of care are clear and consistent as to who best deals with what, while others aren't so obvious. The care of patients with sarcoma may be a good candidate for the poster child of how to confuse us on these questions. I think that even a casual reading of this issue on the management and treatment of sarcoma would convince even the most strident isolationist that successful care of patients with sarcoma is absolutely dependent on a team-based array of specialties and sometimes specialties within specialties.

This issue very well describes a wide arc of what should be known about sarcoma from epidemiology and biology to all the various types of treatment. The concept of well-managed teams is resonant throughout the issue. It also seems clear that improved outcomes are a direct result of the appropriate timing and combination of operative and nonoperative management.

Varying clinical environments have widely variable access to all the specialties required as well as all the levels of expertise within those specialties. Having centers with all the optimal elements is an exceptional benefit to our communities. However, not every patient who presents with a sarcoma knows that when they seek care; so the vast majority of people are seen in care delivery environments that don't have all the bells and whistles. For that reason above all else, every general surgeon—no matter whether she/he thinks she/he will ever attempt to deliver definitive sarcoma care—needs to be fully aware of how to get started when the question of sarcoma is raised and to get the patient to an environment where uncompromised care can take place.

In most places I have worked, I have seen a progressive narrowing of spectrum of comfort level among providers; though to be fair, it is frequently accompanied by an increase in comfort level within that narrower spectrum. There are also increased pressures to keep patients within narrow networks and to ask for additional expertise from certain centers that may be as much, if not more, influenced by their financial

Surg Clin N Am 96 (2016) xiii–xiv
http://dx.doi.org/10.1016/j.suc.2016.07.017
0039-6109/16/© 2016 Published by Elsevier Inc.

surgical.theclinics.com

relationships than their clinical qualifications. We all need to be mindful of the long-term unintended consequences of early missteps in the care of these patients.

Dr Porpiglia, Dr Farma, and their colleagues have put together an excellent collection of reviews that will well help anybody navigate safely through the initial and subsequent more complicated care of patients with sarcoma. We are deeply grateful for their efforts.

Ronald F. Martin, MD, FACS
Colonel (ret.), United States Army Reserve
York Hospital
16 Hospital Drive, Suite A
York, ME 03909, USA

E-mail address:
rmartin@yorkhospital.com

Preface

Current Treatment of Sarcomas

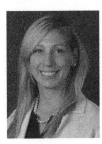 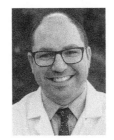

Andrea S. Porpiglia, MD, MS   Jeffrey M. Farma, MD, FACS
Editors

Surgical oncologists face increasing challenges when confronted with treating patients with sarcomas. These are a rare, heterogeneous group of tumors that encompasses over a hundred different histologic subtypes. Sarcomas can present anywhere in the body and affect all age groups. They can be locally aggressive, posing surgical challenges in treatment. Historically, surgery was the mainstay of therapy for most sarcomas. However, through research and clinical trials, radiation and chemotherapy have been incorporated into the treatment algorithm. Furthermore, treatment of these tumors involves a multidisciplinary team approach. In addition, there is much more that needs to be discovered through research and clinical trials to improve outcomes.

The purpose of this issue of *Surgical Clinics of North America* is to provide an up-to-date, multidisciplinary overview of extremity sarcomas, retroperitoneal sarcomas, gastrointestinal stromal tumors, bone sarcomas, and pediatric tumors and to discuss the epidemiology, pathology, and current evidence-based treatment options for patients with these different types of sarcomas. In addition, the issue reviews treatment of recurrent and metastatic sarcomas.

We greatly appreciate the efforts of our nationally recognized sarcoma expert contributing authors, for their time dedicated, experience, and knowledge. We hope

Surg Clin N Am 96 (2016) xv–xvi
http://dx.doi.org/10.1016/j.suc.2016.07.015
0039-6109/16/© 2016 Published by Elsevier Inc.

surgical.theclinics.com

to provide helpful, relevant information for surgeons who may encounter these tumors in hopes of improving knowledge on how we treat sarcoma patients.

It has been a privilege and an honor to be guest editors of this issue.

Andrea S. Porpiglia, MD, MS
Department of Surgery
Crozer Keystone Health Network
2100 Keystone Avenue
1st Floor MOB
Drexel Hill, PA 19026, USA

Jeffrey M. Farma, MD, FACS
Department of Surgical Oncology
Fox Chase Cancer Center
333 Cottman Avenue
Philadelphia, PA 19111, USA

E-mail addresses:
Andrea.porpiglia@crozer.org (A.S. Porpiglia)
Jeffrey.farma@fccc.edu (J.M. Farma)

Epidemiology and Etiology of Sarcomas

Jane Y.C. Hui, MD, MSc, FRCSC

KEYWORDS

• Sarcoma • Epidemiology • Etiology • Li-Fraumeni • Radiation

KEY POINTS

- Sarcomas are rare malignant tumors of mesenchymal origin, accounting for less than 1% of all new cancer diagnoses.
- The extremity (particularly the thigh) is the most common location for soft tissue sarcoma. Bone sarcomas are rare and are more commonly seen in the pediatric population.
- Most sarcomas are sporadic and idiopathic, with no associated inherited genetic defect or environmental factor identified as the cause.
- Genetic syndromes associated with sarcoma development include Li-Fraumeni syndrome, retinoblastoma, neurofibromatosis type 1, and familial adenomatous polyposis syndrome.
- Ionizing radiation is strongly linked to subsequent development of bone sarcoma and soft tissue sarcoma. In cases of prior radiation therapy, the secondary sarcoma develops within the radiation field.

INTRODUCTION

Sarcomas make up a broad group of malignant neoplasms of mesenchymal origin. More than 70 histologic subtypes have been identified. However, sarcomas can be classified into 2 broad categories: (1) soft tissue sarcomas (STS), and (2) sarcomas of the bone. In the former group, sarcomas that have histologic resemblance to fat, muscle, nerve sheath, and blood vessels are included and are named accordingly.

EPIDEMIOLOGY

Sarcomas are rare, making up less than 1% of all new cancer diagnoses. There will have been an estimated 1.66 million new cancer diagnoses in 2015 in the United States, of which, only 11,930 cases will have been STS, and 2970 cases, bone sarcomas.[1]

Disclosure: Dr J. Hui has no commercial or financial conflicts of interest or any funding sources.
Division of Surgical Oncology, Department of Surgery, University of Minnesota, 420 Delaware Street Southeast, Mayo Mail Code 195, Minneapolis, MN 55455, USA
E-mail address: jhui@umn.edu

Surg Clin N Am 96 (2016) 901–914
http://dx.doi.org/10.1016/j.suc.2016.05.005
0039-6109/16/$ – see front matter © 2016 Elsevier Inc. All rights reserved.

Soft Tissue Sarcoma

According to the Surveillance, Epidemiology, and End Results Program of the National Cancer Institute, the incidence of STS is approximately 3.4 per 100,000.[2] The true incidence of STS is likely somewhat underestimated, as some visceral sarcomas are likely counted with their organ of origin rather than with STS. There is a slight male preponderance of 1.4:1.[2] The median age at diagnosis is 59,[2] with a bimodal distribution that peaks in the fifth and eighth decades.[3]

STS occur most commonly on the extremities; upper and lower extremity STS account for 12% and 28%,[4] respectively, of all STS. The thigh is the most common site of STS, accounting for 44% of all extremity STS.[4] The most common type of extremity STS is liposarcoma (LPS).[4] Visceral STS account for 22% of all STS[4] and include gastrointestinal stromal tumors (GIST) and uterine leiomyosarcoma (LMS). GISTs are most commonly located in the stomach (59%), followed by small intestine (31%), with rectal (3.3%), colonic (2.7%), and esophageal (0.6%) locations being rare.[5] The median age at diagnosis for GIST is 62.[5] Retroperitoneal sarcomas account for 16% of all STS, whereas trunk and other sites (including the head and neck) account for 10% and 12%, respectively.[4] Retroperitoneal sarcomas are typically LPS and LMS.

Overall, LPS is the most common type of STS, accounting for approximately 20% to 25% of all STS.[2,4,6] LPS can be further subdivided into well-differentiated LPS (also called *atypical lipomatous tumor*), dedifferentiated LPS, myxoid LPS, and pleomorphic LPS.[7] Other common STS histologic subtypes include LMS (14%) and undifferentiated pleomorphic sarcoma (14%),[4] formerly known as *malignant fibrous histiocytoma*. The histologic distribution of STS among the various sites is found in **Fig. 1**.

Bone Sarcoma

Bone sarcomas are even more uncommon, accounting for 0.2% of all new cancer diagnoses.[2] This disease tends to affect the younger population, most frequently diagnosed in those 20 years or younger.[2] The age at diagnosis also varies with the histologic subtype. Osteosarcoma is the most common bone sarcoma overall and is more frequently seen in adolescents than in adults.[8] Similarly, Ewing sarcoma is more common in children and adolescents[8] but can also be seen in adults. The median age at diagnosis is 15.[8] Although any bone (or even soft tissue) can be involved,

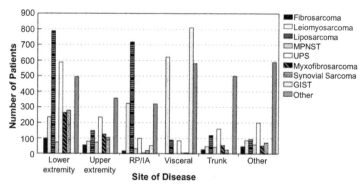

Fig. 1. Histopathology of soft tissue sarcomas by site of disease, N = 10,000. IA, intraabdominal; RP, retroperitoneum; UPS, undifferentiated pleomorphic sarcoma. (*From* Brennan MF, Antonescu CR, Moraco N, et al. Lessons learned from the study of 10,000 patients with soft tissue sarcoma. Ann Surg 2014;260(3):419; with permission.)

Ewing sarcoma is found commonly in the extremities.[8] Ewing sarcoma is most common in Caucasians and is rare in African-American or Asian populations.[8] The primary site of Ewing sarcoma also varies by race. In the Caucasian population, Ewing sarcoma is more frequently identified in the bone (80%) than in soft tissues (20%), whereas in the African-American population, the split is more even, with 55% located in bone and 45% located in the soft tissues.[9]

Although bone sarcoma primarily affects the younger population, certain types have a predilection for the adult population. Chondrosarcoma is typically diagnosed between ages 30 and 60 and is the most common subtype of bone sarcoma in adults.[8] Chordomas are rare, with an incidence of 0.5 per 1 million person-years.[8] The peak incidence of chordomas is between 50 to 60 years of age, and is rarely seen in patients younger than 40.[10] Although primarily thought of as a disease of the sacrum, there is actually a nearly equal distribution of chordoma between skull base (32%), mobile spine (33%), and sacrum (29%).[10]

Cutaneous Sarcoma

Cutaneous sarcomas are far less common than bone sarcomas or STS. The incidence of cutaneous sarcoma is 24.4 per 1 million person-years.[11] Kaposi sarcoma is the most common, making up 71% of cutaneous sarcomas.[11] Dermatofibrosarcoma protuberans is the second most common, constituting 18% of cutaneous sarcomas, with an incidence of 4.5 per 1 million person-years.[11] Dermatofibrosarcoma protuberans is more common in the African-American population than in Caucasians[11] and is most commonly identified on the trunk.[11,12] The mean age at diagnosis is 42.[12] Rare histologic subtypes of cutaneous sarcomas include undifferentiated pleomorphic sarcoma, LMS, and angiosarcoma.[11]

Pediatric Sarcoma

Despite its rarity, sarcomas can have a significant impact on the population, particularly for those younger than 20 years. STS and bone sarcomas are the third and fourth leading cause of cancer death in this age group, respectively.[1] The incidence of bone sarcomas in children is approximately 9.1 per 1,000,000; this has been stable over the last 4 decades.[2] The most commonly seen histologic subtypes are osteosarcoma (5.3 per 1,000,000) and Ewing sarcoma (2.8 per 1,000,000).[2] The childhood incidence of STS is 12.5 per 1,000,000, which has slightly increased over time.[2] The most common histology is rhabdomyosarcoma, with an incidence of 4.9 per 1,000,000.[2]

Pediatric Ewing sarcoma (of both bone and soft tissue) is most commonly identified in the extremities and the pelvis.[13] Specifically, in children ages 1 to 19, 29.4% and 22.8% of Ewing sarcoma are located in the lower extremity and pelvis, respectively.[14] In contrast, the distribution of Ewing sarcoma in infants is relatively even across the various sites: head (17.7%), upper extremity (17.7%), lower extremity (11.8%), pelvis (17.7%), chest (14.7%), abdomen (11.8%), and spine (8.8%).[14]

ETIOLOGY

Although there are some genetic defects and environmental factors that have been linked to the development of sarcoma, the most sarcomas are sporadic and idiopathic. The etiology of most sarcomas remains largely unknown.

Genetic Susceptibility

The genetic defects that lead to sarcoma development can be divided into 2 groups (**Table 1**): (1) simple karyotypic defects, and (2) complex karyotypic defects.[15]

Table 1	
Types of genetic defects that lead to sarcoma development	
Genetic Defect	**Example of Sarcoma Type**
Simple karyotypic defect • Disease-specific chromosomal translocation	• Ewing sarcoma • Alveolar rhabdomyosarcoma • Synovial sarcoma • Dermatofibrosarcoma protuberans • Desmoplastic small round-cell tumor
Complex karyotypic defect • Severe genetic instability • Disturbances in cell cycle genes	• Leiomyosarcoma • Liposarcoma • Undifferentiated pleomorphic sarcoma • Osteosarcoma • Angiosarcoma • Malignant peripheral nerve-sheath tumor

Simple karyotypic defects consist of disease-specific chromosomal translocations that lead to abnormal gene (and protein) function that facilitate sarcoma development. Sarcomas associated with simple karyotypic defects include Ewing sarcoma, alveolar rhabdomyosarcoma, and synovial sarcoma.[15] In Ewing sarcoma, the simple karyotypic defect occurs from the fusion of the DNA-binding domain of *FLI1* (a transcription factor) with the transactivation domain of *EWSR1* (another transcription factor).[15]

In contrast, complex karyotypic defects, such as complex chromosomal rearrangements, lead to disturbances in cell cycle genes and severe genetic instability. Sarcomas borne of this pathway tend to occur in older patients, and have a high frequency of mutations in the p53 and retinoblastoma (Rb) signaling pathways.[15,16] LMS, LPS, angiosarcoma, and osteosarcomas are examples of such tumors.[15] Sarcomas with complex karyotypic defects can also occur as secondary malignancies after prior radiation therapy (RT).

Germline genetic defects are seen in genetic syndromes (**Table 2**). In a single-center review, approximately 3% of STS were linked to a genetic syndrome.[17] The median age of diagnosis was 37 in patients with a genetic syndrome, significantly younger than in the sporadic population, with a median age of diagnosis of 53.[17] In addition, LPS was seen less frequently in patients with genetic syndromes than in patients with sporadic STS.[17]

Li-Fraumeni syndrome
In 1969, Li and Fraumeni[18] described 4 families with development of STS, breast cancer, and other malignant neoplasms in an autosomal dominant fashion.[18] Germline mutations in *TP53* were ultimately identified as the culprit. The loss of p53 protein function impairs the ability of cells with DNA damage to undergo apoptosis.[15] Although germline *TP53* mutations are associated with a variety of cancer types, sarcomas account for 25% of the cancer diagnoses in these patients.[19] Patients with *TP53* mutation–associated sarcoma tend to be younger than patients with sporadic sarcoma. The histology of *TP53* mutation–associated sarcomas tend to also be different from sporadic sarcoma. These differences are illustrated in **Fig. 2**. Patients with *TP53* mutations are more likely to have osteosarcoma at any age, and rhabdomyosarcoma at age less than 5, than those without germline *TP53* mutations.[19] Furthermore, LMS and LPS are less commonly seen in *TP53* mutation carriers (12%) than in sporadic sarcoma patients (52%).[19] Li-Fraumeni is rare; only 3.6% of adult-onset sarcoma patients carry a germline *TP53* mutation.[20] Thus, specific clinical criteria (the Chompret criteria) have been developed to guide germline *TP53* mutation

Table 2
Genetic syndromes and their associated sarcomas

Genetic Syndrome	Mutation	Associated Sarcoma
Li-Fraumeni syndrome	TP53	• Osteosarcoma • Rhabdomyosarcoma • Liposarcoma
Retinoblastoma	RB1	• Osteosarcoma • Chondrosarcoma • Ewing sarcoma • Uterine leiomyosarcoma • Fibrosarcoma • Rhabdomyosarcoma
Neurofibromatosis type 1	NF-1	• Rhabdomyosarcoma • Gastrointestinal stroma tumor • Malignant peripheral nerve sheath tumor
Familial adenomatous polyposis	APC	Desmoid tumor
Familial gastrointestinal stromal tumors	KIT PDGFRA	Gastrointestinal stromal tumor
Carney-Stratakis syndrome	SDH	Gastrointestinal stromal tumor
Bloom's syndrome	BLM	Osteosarcoma
Werner's syndrome	WRN	Osteosarcoma
Rothmund-Thomson syndrome	RECQ4	Osteosarcoma

screening. Other malignancies within the Li-Fraumeni tumor spectrum include brain tumors, premenopausal breast cancer, adrenocortical carcinoma, leukemia, and bronchoalveolar cancer.[21–23]

Only a small proportion of sarcomas that are associated with an aberrant p53 pathway develop as a result of a germline TP53 mutation. An alternate loss of the p53 protein has been characterized by the amplification of the MDM2 gene product. The protein product of the MDM2 gene functions to bind the p53 protein and to inhibit the transcriptional activity of TP53,[24] thus resulting in a functional loss of TP53 activity. This interaction has been found in retroperitoneal LPS, in which MDM2 and TP53 expression were seen in both well-differentiated and dedifferentiated LPS but were absent in myxoid and round cell LPS.[25] Additionally, well-differentiated LPS can be distinguished diagnostically from lipomas by MDM2 expression, as lipomas do not overexpress MDM2.[25,26]

Retinoblastoma

Hereditary retinoblastoma (Rb) is caused by a germline mutation in the RB1 gene, with high penetrance. Approximately 80% to 90% of carriers subsequently have ocular tumors.[16] The RB1 gene is a tumor-suppressor gene, which encodes the Rb protein. Rb normally functions as a cell cycle regulator by blocking entry to the S phase of the cell cycle.[16] Sarcomas occur in Rb survivors as a result of 2 contributing factors: (1) genetic susceptibility, and (2) prior RT for the Rb.[16,27] Bone sarcomas account for 25% to 30% of secondary cancers in Rb survivors; they tend to develop at around age 10 to 20 and are thought to be a result of RT and the high accumulative doses of alkylating chemotherapy given for the Rb, although up to 40% of these tumors occur outside of the radiation field.[16] Osteosarcoma is the most common sarcoma of the bone in this population.[16] Other histologic subtypes of bone sarcomas seen are chondrosarcoma and Ewing sarcoma.[16] STS generally develop later than bone

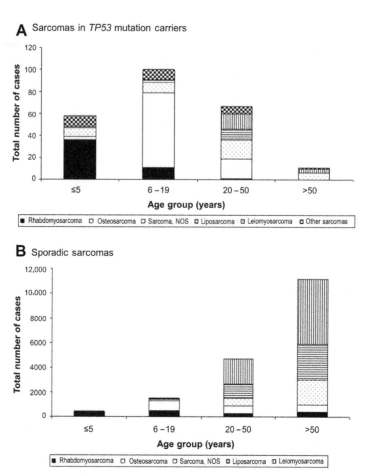

Fig. 2. Distribution of different histologic subtypes by age group, in (A) *TP53* mutation carriers from the International Agency for Research on Cancer *TP53* database, and (B) sporadic sarcoma patients from the Surveillance, Epidemiology, and End Results database. NOS, not otherwise specified. (*From* Ognjanovic S, Olivier M, Bergemann TL, et al. Sarcomas in TP53 germline mutation carriers: a review of the IARC TP53 database. Cancer 2012;118(5):1391; with permission.)

sarcomas, occurring from within 10 years to 50 years after Rb diagnosis. STS make up 12% to 32% of secondary cancers in Rb survivors.[16] The most commonly identified STS in this setting are uterine LMS.[16]

Neurofibromatosis type 1

Neurofibromatosis type 1 (NF-1) is also known as von Recklinghausen disease, with an incidence of 1 in 3000 live births, although the phenotype is variable.[28] The *NF-1* gene is a tumor-suppressor gene. It normally encodes the protein neurofibromin, a negative regulator of the RAS-MAPK pathway.[28] NF-1 is characterized by specific clinical features consisting of neurofibromas (benign tumors arising from Schwann cells), café-au-lait spots, neurofibromas, axillary or inguinal freckling, optic glioma, bony dysplasia, and Lisch nodules.[28,29] The prevalence of rhabdomyosarcoma in children with NF-1 is 0.02% to 0.03%, which is 20 times higher than in the general population.[28] Rhabdomyosarcoma associated with NF-1 commonly develops in the bladder and prostate.[28] There are also STS that are associated with NF-1 in adults, GIST and malignant peripheral nerve sheath tumor (MPNST). The lifetime risk of GIST development for NF-1 patients is 6%.[28] Unlike sporadic GISTs, which tend to be solitary gastric tumors, GISTs of NF-1 patients manifest as multifocal disease and are more commonly found in the small intestine.[28] The annual incidence of MPNST in NF-1 patients is 0.16%, significantly higher than that of the general population (0.001%).[28] These tumors arise typically from preexisting plexiform neurofibromas and have a poorer overall survival than sporadic MPNST.[28]

Familial adenomatous polyposis
In familial adenomatous polyposis (FAP), a germline mutation in the adenomatous polyposis coli (APC) gene results in the development of innumerable colorectal adenomas that ultimately lead to colorectal carcinoma. However, in addition to colorectal carcinoma, a subset (approximately 10%)[30,31] of FAP patients are also at risk for desmoid tumors. Desmoid tumors can also occur sporadically but are 850 to 1000 times more likely to occur in FAP patients.[32,33] Desmoid tumors are myofibroblastic tumors that are histologically benign but can be locally aggressive. These tumors commonly occur in the abdominal wall or within the mesentery but can also be found on other extra-abdominal musculoaponeurotic tissues such as the chest wall or inguinal region. Although the etiology of desmoid tumors is unclear, some risk factors have been suggested, such as trauma (ie, surgery),[30–32] pregnancy,[34] and female gender.[32] Desmoid tumors are also associated with a mutation 3′ to codon 1399[32] and codon 1444[31] of the APC gene.[31,32]

Gastrointestinal stromal tumors
GIST is the most common mesenchymal tumor in the gastrointestinal tract and arises from the interstitial cells of Cajal. The first associated genetic mutation associated with GIST was an activating KIT mutation.[35] Unlike TP53, RB1, or NF-1, KIT is a protooncogene. KIT mutation results in the gain of function of a tyrosine kinase receptor and subsequent downstream signaling that supports cell proliferation. KIT mutations (particularly exons 8, 9, 11, 13, and 17) are seen in 70% to 80% of GIST.[36] Subsequently, activating PDGFRA (platelet-derived growth factor receptor alpha) mutations (exons 12, 14, 18) were also identified, accounting for 5% to 15% of all GIST.[36] Although most GISTs are sporadic (with somatic KIT or PDGFRA mutations), a small subset occurs as familial GIST, with germline KIT or PDGFRA mutations, resulting in an inherited predisposition to GIST development.[36–38] More recently, mutations of succinate dehydrogenase (SDH) have been implicated in patients with wild type KIT and PDFGRA GISTs. A germline mutation in the SDH enzyme subunits results in Carney-Stratakis syndrome. These patients present with multifocal GISTs, paragangliomas, and pheochromocytomas.[36,39]

Bloom's syndrome, Werner's syndrome, and Rothmund-Thomson syndrome
Bloom's syndrome was first described as a case of congenital telangiectatic erythema in a patient with dwarfism.[40] It is an extremely rare autosomal recessive disorder that is more common in the Ashkenazi Jewish population.[41] Clinical characteristics include intrauterine growth restriction, growth deficiency that is persistent into childhood and adulthood, telangiectatic erythema that resembles lupus erythematosus in sun-exposed areas, and the development of malignancies.[42] A germline mutation in the BLM gene on chromosome 15 has been identified. BLM normally encodes for a DNA helicase in the RecQ family, which maintains genomic stability.[41,43] Patients

are at increased risk of all types of malignancies,[41] including osteosarcoma, which is more common in pediatric patients with Bloom's syndrome.[42]

Werner's syndrome is marked by a germline mutation in the *WRN* gene on chromosome 8.[41] A founder mutation in the *WRN* gene has been identified in the Japanese population.[41] Like Bloom's syndrome, Werner's syndrome is an autosomal recessive disorder, is extremely rare, and is a result of a mutant DNA helicase in the RecQ family.[41] However, unlike Bloom's syndrome, patients with Werner's syndrome are phenotypically normal until adolescence, when an absence of a growth spurt is noted; thus, adults with Werner's syndrome are typically of short stature.[41] Werner's syndrome was first described in 1904 in a family with symptoms of early-onset of age-related diseases, similar to premature aging. The syndrome is associated with early-onset arteriosclerosis, diabetes mellitus, hyperlipidemia, osteoporosis, malignancy of epithelial and mesenchymal origins.[44] In a review of Japanese case reports, common malignancies were reported to be osteosarcoma, thyroid cancer, and malignant melanoma.[44,45]

A third syndrome associated with a mutant DNA helicase of the RecQ family is the Rothmund-Thomson syndrome.[41] Most cases of Rothmund-Thomson syndrome are caused by a germline mutation in the *RECQ4* gene on chromosome 8.[41] Patients with Rothmund-Thomson syndrome have characteristic poikiloderma, alopecia, and juvenile cataracts.[41,46] They, too, are at increased risk of malignancy development, also most notably osteosarcoma.[47]

Ionizing Radiation

Ionizing radiation has been found to increase the risk of subsequent sarcoma development.[48–51] Those with ionizing radiation exposure include atomic bomb survivors and patients previously treated with RT. In the Life Span Study of Japanese atomic bomb survivors of Hiroshima and Nagasaki, increased cases of bone sarcoma (particularly osteosarcoma) and STS (most commonly leiomyosarcoma) have been reported.[52,53]

In 1948, diagnostic criteria were outlined for a radiation-induced sarcoma,[50] which were subsequently modified by Arlen and colleagues[51] (**Box 1**). Briefly, the diagnosis requires prior RT with a new sarcoma arising within the radiation field at least 3 years later. The most common prior cancers associated with subsequent radiation-induced sarcomas are breast cancer and non-Hodgkin's lymphoma[17,49,54]; therefore, these secondary sarcomas tend to occur on the chest wall or upper extremity.[17,49] Another common prior cancer is prostate cancer.[55] Most of these sarcomas are high grade[49] and are commonly undifferentiated pleomorphic sarcoma, angiosarcoma, undifferentiated spindle cell carcinoma, or leiomyosarcoma.[17,49,55] Liposarcoma, normally a common histologic subtype of STS, is less frequent among radiation-induced

---

Box 1
The modified Cahan criteria: diagnosis of a radiation-induced sarcoma.

1. Previous receipt of radiation therapy (RT) for benign or malignant disease.

2. Subsequent sarcoma development within the RT field.

3. Sarcoma is histologically different from the primary cancer for which the RT was given.

4. Latent period of 3 years (between RT and sarcoma development).

Data from Cahan WG, Woodard HQ, et al. Sarcoma arising in irradiated bone; report of 11 cases. Cancer 1948;1(1):3–29; and Arlen M, Higinbotham NL, Huvos AG, et al. Radiation-induced sarcoma of bone. Cancer 1971;28(5):1087–99.

sarcomas.[17,49] The median latent period between receipt of RT and subsequent sarcoma development in general is approximately 16 years.[49]

Prior breast cancer

Breast cancer is commonly treated with breast conservation therapy, consisting of a segmental mastectomy followed by adjuvant RT. This treatment strategy is equivalent in efficacy to mastectomy for early-stage breast cancer management. There have been reports of subsequent radiation-induced sarcomas in treated breast cancer patients.[56–61] The first case of radiation-induced angiosarcoma was reported in 1981.[62] Angiosarcoma is the classical sarcoma subtype associated with radiation for breast cancer. The clinical presentation consists of discolored cutaneous lesions along the surgical scar within the radiation field. These tumors also tend to be high grade.[54,60] The mean latency period between treatment of the breast cancer with RT and onset of the angiosarcoma is between 6 and 8 years.[57,60,63] Angiosarcoma of the breast can also be a sporadic disease, albeit rare. Patients with angiosarcoma who received prior RT are significantly older than RT-naïve angiosarcoma patients, although no differences were observed between the 2 groups of patients in terms of tumor size or grade.[60] Other STS types that have been seen after RT-treated breast cancer are undifferentiated pleomorphic sarcoma and fibrosarcoma.[57,61] The risk of STS development is 30 times higher after RT doses in excess of 44 Gy than after doses less than 15 Gy.[61] RT, however, has not been found to increase the risk of STS development outside the field of radiation.[57]

Another described sarcoma after the treatment of breast cancer is lymphangiosarcoma, so-called Stewart-Treves syndrome. This syndrome is a rare disease[17,59] with a poor prognosis. Although classically associated with chronic lymphedema after radical mastectomy, this syndrome can be applied to lymphangiosarcoma that develops from chronic lymphedema of any reason, such as, filariasis, venous stasis, trauma, or groin dissection for melanoma, cervical, or penile cancer.[64]

Despite the descriptions of STS development after treatment of breast cancer, it should be noted that the absolute incidence of these secondary cancers is extremely low (31 STS per 100,000 person-years and 7 angiosarcomas per 100,000 person-years). Reports of these extremely rare secondary sarcomas do not outweigh the benefits gained from adjuvant RT in the treatment of breast cancer, that is, a significant reduction in the risk of local recurrence.

Other Environmental Factors

The strongest link in the environment for sarcoma development is with ionizing radiation, described above. However, other environmental factors have been examined. Exposure to vinyl chloride has been found to increase the risk of angiosarcoma of the liver. Vinyl chloride was used in the plastics industry extensively in the 1970s. The mean latency period from exposure to hepatic angiosarcoma development was 36 years.[65] Other occupational exposures have been examined in an epidemiologic study in Europe, suggesting an increased risk of bone sarcoma development in blacksmiths, carpenters, bricklayers, and toolmakers, although no specific chemical was identified or implicated.[66] Finally, certain viruses, particularly in the setting of immunosuppression, have been implicated in the development of STS. The most well known is the association between Kaposi sarcoma and the Kaposi sarcoma–associated herpesvirus, also known as *the human herpesvirus 8*, in patients with human immunodeficiency virus–1.[67] Kaposi sarcomas are also seen in patients who are immunosuppressed in the absence of human immunodeficiency viral infection, including posttransplant patients[68–71] and, rarely, even patients with ulcerative colitis treated with immunosuppressive agents.[72,73] In particular, the incidence of Kaposi sarcoma was found to be increased in post–renal transplant patients during immunosuppression but not after transplant failure, when immunosuppression was reduced or ceased.[74] There are also rare reports of an association between the Epstein-Barr virus and smooth muscle tumors, including LMS, which also appears to be related to immunosuppression.[75–78]

SUMMARY

Bone and soft tissue sarcomas are rare malignancies with largely unknown etiology. Most of these tumors are sporadic, although small subsets can be associated with genetic susceptibility and environmental factors. Genetic syndromes associated with sarcoma development include Li-Fraumeni syndrome, retinoblastoma, neurofibromatosis-1, and familial adenomatous polyposis syndrome. Ionizing radiation is the strongest environmental factor leading to subsequent sarcoma development, particularly RT in a medical setting.

REFERENCES

1. Siegel RL, Miller KD, Jemal A. Cancer statistics, 2015. CA Cancer J Clin 2015; 65(1):5–29.
2. Howlader N, Noone AM, Krapcho M, et al. SEER cancer statistics review, 1975-2012. Based on November 2014 SEER data submission, posted to the SEER web site. 2015. Available at: http://seer.cancer.gov/csr/1975_2012/. Accessed December 22, 2015.
3. Bauer HC, Trovik CS, Alvegard TA, et al. Monitoring referral and treatment in soft tissue sarcoma: study based on 1,851 patients from the Scandinavian Sarcoma Group Register. Acta Orthop Scand 2001;72(2):150–9.
4. Brennan MF, Antonescu CR, Moraco N, et al. Lessons learned from the study of 10,000 patients with soft tissue sarcoma. Ann Surg 2014;260(3):416–22.
5. Guller U, Tarantino I, Cerny T, et al. Population-based SEER trend analysis of overall and cancer-specific survival in 5138 patients with gastrointestinal stromal tumor. BMC Cancer 2015;15:557.
6. Toro JR, Travis LB, Wu HJ, et al. Incidence patterns of soft tissue sarcomas, regardless of primary site, in the surveillance, epidemiology and end results program, 1978-2001: an analysis of 26,758 cases. Int J Cancer 2006;119(12): 2922–30.
7. Fletcher CD, Bridge JA, Hogendoorn PC, et al. WHO Classification of Tumours of Soft Tissue and Bone. Lyon (France): International Agency for Research on Cancer (IARC); 2013.
8. The ESMO/European Sarcoma Network Working Group. Bone sarcomas: ESMO clinical practice guidelines for diagnosis, treatment and follow-up. Ann Oncol 2014;25(Suppl 3):iii113–23.
9. Worch J, Matthay KK, Neuhaus J, et al. Ethnic and racial differences in patients with Ewing sarcoma. Cancer 2010;116(4):983–8.
10. McMaster ML, Goldstein AM, Bromley CM, et al. Chordoma: incidence and survival patterns in the United States, 1973-1995. Cancer Causes Control 2001; 12(1):1–11.
11. Rouhani P, Fletcher CD, Devesa SS, et al. Cutaneous soft tissue sarcoma incidence patterns in the U.S. : an analysis of 12,114 cases. Cancer 2008;113(3): 616–27.

12. Kuzel P, Metelitsa AI, Dover DC, et al. Epidemiology of dermatofibrosarcoma protuberans in Alberta, Canada, from 1988 to 2007. Dermatol Surg 2012;38(9): 1461–8.
13. Lee J, Hoang BH, Ziogas A, et al. Analysis of prognostic factors in Ewing sarcoma using a population-based cancer registry. Cancer 2010;116(8):1964–73.
14. Wong T, Goldsby RE, Wustrack R, et al. Clinical features and outcomes of infants with Ewing sarcoma under 12 months of age. Pediatr Blood Cancer 2015;62(11): 1947–51.
15. Helman LJ, Meltzer P. Mechanisms of sarcoma development. Nat Rev Cancer 2003;3(9):685–94.
16. Kleinerman RA, Schonfeld SJ, Tucker MA. Sarcomas in hereditary retinoblastoma. Clin Sarcoma Res 2012;2(1):15.
17. Penel N, Grosjean J, Robin YM, et al. Frequency of certain established risk factors in soft tissue sarcomas in adults: a prospective descriptive study of 658 cases. Sarcoma 2008;2008:459386.
18. Li FP, Fraumeni JF Jr. Soft-tissue sarcomas, breast cancer, and other neoplasms. A familial syndrome? Ann Intern Med 1969;71(4):747–52.
19. Ognjanovic S, Olivier M, Bergemann TL, et al. Sarcomas in TP53 germline mutation carriers: a review of the IARC TP53 database. Cancer 2012;118(5):1387–96.
20. Mitchell G, Ballinger ML, Wong S, et al. High frequency of germline TP53 mutations in a prospective adult-onset sarcoma cohort. PLoS One 2013;8(7):e69026.
21. Chompret A, Abel A, Stoppa-Lyonnet D, et al. Sensitivity and predictive value of criteria for p53 germline mutation screening. J Med Genet 2001;38(1):43–7.
22. Bougeard G, Sesboue R, Baert-Desurmont S, et al. Molecular basis of the Li-Fraumeni syndrome: an update from the French LFS families. J Med Genet 2008;45(8):535–8.
23. Tinat J, Bougeard G, Baert-Desurmont S, et al. 2009 version of the Chompret criteria for Li Fraumeni syndrome. J Clin Oncol 2009;27(26):e108–9 [author reply: e110].
24. Oliner JD, Pietenpol JA, Thiagalingam S, et al. Oncoprotein MDM2 conceals the activation domain of tumour suppressor p53. Nature 1993;362(6423):857–60.
25. Pilotti S, Torre GD, Lavarino C, et al. Distinct mdm2/p53 expression patterns in liposarcoma subgroups: implications for different pathogenetic mechanisms. J Pathol 1997;181(1):14–24.
26. Ito M, Barys L, O'Reilly T, et al. Comprehensive mapping of p53 pathway alterations reveals an apparent role for both SNP309 and MDM2 amplification in sarcomagenesis. Clin Cancer Res 2011;17(3):416–26.
27. Kleinerman RA, Tucker MA, Tarone RE, et al. Risk of new cancers after radiotherapy in long-term survivors of retinoblastoma: an extended follow-up. J Clin Oncol 2005;23(10):2272–9.
28. Brems H, Beert E, de Ravel T, et al. Mechanisms in the pathogenesis of malignant tumours in neurofibromatosis type 1. Lancet Oncol 2009;10(5):508–15.
29. Korf BR. Neurofibromatosis. Handb Clin Neurol 2013;111:333–40.
30. Gurbuz AK, Giardiello FM, Petersen GM, et al. Desmoid tumours in familial adenomatous polyposis. Gut 1994;35(3):377–81.
31. Nieuwenhuis MH, Lefevre JH, Bulow S, et al. Family history, surgery, and APC mutation are risk factors for desmoid tumors in familial adenomatous polyposis: an international cohort study. Dis Colon Rectum 2011;54(10):1229–34.
32. Sinha A, Tekkis PP, Gibbons DC, et al. Risk factors predicting desmoid occurrence in patients with familial adenomatous polyposis: a meta-analysis. Colorectal Dis 2011;13(11):1222–9.

33. Fallen T, Wilson M, Morlan B, et al. Desmoid tumors – a characterization of patients seen at Mayo Clinic 1976-1999. Fam Cancer 2006;5(2):191–4.
34. Burtenshaw SM, Cannell AJ, McAlister ED, et al. Toward observation as first-line management in abdominal desmoid tumors. Ann Surg Oncol 2016;23(7):2212–9.
35. Hirota S, Isozaki K, Moriyama Y, et al. Gain-of-function mutations of c-kit in human gastrointestinal stromal tumors. Science 1998;279(5350):577–80.
36. Patil DT, Rubin BP. Genetics of gastrointestinal stromal tumors: a heterogeneous family of tumors? Surg Pathol Clin 2015;8(3):515–24.
37. Neuhann TM, Mansmann V, Merkelbach-Bruse S, et al. A novel germline KIT mutation (p.L576P) in a family presenting with juvenile onset of multiple gastrointestinal stromal tumors, skin hyperpigmentations, and esophageal stenosis. Am J Surg Pathol 2013;37(6):898–905.
38. Nishida T, Hirota S, Taniguchi M, et al. Familial gastrointestinal stromal tumours with germline mutation of the KIT gene. Nat Genet 1998;19(4):323–4.
39. Gaal J, Stratakis CA, Carney JA, et al. SDHB immunohistochemistry: a useful tool in the diagnosis of Carney-Stratakis and Carney triad gastrointestinal stromal tumors. Mod Pathol 2011;24(1):147–51.
40. Bloom D. Congenital telangiectatic erythema resembling lupus erythematosus in dwarfs; probably a syndrome entity. AMA Am J Dis Child 1954;88(6):754–8.
41. Hickson ID. RecQ helicases: caretakers of the genome. Nat Rev Cancer 2003;3(3):169–78.
42. German J. Bloom's syndrome. XX. The first 100 cancers. Cancer Genet Cytogenet 1997;93(1):100–6.
43. Ellis NA, Groden J, Ye TZ, et al. The Bloom's syndrome gene product is homologous to RecQ helicases. Cell 1995;83(4):655–66.
44. Yamamoto K, Imakiire A, Miyagawa N, et al. A report of two cases of Werner's syndrome and review of the literature. J Orthop Surg (Hong Kong) 2003;11(2):224–33.
45. Goto M, Miller RW, Ishikawa Y, et al. Excess of rare cancers in Werner syndrome (adult progeria). Cancer Epidemiol Biomarkers Prev 1996;5(4):239–46.
46. Simon T, Kohlhase J, Wilhelm C, et al. Multiple malignant diseases in a patient with Rothmund-Thomson syndrome with RECQL4 mutations: Case report and literature review. Am J Med Genet A 2010;152A(6):1575–9.
47. Hicks MJ, Roth JR, Kozinetz CA, et al. Clinicopathologic features of osteosarcoma in patients with Rothmund-Thomson syndrome. J Clin Oncol 2007;25(4):370–5.
48. Henderson TO, Whitton J, Stovall M, et al. Secondary sarcomas in childhood cancer survivors: a report from the Childhood Cancer Survivor Study. J Natl Cancer Inst 2007;99(4):300–8.
49. Riad S, Biau D, Holt GE, et al. The clinical and functional outcome for patients with radiation-induced soft tissue sarcoma. Cancer 2012;118(10):2682–92.
50. Cahan WG, Woodard HQ, Higinbotham NL, et al. Sarcoma arising in irradiated bone; report of 11 cases. Cancer 1948;1(1):3–29.
51. Arlen M, Higinbotham NL, Huvos AG, et al. Radiation-induced sarcoma of bone. Cancer 1971;28(5):1087–99.
52. Samartzis D. Exposure to ionizing radiation and development of bone sarcoma: new insights based on atomic-bomb survivors of Hiroshima and Nagasaki. J Bone Joint Surg Am 2011;93(11):1008.
53. Samartzis D, Nishi N, Cologne J, et al. Ionizing radiation exposure and the development of soft-tissue sarcomas in atomic-bomb survivors. J Bone Joint Surg Am 2013;95(3):222–9.

54. Brady MS, Gaynor JJ, Brennan MF. Radiation-associated sarcoma of bone and soft tissue. Arch Surg 1992;127(12):1379–85.
55. Cha C, Antonescu CR, Quan ML, et al. Long-term results with resection of radiation-induced soft tissue sarcomas. Ann Surg 2004;239(6):903–10.
56. Karlsson P, Holmberg E, Johansson KA, et al. Soft tissue sarcoma after treatment for breast cancer. Radiother Oncol 1996;38(1):25–31.
57. Mery CM, George S, Bertagnolli MM, et al. Secondary sarcomas after radiotherapy for breast cancer: sustained risk and poor survival. Cancer 2009; 115(18):4055–63.
58. D'Angelo SP, Antonescu CR, Kuk D, et al. High-risk features in radiation-associated breast angiosarcomas. Br J Cancer 2013;109(9):2340–6.
59. Kirova YM, Gambotti L, De Rycke Y, et al. Risk of second malignancies after adjuvant radiotherapy for breast cancer: a large-scale, single-institution review. Int J Radiat Oncol Biol Phys 2007;68(2):359–63.
60. Vorburger SA, Xing Y, Hunt KK, et al. Angiosarcoma of the breast. Cancer 2005; 104(12):2682–8.
61. Rubino C, Shamsaldin A, Le MG, et al. Radiation dose and risk of soft tissue and bone sarcoma after breast cancer treatment. Breast Cancer Res Treat 2005; 89(3):277–88.
62. Maddox JC, Evans HL. Angiosarcoma of skin and soft tissue: a study of forty-four cases. Cancer 1981;48(8):1907–21.
63. Depla AL, Scharloo-Karels CH, de Jong MA, et al. Treatment and prognostic factors of radiation-associated angiosarcoma (RAAS) after primary breast cancer: a systematic review. Eur J Cancer 2014;50(10):1779–88.
64. Sharma A, Schwartz RA. Stewart-Treves syndrome: pathogenesis and management. J Am Acad Dermatol 2012;67(6):1342–8.
65. Collins JJ, Jammer B, Sladeczek FM, et al. Surveillance for angiosarcoma of the liver among vinyl chloride workers. J Occup Environ Med 2014;56(11):1207–9.
66. Merletti F, Richiardi L, Bertoni F, et al. Occupational factors and risk of adult bone sarcomas: a multicentric case-control study in Europe. Int J Cancer 2006;118(3): 721–7.
67. Newton R, Carpenter L, Casabonne D, et al. A prospective study of Kaposi's sarcoma-associated herpesvirus and Epstein-Barr virus in adults with human immunodeficiency virus-1. Br J Cancer 2006;94(10):1504–9.
68. Carenco C, Faure S, Ursic-Bedoya J, et al. Solid, non-skin, post-liver transplant tumors: key role of lifestyle and immunosuppression management. World J Gastroenterol 2016;22(1):427–34.
69. Rossetto A, Tulissi P, De Marchi F, et al. De Novo solid tumors after kidney transplantation: is it time for a patient-tailored risk assessment? Experience from a single center. Transplant Proc 2015;47(7):2116–20.
70. Hosseini-Moghaddam SM, Soleimanirahbar A, Mazzulli T, et al. Post renal transplantation Kaposi's sarcoma: a review of its epidemiology, pathogenesis, diagnosis, clinical aspects, and therapy. Transpl Infect Dis 2012;14(4):338–45.
71. Engels EA, Pfeiffer RM, Fraumeni JF Jr, et al. Spectrum of cancer risk among US solid organ transplant recipients. JAMA 2011;306(17):1891–901.
72. Svrcek M, Tiret E, Bennis M, et al. KSHV/HHV8-associated intestinal Kaposi's sarcoma in patient with ulcerative colitis receiving immunosuppressive drugs: report of a case. Dis Colon Rectum 2009;52(1):154–8.
73. Rodriguez-Pelaez M, Fernandez-Garcia MS, Gutierrez-Corral N, et al. Kaposi's sarcoma: an opportunistic infection by human herpesvirus-8 in ulcerative colitis. J Crohns Colitis 2010;4(5):586–90.

74. van Leeuwen MT, Webster AC, McCredie MR, et al. Effect of reduced immuno-suppression after kidney transplant failure on risk of cancer: population based retrospective cohort study. BMJ 2010;340:c570.

75. Miettinen M. Smooth muscle tumors of soft tissue and non-uterine viscera: biology and prognosis. Mod Pathol 2014;27(Suppl 1):S17–29.

76. Hussein K, Rath B, Ludewig B, et al. Clinico-pathological characteristics of different types of immunodeficiency-associated smooth muscle tumours. Eur J Cancer 2014;50(14):2417–24.

77. Nur S, Rosenblum WD, Katta UD, et al. Epstein-Barr virus-associated multifocal leiomyosarcomas arising in a cardiac transplant recipient: autopsy case report and review of the literature. J Heart Lung Transplant 2007;26(9):944–52.

78. Rogatsch H, Bonatti H, Menet A, et al. Epstein-Barr virus-associated multicentric leiomyosarcoma in an adult patient after heart transplantation: case report and review of the literature. Am J Surg Pathol 2000;24(4):614–21.

Bone and Soft Tissue Pathology
Diagnostic and Prognostic Implications

Julie Gibbs, MD[a], Evita Henderson-Jackson, MD[a,b],
Marilyn M. Bui, MD, PhD[a,b],*

KEYWORDS

- Soft tissue • Bone • Sarcoma • Diagnosis • Prognosis • Pathology • Molecular

KEY POINTS

- A multidisciplinary team approach is necessary for optimal treatment of sarcomas, and the role of pathology is important for each member to be familiar with.
- Recent advances in immunohistochemical markers, cytogenetics, and molecular pathology techniques have lead to more accurate diagnoses and have improved the management of sarcomas.
- The current pathological definitions, classification and grading systems, and ancillary techniques are summarized here for some of the more common soft tissue and bone tumors.

INTRODUCTION

Most soft tissue and bone tumors are benign, requiring only conservative management. Soft tissue and bone sarcomas, on the other hand, require a multidisciplinary team approach for optimal diagnosis and management.[1–3] They are rare malignant neoplasms, accounting for less than 1% of all adult and up to 20% of all pediatric malignancies, and may be classified according to the type of tissue that they most closely histologically resemble.[3,4] The large majority are soft tissue sarcomas, most of which originate within the soft tissue of extremities, while the remaining approximately 10% are bone sarcomas.[3,5,6] Numerous advances in immunohistochemical markers, cytogenetics, and molecular pathology techniques have led to more accurate diagnoses and have improved the management of sarcomas over the past decade.[7–10] However, sarcomas are rare and diverse, often with overlapping histologic and

The authors have nothing to disclose.

[a] Department of Pathology and Cell Biology, University of South Florida Morsani College of Medicine, 12901 Bruce B. Downs Boulevard, Tampa, FL 33612, USA; [b] Department of Anatomic Pathology, H. Lee Moffitt Cancer Center & Research Institute, 12902 Magnolia Drive, Tampa, FL 33612, USA

* Corresponding author. Department of Anatomic Pathology, H. Lee Moffitt Cancer Center & Research Institute, 12902 Magnolia Drive, Tampa, FL 33612.

E-mail address: Marilyn.Bui@Moffitt.org

Surg Clin N Am 96 (2016) 915–962
http://dx.doi.org/10.1016/j.suc.2016.06.003
0039-6109/16/$ – see front matter © 2016 Elsevier Inc. All rights reserved.

surgical.theclinics.com

immunophenotypical features, making them a challenging group of tumors to accurately diagnose. Numerous online references and algorithmic clinical guidelines (**Table 1**), such as those created by the National Comprehensive Cancer Network (NCCN), are also readily available to help guide the diagnosis and management of soft tissue and bone tumors.[11–18]

All members of a multidisciplinary team should have an understanding of the role of pathology, including the availability of ancillary studies, in order to optimize patient care. Clinical and radiologic information plays a key role in the initial workup and is often followed by tissue sampling, such as fine-needle aspiration (FNA), image-guided biopsy, or open biopsy, for definitive pathologic diagnosis before therapy or surgical resection. Although core biopsy with image guidance is the most accepted method for initial sampling of suspected sarcomas, FNA is especially useful in the evaluation of possible recurrent or metastatic disease. The appropriate selection of a sampling technique improves the accuracy and timeliness of the definitive pathologic diagnosis.[1,11] Ancillary techniques, including immunohistochemical studies and molecular studies, then facilitate in the definitive diagnosis of most sarcomas.[7,10]

This article begins with a brief summary of the changes included in recently updated World Health Organization (WHO) classification series of soft tissue and bone tumors. Although a comprehensive discussion of every currently recognized bone and soft tissue tumor and variant is not possible to cover in this article, the authors aim to discuss the key pathologic findings, grading and staging systems, and prognostic implications of some of the more common malignant, intermediate, and benign soft tissue and bone tumors.

WORLD HEALTH ORGANIZATION 2013 UPDATE

The most recently updated WHO classification series of soft tissue and bone tumors includes several newly recognized entities and reflects changes that have resulted from improved understanding of tumor characteristics.[19–22] In summary, compared with the previous 2002 edition, this updated version better defines diagnostic criteria, allowing for more reproducible diagnoses, with some additional changes in the classification of various tumors. It incorporates updated molecular and genetic characteristics of tumors, shedding more light on possible factors influencing the pathogenesis of some previously obscure entities.[20]

The update includes discussions that explain why some of the definitions of certain entities have changed. For example, the term atypical lipomatous tumor is preferred over well-differentiated liposarcoma, because they have no metastatic potential. The later term is now reserved, according to clinical judgment, for tumors that are impossible to completely surgically excise with adequate margins, because they are

Table 1		
Selected examples of online references for pathology and clinical guidelines or information		
Pathology	College of American Pathologists	http://www.cap.org/web/home/resources/cancer-reporting-tools/
	Tampa Path	http://tampapath.com
	BoneTumor.org	http://www.bonetumor.org/
	Pathology Outlines	http://www.pathologyoutlines.com/softtissue.html
Clinical oncology	NCCN	https://www.nccn.org/
	European Society for Medical Oncology	http://www.esmo.org/
	American Cancer Society	http://www.cancer.org

locally aggressive and likely to eventually have uncontrollable recurrent disease. In the fibroblastic/myofibroblastic section, solitary fibrous tumors (SFT) and hemangiopericytomas (HPC), previously considered separate entities, have been combined into one entity, now diagnosed as SFT. Similarly, the term Ewing sarcoma/primitive neuroectodermal tumor is no longer used and is now diagnosed, more simply, as Ewing sarcoma, since molecular analysis has supported the current understanding that they are the same entity with varying degrees of neuroectodermal differentiation, accounting for the histologic differences.[20,23]

Undifferentiated sarcomas, historically also known as malignant fibrous histiocytomas (MFHs), were moved out of the fibrohistiocytic section, forming a new section of undifferentiated/unclassified sarcomas.[19] These undifferentiated sarcomas are a diagnosis of exclusion and should be reported as undifferentiated spindle cell sarcoma, undifferentiated pleomorphic sarcoma, undifferentiated round cell sarcoma, undifferentiated epithelioid sarcoma (ES), or undifferentiated sarcoma, not otherwise specified (NOS). Myofibroma and angiomyolipoma were both moved into the perivascular section, from the fibroblastic and smooth muscle sections, respectively. In addition, the mixed-type liposarcoma subtype has been removed, whereas extraskeletal myxoid chondrosarcoma and angiomatoid fibrous histiocytoma have been reclassified as tumors of uncertain differentiation, because of their unclear line of differentiation when analyzed by presently available technology.[20]

Newly recognized entities or variants have also been added, such as the new spindle cell/sclerosing variant of rhabdomyosarcoma and the pseudomyogenic hemangioendothelioma. Entirely new sections have been added to include tumors such as gastrointestinal stromal tumors (GIST) and nerve sheath tumors. A few bone tumors and variants were also added, including the benign notochordal cell tumor and primary non-Hodgkin lymphoma of bone, whereas other entities, such as schwannoma and leiomyoma of bone, were removed. In addition, the controversial issue regarding the coexistence of several grading systems of soft tissue tumors is discussed, focusing on the 2 most common grading systems in regards to their main advantages and limitations.[20,22,24]

PATHOLOGIC GRADING OF SOFT TISSUE SARCOMAS

Soft tissue sarcomas are a heterogeneous and diverse group of tumors proven very difficult to uniformly grade. However, in 1984, Costa and colleagues[25] introduced a grading system known as the National Cancer Institute system. However, the grading system proposed by French Federation of Cancer Centers (Federation Nationale des Centres de Lutte Contre le Cancer, FNCLCC) popular in Europe is the most widely used system.[26] In addition, it has been validated by the largest number of patients studied, and its reproducibility has been tested with a large number of pathologists.[27,28] The FNCLCC grading system of soft tissue sarcomas is based on the total score obtained from the summation of points for 3 factors: differentiation, mitotic rate, and tumor necrosis (**Box 1**).[29] For each soft tissue sarcoma type, points are assigned (1–3) for level of differentiation (**Box 2**), mitotic count, and tumor necrosis. The sum of the points is then categorized as either grade 1 (2–3 points), grade 2 (4–5 points), or grade 3 (6–8 points). The mitotic count refers to the number of mitotic figures counted in 10 high-power fields (HPF; field size of 0.174 mm^2). It is not practical to grade soft tissue sarcomas status after chemotherapy or radiation because treatment tends to affect the mitotic counts, increase necrosis, and sometimes seemingly induce differentiation or cause selection for more differentiated components.[29] Other histopathologic features not used in the grading system that are prognostically important include

---

Box 1
The French Federation of Cancer Centers grading system

Tumor differentiation (see Box 2)

Score 1: Sarcomas resembling normal tissue

Score 2: Sarcomas with defined histologic differentiation

Score 3: Undifferentiated sarcomas or sarcomas of uncertain histologic differentiation

Mitotic count

Score 1: 0–9/10 HPF

Score 2: 10–19/10 HPF

Score 3: ≥20/10 HPF

Tumor necrosis

Score 1: Absent

Score 2: <50%

Score 3: ≥50%

Histologic grade

Tumor differentiation + Mitotic count + Tumor necrosis (sum of scores)

Grade 1: 2–3

Grade 2: 4–5

Grade 3: 6–8

Adapted from Guillou L, Coindre JM, Bonichon F, et al. Comparative study of the National Cancer Institute and French Federation of Cancer Centers Sarcoma Group grading systems in a population of 410 adult patients with soft tissue sarcoma. J Clin Oncol 1997;15(1):350–62; and Coindre JM. Grading of soft tissue sarcomas: review and update. Arch Pathol Lab Med 2006;130(10):1449.

---

surgical margin status and presence of vascular invasion.[30] For some histologic types of sarcoma, grade is of no prognostic value, such as in malignant peripheral nerve sheath tumor (MPNST), and its use is not recommended for angiosarcoma, extraskeletal myxoid chondrosarcoma, alveolar soft part sarcoma (ASPS), clear cell sarcoma, and ES.[31–35] Separate from grading, a classification based on biological behavior of soft tissue tumors is provided within the WHO classification series of soft tissue and bone tumors.[22] The soft tissue tumor types are divided into benign, intermediate (locally aggressive or rarely metastasizing), and malignant.

PATHOLOGICAL STAGING OF SOFT TISSUE SARCOMAS

The current American Joint Committee for Cancer (AJCC) Staging System for Soft Tissue Sarcomas manual incorporates the tumor stage, extent of tumor, and tumor grade.[36] This TNM system evaluates tumor size (whether greater than 5 cm or not), depth (whether suprafascial or infrafascial), and localized or disseminated (presence or absence of lymph node or distant metastases) (**Table 2**).

PATHOLOGIC GRADING OF BONE TUMORS

Bone tumors comprise a diverse group of neoplasms that are either cartilaginous, osteogenic, fibrogenic, fibrohistiocytic, hematopoietic, or of other mesenchymal tissue differentiation. The grading of bone neoplasms is largely driven by the histologic diagnosis, and

---

Box 2
Tumor differentiation score (according to histologic type in updated version of the FNCLCC system)

Score 1

Well-differentiated (liposarcoma, fibrosarcoma, MPNST, leiomyosarcoma, chondrosarcoma)

Score 2

Myxoid (liposarcoma, MFH, and chondrosarcoma), conventional (fibrosarcoma, MPNST, leiomyosarcoma, and angiosarcoma), well-differentiated malignant HPC, typical storiform/pleomorphic MFH

Score 3

Round cell liposarcoma, pleomorphic liposarcoma, dedifferentiated liposarcoma, poorly differentiated fibrosarcoma, poorly differentiated MPNST, epithelioid MPNST, malignant Triton tumor, conventional malignant HPC, giant-cell and inflammatory MFH, poorly differentiated/pleomorphic/epithelioid leiomyosarcoma, synovial sarcoma, embryonal/alveolar/pleomorphic rhabdomyosarcoma, mesenchymal chondrosarcoma, poorly differentiated/epithelioid angiosarcoma, extraskeletal osteosarcoma, Ewing sarcoma, ASPS, ES, malignant rhabdoid tumor, clear cell sarcoma, undifferentiated sarcoma

Adapted from Guillou L, Coindre JM, Bonichon F, et al. Comparative study of the National Cancer Institute and French Federation of Cancer Centers Sarcoma Group grading systems in a population of 410 adult patients with soft tissue sarcoma. J Clin Oncol 1997;15(1):352.

---

based on the system advocated by Broders, which assesses cellularity and nuclear features.[37] Generally, the more cellular the tumor is, the higher the grade. Nuclear membrane irregularities, nuclear enlargement, and nuclear hyperchromasia correlate with grade.[22] Mitotic figures and necrosis are other histologic features helpful in grading. According

---

Table 2
American Joint Committee on Cancer version 7 staging for soft tissue sarcomas

Primary tumor (T)	
TX	Primary tumor cannot be assessed
T0	No evidence of primary tumor
T1	Tumor 5 cm or less in greatest dimension
T1a	Superficial tumor
T1b	Deep tumor
T2	Tumor more than 5 cm in greatest dimension
T2a	Superficial tumor
T2b	Deep tumor
Regional lymph nodes (N)	
NX	Lymph nodes cannot be assessed
N0	No regional lymph node metastasis
N1	Regional lymph node metastasis
Distant metastasis (M)	
M0	No distant metastasis
M1	Distant metastasis

Used with the permission of the American Joint Committee on Cancer (AJCC), Chicago, Illinois. The original source for this material is the AJCC Cancer Staging Manual, Seventh Edition (2010) published by Springer Science and Business Media LLC, www.springer.com.

to the AJCC Cancer Staging manual, a 4-grade system is recommended; however, G1, G2 are regarded as low grade, whereas G3, G4 are regarded as high grade (**Box 3**).[36]

Chondrosarcomas are graded based on cellularity, cytologic atypia, and mitotic activity. Grade 1 chondrosarcoma is histologically similar to enchondroma, but shows radiographic or histologic evidence of aggressive growth. Grade 2 chondrosarcomas are more cellular than grade 1 chondrosarcomas; have more cytologic atypia, greater hyperchromasia, and nuclear size; or have prominent myxoid change. Grade 3 chondrosarcomas are hypercellular with significant nuclear pleomorphism and prominent mitotic activity.[38]

Chordomas are locally aggressive with a propensity for metastasis and are not graded. Adamantinomas are considered low grade. Sarcomas of types that occur in both bone and soft tissue (eg, mesenchymal chondrosarcoma, leiomyosarcoma, undifferentiated pleomorphic sarcoma) are graded according to the FNCLCC system.

PATHOLOGIC STAGING OF BONE TUMORS

As with soft tissue sarcomas, the AJCC Cancer Staging manual staging of bone tumors incorporates grade of the tumor and the extent of disease. It includes a 4-grade

---

Box 3
Bone tumor grading

Grade 1

Low-grade central osteosarcoma

Clear cell chondrosarcoma

Grade 1 chondrosarcoma

Parosteal osteosarcoma

Adamantinoma

Grade 2

Periosteal osteosarcoma

Grade 2 chondrosarcoma

Grade 3

Conventional osteosarcoma

Telangiectactic osteosarcoma

Small cell osteosarcoma

Secondary osteosarcoma

High-grade surface osteosarcoma

Malignant giant cell tumor

Ewing sarcoma

Grade 3 chondrosarcoma

Mesenchymal chondrosarcoma

Dedifferentiated chondrosarcoma

From Randall LR. Approach to the diagnosis of bone and soft tissue tumors – clinical, radiologic, and classification aspects. In: Folpe AL, Inwards CY, eds. Bone and soft tissue pathology. Philadelphia: Saunders/Elsevier; 2010; with permission.

system based on differentiation that can be converted into high grade and low grade. In other words, grade 1 tumors = low grade and grade 2 to 3 tumors = high grade.[36,39] The TNM system evaluates tumor size (whether greater than 8 cm or not) with or without discontinuous tumors in the primary bone site, and localized or disseminated (presence or absence of lymph node or distant metastases) (**Table 3**).

OVERVIEW OF THE PATHOLOGIC ASPECT OF DIAGNOSIS, PROGNOSIS, AND THERANOSTICS

Although soft tissue and bone tumors are classified by the histologic differentiation in the medical textbooks, the tumors encountered by pathologists present with various histologic findings, such as spindled cells, round cells, epithelioid cells, pleomorphic cells, giant cells, myxoid, fibrous, choroid, osteoid, and so forth. The pathologist then formulates a list of pertinent differential diagnoses, using the histologic information, in conjunction with clinical and radiological information, followed by ancillary techniques, such as immunohistologic, flow cytometry, cytogenetic, and molecular techniques, to define the histologic lineage and determine an accurate diagnosis. Biomarker studies of the tumor may also provide insight into response to therapy or prognosis.

The survival of patients with any high-grade or metastatic sarcoma is usually poor and with limited therapeutic options. The urgent need for improved targeted therapies for these rare aggressive tumors has led to chemotherapy-predictive (theranostic) molecular profiling services, particularly for patients with aggressive cancers and advanced stage of disease. Molecular profiling to uncover potential theranostic biomarkers are being evaluated with the use of various methods, such as immunohistochemistry, fluorescence in situ hybridization (FISH), polymer chain reaction

Table 3	
American Joint Committee on Cancer staging version 7 for bone tumors	
Primary tumor	
TX	Primary tumor cannot be assessed
T0	No evidence of primary tumor
T1	Tumor ≤8 cm in greatest dimension
T2	Tumor >8 cm in greatest dimension
T3	Discontinuous tumors in primary bone site
Regional lymph nodes	
NX	Lymph nodes cannot be assessed
N0	No regional lymph node metastasis
N1	Regional lymph node metastasis
Distant metastasis	
MX	Distant metastasis cannot be assessed
M0	No distant metastasis
M1	Distant metastasis
M1a	Lung
M1b	Other distant sites

Used with the permission of the American Joint Committee on Cancer (AJCC), Chicago, Illinois. The original source for this material is the AJCC Cancer Staging Manual, Seventh Edition (2010) published by Springer Science and Business Media LLC, www.springer.com.

(PCR)-based panels, comparative genome hybridization, whole-genome transcriptome analysis, and next-generation exome sequencing, among others.[40,41] Analysis of the molecular profile findings has the potential to provide therapeutic targets, such those involved in cell cycle regulation, DNA replication, the receptor tyrosine kinase pathway, among others, predicting susceptibilities to certain chemotherapeutic agents, and ultimately individualizing therapy.[40–42]

MALIGNANT SOFT TISSUE AND BONE TUMORS
Liposarcoma

Malignant liposarcomas include dedifferentiated liposarcoma, myxoid liposarcoma, and pleomorphic liposarcoma.[6,22] Atypical lipomatous tumors (ALT) may undergo dedifferentiation resulting in a nonlipogenic sarcomatous component, consistent with dedifferentiated liposarcoma (**Fig. 1**). Typically the nonlipogenic sarcomatous component, of variable grade, is at least several millimeters in diameter and is either associated with a primary ALT/well-differentiated liposarcoma or in a recurrence.[43,44] Myxoid liposarcomas, formerly also known as round cell liposarcomas, account for up to 20% of all liposarcomas and are composed of primitive mesenchymal cells, with a variable number of signet-ring cell lipoblasts, within an abundant myxoid stroma, characteristically with a delicate arborizing vascular pattern.[22,45] Pleomorphic liposarcoma is the most rare subtype and contains a variable amount of pleomorphic lipoblasts, with no associated well-differentiated component.

Dedifferentiation occurs in up to 10% of well-differentiated liposarcomas, with 90% observed at the time of initial diagnosis, and 10% presenting as a recurrence.[2,46] The concept of low-grade dedifferentiation has been increasingly recognized, which can present as an area resembling low-grade myxofibrosarcoma, well-differentiated fibrosarcoma, dermatofibrosarcoma, or even desmoid-type fibromatosis,[47] Myxoid liposarcomas (**Fig. 2**) are the second most common subtype of liposarcoma, comprising one-third of all liposarcomas, whereas pleomorphic liposarcomas account for only about 5% of all liposarcomas.[2,3,17] Dedifferentiated liposarcomas occur most often in the retroperitoneum, whereas myxoid and pleomorphic liposarcomas most frequently affect the deep tissues of the extremities.

Ancillary studies

Dedifferentiated liposarcoma is characterized by the presence of a supernumerary ring or giant rod chromosome containing amplified 12q13 to 15 region segments,

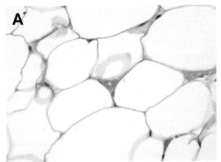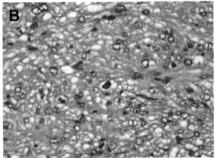

Fig. 1. Well-differentiated component, high power (*A*) (hematoxylin-eosin, original magnification ×40), of a dedifferentiated liposarcoma (*B*), high power (hematoxylin-eosin, original magnification ×20).

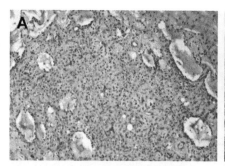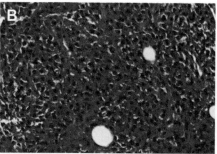

Fig. 2. A myxoid liposarcoma, low power (*A*) (hematoxylin-eosin, original magnification ×4) and high power (*B*), the latter showing a round cell histologic appearance (hematoxylin-eosin, original magnification ×20).

with several oncogenes identified within this region, including MDM2, CDK4, HMGA2, CHOP (DDIT3), and GLI1, among others.[47,48] MDM2 and CDK4 testing is very useful in the diagnosis of dedifferentiated liposarcomas or atypical lipomatous tumor, and they are usually negative in myxoid and pleomorphic liposarcomas. Poorly differentiated sarcomas with no identifiable atypical lipogenic component can be diagnosed as dedifferentiated liposarcoma on the basis of MDM2.[47] Gene amplification or protein overexpression of these markers can be detected by molecular studies, including FISH and immunohistochemistry. Greater than 90% of myxoid liposarcomas harbor the t(12;16)(q13;p11) karyotypic hallmark, which leads to the fusion of the FUS (TLS) and DDIT3 (CHOP) genes, generating a FUS/DDIT3 hybrid protein.[22,49–51]

Prognostic implications

Anatomic location is the most important known prognostic factor in dedifferentiated liposarcomas, with retroperitoneum tumors having the worst clinical behavior. The retroperitoneum is the most common primary location, and the lungs are the most common metastatic site.[44] Histologic grade, presence of necrosis, and TP53 overexpression are also associated with a less favorable prognosis.[49,52] Complex karyotypic aberrations and TP53 mutations are relatively uncommon in dedifferentiated liposarcomas, when compared with other high-grade sarcomas, which may contribute to the greater overall survival.[2,23,53,54] TP53 mutations are much more common in pleomorphic liposarcomas.[47] Myxoid liposarcoma is usually the least aggressive subtype, with less than 10% of low-grade tumors progressing to metastatic disease. In addition to histologic grade, TP53 and CDKN2A mutations are unfavorable prognostic markers for myxoid liposarcoma.[10,22,53,55] Likely oncogenic roles have been demonstrated for MDM2, CDK4, HMGA2, and TSPAN31 in dedifferentiated liposarcoma (and atypical lipomatous tumor/well-differentiated liposarcoma). Amplification of the fibroblast growth factor receptor substrate 2 gene in dedifferentiated (and well-differentiated) liposarcomas has also been recently described.[56]

Fibrosarcoma

Malignant fibrosarcomas include adult fibrosarcoma, myxofibrosarcoma, low-grade fibromyxoid sarcoma, and sclerosing epithelioid fibrosarcoma. Adult fibrosarcoma is a malignant fibroblastic tumor with variable collagen production, classically demonstrating herringbone architecture. They are thought to account for 1% to 3% of all adult sarcomas,[5,22] typically involving deep soft tissue of the extremities, trunk, or head and neck regions.[3,5] Myxofibrosarcomas (**Fig. 3**) have a variable amount of myxoid stroma, pleomorphic nuclei, characteristically with a curvilinear vascular pattern. They are more

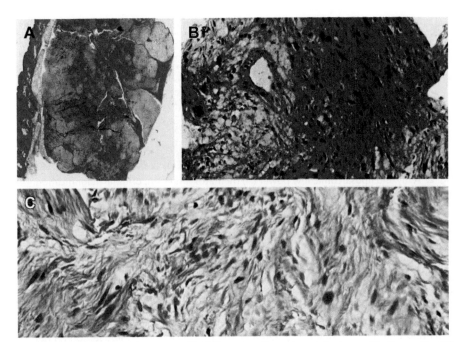

Fig. 3. Myxofibrosarcoma, low power (*A, B*) (hematoxylin-eosin, original magnifications ×2, ×10) and high power (*C*) (hematoxylin-eosin, original magnification ×40).

common in elderly patients and most commonly arise in the extremities.[3,17] Low-grade fibromyxoid sarcomas are composed of blander-appearing spindled cells with admixed myxoid and collagenous stromal areas, a whorled pattern of growth, and a curvilinear vascular pattern. Sclerosing epithelioid fibrosarcomas have a densely sclerotic stroma with cords and nests of epithelioid fibroblasts.

Histopathology and ancillary studies

The spindled cells in adult fibrosarcoma are characteristically angled in a herringbone or chevronlike pattern with hyperchromatic nuclei, variably prominent nucleoli, and scant cytoplasm. The neoplastic cells may phenotypically show myofibroblastic differentiation with SMA positivity. To date, there are no characteristic molecular studies to help definitively diagnose difficult cases of adult fibrosarcomas; however, disruption of one or more genes in the 2q14 to 22 region have been described as possibly contributing to the pathogenesis of at least some cases.[17,51,57,58] Infantile fibrosarcomas are histologically identical to adult fibrosarcomas, but they carry a distinctive translocation, t(12;15)(p13;q26), resulting in the ETV6-NTRK3 fusion, which can be detected by FISH or PCR.[51] Low-grade fibromyxoid sarcoma consistently has either a t(7;16) or t(11;16) translocation, resulting in an FUS-CREB3L2 or FUS-CREB3L1 gene fusion, respectively.[51] A few low-grade fibromyxoid sarcomas have been shown to have the EWSR1-CRE-B3L1 gene fusion; however, EWSR1 gene rearrangements are much more frequent in sclerosing ES. Low-grade fibromyxoid sarcomas and sclerosing ES also share mucin 4 immunoreactivity.[51]

Prognostic implications

The reported recurrence rates for adult fibrosarcomas and myxoinflammatory fibromyxoid sarcomas after complete excision range anywhere from 12% to 80%. Lung and bone are most common sites of metastasis for adult fibrosarcoma, and local bone and lymph node involvement is more common in myxoinflammatory fibroblastic sarcoma.[3,53] High histologic grade, mitotic rates of greater than 20 per 10 HPF, and minimal amount of collagen are associated with a worse prognosis in adult fibrosarcomas.[22] Infantile fibrosarcomas have an overall much more favorable prognosis, only rarely metastasizing, and even with cases of spontaneous regression reported,[22,59,60] although retroperitoneal location may be associated with a worse prognosis.[60]

Undifferentiated Sarcomas

The undifferentiated/unclassified sarcoma category was created as category of differentiation for any undifferentiated soft tissue sarcoma (USTS) and can be divided into subtypes based on morphologic findings as either undifferentiated spindle cell sarcoma, undifferentiated pleomorphic sarcoma, undifferentiated round cell sarcoma, undifferentiated ES, or undifferentiated sarcoma, NOS (**Fig. 4**). These USTS were previously included in the fibrohistiocytic section as "undifferentiated pleomorphic sarcoma," historically also known as "malignant fibrous histiocytoma", as they were previously thought to likely be of fibrohistiocytic differentiation. They lack a defined line of differentiation with the use of currently available technology and should be a diagnosis of exclusion. USTS usually occur in adults over the age of 40, accounting for up to 20% of all sarcomas and one-fourth of radiation-related sarcomas.[22] Most USTS arise within deep soft tissue of extremities, with some occurring in the trunk region, and less than 10% occurring superficially within subcutaneous tissue.[22]

Ancillary studies

Tumors should be sampled generously, and ancillary techniques must be used in order to rule out a defined line of differentiation. USTS may show a small number of cells expressing keratins, smooth muscle markers, epithelial membrane antigen (EMA), CD99, or CD34, insufficient for definitive differentiation.[22] Molecular studies have shown several genomic imbalances and alterations of TP53, CDKN2, and RB1, which may play a role in the development of USTS, but further studies are required to more clearly understand this relationship.[22,51]

Prognostic implications

USTS are aggressive tumors with a 50% to 60% overall 5-year survival.[61] Genetic analysis could be particularly beneficial for the possible identification of a

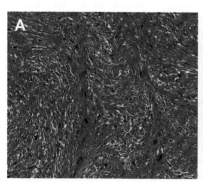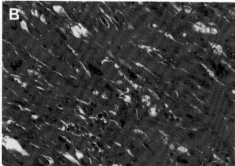

Fig. 4. USTS, low power (A) (hematoxylin-eosin, original magnification ×2) and high power (B) (hematoxylin-eosin, original magnification ×40).

dedifferentiated liposarcoma, which carries a more favorable prognosis. Undifferentiated round cell sarcomas occasionally have gene rearrangements involving the fusion of the EWSR1 gene with a non-Ewing sarcoma tumor gene, sometimes showing a possible close molecular link with Ewing sarcoma, and are usually even treated the same as Ewing sarcoma clinically.[22,62,63]

Angiosarcoma

Angiosarcoma of soft tissue is a rare malignant vascular tumor, which variably resembles normal endothelial cells. Most angiosarcomas present as a primary cutaneous tumor, and they less often present as a deep soft tissue mass.[3,5,17] Several mechanisms of pathogenesis have been suggested because they are known to be associated with radiation therapy; tumor syndromes, such as neurofibromatosis (NF); and foreign material, including grafts. They typically have areas of spindled cells and areas of epithelioid cells, with high nuclear grade, arranged in sheets or chords, and irregularly intercommunicating vascular channels. Epithelioid angiosarcoma is a variant composed predominantly of epithelioid cells with vesicular nuclei and abundant eosinophilic cytoplasm.

Ancillary studies
Immunohistochemical studies for CD34, CD31, and von Willebrand factor (vWF) support the diagnosis of angiosarcoma. vWF is the most specific, but least sensitive marker, whereas CD34 is the least specific and most sensitive marker. CD31 has both excellent sensitivity and specificity. New vascular markers that are useful in diagnosing angioarcoma include FLI1 and ERG. High levels of MYC (8q24) amplification and occasional FLT gene abnormalities have been reported in radiation-induced angiosarcomas, whereas neither have been associated with primary angiosarcomas or even radiation-associated vascular lesions.[7,22,51]

Prognostic implications
Angiosarcomas are highly aggressive with frequent local recurrences. The most common site of metastatic disease is the lung, but may often also involve lymph nodes, bone, and soft tissue. Large tumor size, retroperitoneal location, older age, and high Ki-67 proliferative index are associated with a worse prognosis.[22]

Epithelioid Hemangioendothelioma

Epithelioid hemangioendothelioma (EHE) is a malignant vascular tumor that is most commonly seen in adolescents and adults, usually presenting as a mildly painful soft tissue mass within the upper extremities. Histologic evaluation reveals angiocentric cords of epithelioid endothelial cells with eosinophilic cytoplasm containing frequent vacuoles (**Fig. 5**), within a myxo-hyalinized stroma, usually with complete obliteration of the associated vascular lumens.[22]

Ancillary studies
EHE should be immunoreactive with vascular markers such as CD34, CD31, FLI1, and ERG transcription factor. They may also show epithelial marker expression, often with keratin 7, 8, 18, or EMA.[22] Approximately 90% of EHE cases harbor the characteristic WWTR1-CAMTA1 fusion,[22,64] which leads to overexpression of both genes. The WWTR1 protein is known to be expressed by many cell types, but the CAMTA1 protein expression is usually limited to the brain. A recent study used a new polyclonal antibody, different than a previously studied one, directed against the C-terminus of CAMTA1, with findings suggesting that it may be a useful diagnostic marker for EHE.[64]

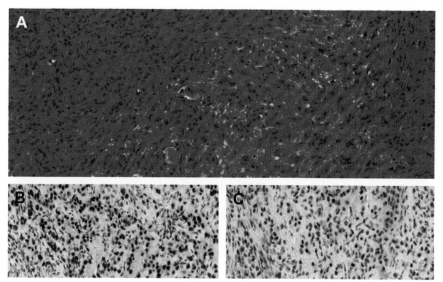

Fig. 5. EHE (*A*), low power (hematoxylin-eosin, original magnification ×10), showing nuclear immunoreactivity for ERG (*B*) and FLI1 (*C*) (original magnification ×10).

Prognostic implications

Risk stratification may be useful for categorizing these tumors into low-risk or high-risk groups, with high-risk features including tumor diameter greater than 3 cm and greater than 3 mitoses per 50 HPF. One study showed the disease-free survival at 5 years for patients with these high-risk features as nearly 60%, whereas the lack of these features showed a 100% survival at 5 years.[22,65]

Leiomyosarcoma

Leiomyosarcomas are malignant tumors that have distinct smooth muscle features. They account for a large portion of retroperitoneal sarcomas and less commonly arise within the extremities.[6,22] They are also the most common sarcoma that can arise from large blood vessel walls. They are more commonly seen in women, usually presenting as a large, variably painful, retroperitoneal or pelvic tumor.[61] If associated with a large vessel, the most common sites are the inferior vena cava and the large vessels of the lower extremities.[3,17] If the upper portion of the inferior vena cava is involved, an obstruction may result in Budd-Chiari syndrome.[66,67] Involvement of the middle portion may lead to renal vein obstruction and renal dysfunction, while involvement of the lower portions of the vessel may cause lower extremity edema.[22]

Classically, leiomyosarcomas exhibit a fascicular growth pattern, with cellular bundles of spindled cells, which are well delineated from and intersect with other bundles of spindled cells (**Fig. 6**). The cells typically have hyperchromatic and elongated nuclei with blunted ends, commonly with indentations and often with notable pleomorphism. Brisk mitoses and areas of tumor necrosis are commonly present, especially in larger tumors.[22]

Ancillary studies

Immunohistochemical studies for smooth muscle markers, such as smooth muscle actin (SMA), desmin, and caldesmin should be positive. Most reported karyotypes performed on leiomyosarcomas have shown complex karyotypes with no consistent

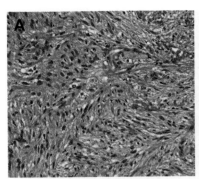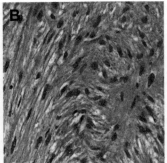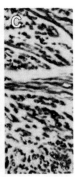

Fig. 6. Leiomyosarcoma, low power (*A*) (hematoxylin-eosin, original magnification ×10) and high power (*B*) (hematoxylin-eosin, original magnifications ×20), showing strong diffuse immunoreactivity to desmin (*C*) (Original magnification ×10).

aberrations. The RB1 gene has been frequently implicated in the pathogenesis of leiomyosarcomas with frequent abnormalities observed during analysis of the Rb-cyclinD pathway. TP53 and MDM2 are less frequently seen, but may have prognostic value, correlating with a worse prognosis.[8,51]

Prognostic implications

Retroperitoneal leiomyosarcomas are often larger than 10 cm at the time of diagnosis and may be extremely difficult to excise, commonly resulting in both local and distant metastases.[3,22,68] On the other hand, nonretroperitoneal leiomyosarcomas are generally smaller at presentation and more amenable to surgical resection with more favorable overall outcomes.[17,69] Greater histologic grade, osseous invasion, and vascular involvement are poor prognostic factors.[61] Potential therapeutic targets, such as FOXM1, are under investigation, which may have the ability to decrease the cell proliferation and increase chemosensitivity for LMS.[70]

Rhabdomyosarcoma

Rhabdomyosarcomas are malignant mesenchymal tumors that exhibit skeletal muscle differentiation. Currently, the 4 recognized subtypes include the embryonal, alveolar, pleomorphic, and spindle-cell/sclerosing rhabdomyosarcomas.[20] Embryonal rhabdomyosarcoma phenotypically and biologically resembles embryonic skeletal muscle and includes the botryoid and anaplastic variants. A spindle cell variant was previously included, but is now considered a separate subtype of rhabdomyosarcoma.[71,72] Alveolar rhabdomyosarcoma is another primitive soft tissue sarcoma, with partial skeletal muscle differentiation, which cytologically more closely resembles lymphoma.[73–76] Pleomorphic rhabdomyosarcomas should have no embryonal or alveolar components and consist of bizarre polygonal, spindled, or round cells, which have evidence of skeletal muscle differentiation.[22]

Rhabdomyosarcomas account for the largest number of sarcoma cases among children and adolescents, affecting 4 to 5 per every million US children under the age of 15.[3,53,77,78] Embryonal rhabdomyosarcoma is the most common subtype with nearly 50% occurring in children less than 5 years of age, and with a slight male predominance.[3,77,78] Alveolar rhabdomyosarcoma most often occurs in adolescents and young adults, whereas pleomorphic rhabdomyosarcoma occurs almost exclusively in adults.[3,22,78] Clinical symptoms are usually related to local mass affect and obstruction of nearby structures. The botyroid variant typically presents within hollow viscera (eg, gallbladder or urinary bladder) and has a unique appearance consisting of a cluster of variably sized tumor nodules.[22]

The most primitive histologic appearance of rhabdomyosarcoma consists of stellate rhabdomyoblasts with central oval nuclei and slightly amphophilic to eosinophilic cytoplasm. As the cells acquire greater differentiation toward mature skeletal muscle, their cytoplasm becomes eosinophilic and they become more elongated. Terminal differentiation is indicated by cross-striation and multinucleation.[22] Of note, cross-striations are a helpful diagnostic histologic feature, but are exceedingly rare in pleomorphic rhabdomyosarcomas. Alveolar rhabdomyosarcomas may present with typical morphologic features, with nested tumor cells separated by fibrovascular septa, a solid pattern, or with mixed alveolar and embryonal features.[22,75,78]

Ancillary studies

Desmin and actin immunoreactivity is acquired early on by rhabdomyoblasts. Markers for skeletal muscle differentiation, such as Myo-D or myogenin, typically show a diffusely strong nuclear staining pattern, but primitive tumors may show only focal or negative immunoreactivity. Most embryonal rhabdomyosarcomas have a loss in the chromosomal region 11p15, a region also affected by the inherited Beckwith-Wiedemann syndrome. Cytogenetic analysis of alveolar rhabdomyosarcomas revealed a specifically associated translocation, t(2;13)(q35;q14), in greater than 75%, and a t(1;13)(p36;q14) in a smaller subset, involving the PAX3 gene (chromosome 2) or the PAX7 gene (chromosome 1) and the FKHR gene on chromosome 13, forming chimeric genes, resulting in chimeric fusion proteins.[51,79–81] Chromosome analyses of pleomorphic rhabdomyosarcoma cases have shown complex karyotypes, but they lack a known recurrent genetic alteration.[23,80]

Prognostic implications

Pathologic stage, histologic classification, patient age, and site of origin help determine the prognosis of embryonal and alveolar rhabdomyosarcomas. The botyroid variant of embryonal rhabdomyosarcoma and the spindle-cell/sclerosing rhabdomyosarcoma subtype typically have more favorable outcomes, whereas alveolar and pleomorphic rhabdomyosarcomas are more aggressive subtypes. Some evidence has suggested an improved outcome with PAX7/FKHR-positive tumors when compared with PAX3/FKHR tumors.[8–10,46,54,58,79,80,82–86] In addition, a recent meta-analysis showed indications suggestive of PAX3-FOXO1 being an unfavorable prognostic factor; however, no statistically significant difference in overall survival was found.[81,87]

Synovial Sarcoma

Synovial sarcoma is currently a tumor of uncertain differentiation that shows variable epithelioid differentiation, with no identified epithelial origin to date. Despite the name, it has no association with synovial tissue. Synovial sarcoma has distinct morphologic and genetic findings, including spindled cells, often with an epithelioid component, and the chromosomal translocation t(X;18)(p11;q11). They account for up to 10% of soft tissue sarcomas and may occur at any age, most often between the ages of 15 and 40.[3,7,18,22] They can present at any site, usually as a slowly growing mass, the large majority of which develop within the deep soft tissue of the extremities, primarily near the knee region, and less than 5% occurring within a joint or bursa.[17,22] The patient may report a history of a slow-growing mass, often first noted greater than 2 years before presentation. Synovial sarcomas may be monophasic (**Fig. 7**), appearing as uniform sheets of spindled cells with ovoid pale-staining nuclei and inconspicuous nucleoli, or can be biphasic, which also includes an epithelial component. The

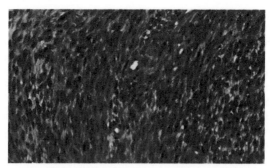

Fig. 7. Synovial sarcoma, high power, showing monophasic spindle cell component (hematoxylin-eosin, original magnification ×20).

epithelial component may even predominate over the spindle cell component and can be glandular, chordlike, or nested.[22]

The epithelial components of synovial sarcomas typically express cytokeratins (CKs) and EMA immunoreactivity. Immunohistochemical staining for Bcl2, CD99, and calponin is typically also positive, whereas S100 may be positive in as many as 30% of synovial sarcomas. The TLE1 (transducer-like enhancer of split 1) has a moderate-to-strong nuclear staining pattern in the majority (80%–90%) of synovial sarcomas, although it is not entirely specific, showing immunoreactivity in other soft tissue tumors, such as nerve sheath tumors and in SFT.[88,89] The cytogenetic hallmark for a synovial sarcoma is the recurrent reciprocal t(X;18)(p11;q11), which is present in greater than 90% of reported cases, involving the fusion of the SYT (18q11) gene with either the SSX1, SSX2, or SSX4 gene,[51] resulting in the respective fusion protein. FISH studies and real-time (RT) -PCR are widely used to detect these molecular findings and can provide a relatively rapid and definitive diagnosis for synovial sarcomas.[51,58] A relatively new immunohistochemical marker for SYT, when strongly and diffusely positive, may be useful in the rapid diagnosis of synovial sarcoma, especially when material is insufficient for PCR or FISH analysis.[90]

Prognostic implications

Tumor size greater than 5 cm, greater than 10 mitoses per HPF, the presence of extensive (>50%) necrosis, the presence of rhabdoid cells, and poorly differentiated variants are all poor prognostic factors. On the other hand, tumors less than 5 cm, young patient age, and the SS18/SSX2 are associated more favorable outcomes. The reported 10-year survival rates vary widely, ranging from about 20% to 75%.[17,22,51,72,91]

Alveolar Soft Part Sarcoma

ASPS accounts for less than 1% of all soft tissue sarcomas, affecting mostly adolescents and young adults. Morphologically, it is composed of fairly monotonous, large, round, or polygonal epithelioid cells containing abundant eosinophilic, granular cytoplasm, arranged in an organoid or nested pattern, usually separated by thin sinusoidal vessels.

Central necrosis of the nested cells may give the appearance of an alveolar pattern, hence the name. Nearly half of ASPS originate within the deep soft tissue of the thigh or buttock, and they typically present as a slowly growing painless mass.

Ancillary studies

The immunohistochemical marker TFE3 shows at least moderate nuclear reactivity in most cells, but is not entirely specific. Periodic acid–Schiff (PAS) with diastase is a useful special stain, which can highlight intracytoplasmic crystal formations that are also immunoreactive for MCT1 and CD147. Molecular evaluation for the detection of the ASPL/TFE3 fusion protein is highly sensitive and specific for ASPS and results from the classic t(X;17)(p11;q25) translocation, although it has also been identified in a small subset of renal cell carcinomas.[51]

Prognostic implications
ASPS is a slow-growing tumor, with an infrequent local recurrence rate; however, early and late metastatic disease is common. Patients often already have distant metastatic disease on initial presentation, usually involving lung, bone, or brain.[2,22,84] The most influential poor prognostic factors include increased patient age, larger tumor size, and the presence of metastasis at presentation.[22]

Clear Cell Sarcoma of Soft Tissue

Clear cell sarcoma of soft tissue, also known as melanoma of soft parts, is a soft tissue sarcoma with melanocytic differentiation that usually involves aponeurosis and tendons. Greater than 90% present as slow-growing, deep-seated extremity tumors, most often affecting young adults. They are composed of polygonal or spindled cells with abundant clear to eosinophilic cytoplasm, arranged in a nested or fascicular pattern, separated by fibrous septa. Mitotic activity and nuclear polymorphism are usually relatively low, but marked pleomorphism and brisk mitotic activity may be seen.[22]

Ancillary studies
Almost all cases of clear cell sarcoma are positive for melanocytic markers, such as S100, HMB45, and Melan-A. Melanosomes are almost always present, varying in their degree of maturation. The hallmark cytogenetic finding is the reciprocal translocation t(12;22)(q13;q12), which results in the EWS/ATF1 fusion.[10,51,83]

Prognostic implications
Overall prognosis is poor, especially with larger tumor size and the presence of necrosis. The 5-year survival is less than 70%, but the 10-year disease-free survival is only about 33%, because the development of late recurrences or metastatic disease is common.[22,51,83,92]

Desmoplastic Small Round Cell Tumor

Desmoplastic small round cell tumor (DSRCT) is a tumor of uncertain differentiation that is composed usually of small round cells with prominent stromal desmoplasia, harboring the consistent presence of the t(11:22)(p13;q12) translocation.[7,23,51,83,93] DSRCT primarily affects children and young adults, with a male predominance, and very often presents with widespread abdominal serosal involvement.[20,83] Morphologic evaluation of the tumor cells typically shows small, uniform cells with hyperchromatic nuclei, dispersed chromatin, and inconspicuous nucleoli, with a high nuclear-to-cytoplasmic ratio, indistinct cell borders, and frequent mitoses.

Ancillary studies
Immunohistochemical studies are usually helpful, with the majority of DSRCT, which show positive immunoreactivity for CKs, EMA, desmin, and WT1. SMA is typically positive in the stromal component. The characteristic t(11:22)(p13;q12) translocation results in the EWS/WT1 fusion, and the resulting chimeric fusion transcript may also be detected with excellent sensitivity and specificity for diagnosis.[7,8,51,58,83,93]

Prognostic implications

Unfortunately, the overall clinical outcomes for this rare entity remain poor, even with aggressive therapy.[94,95] Surgical excision with combination of chemotherapy and possibly the utilization of whole abdominopelvic radiation therapy may significantly improve survival outcomes for abdominal and pelvic DSRCT.[94–96]

Ewing Sarcoma

Ewing sarcoma is considered to be of neuroectodermal origin. The term primitive neuroectodermal tumor is no longer used, because molecular analysis helped show it was a histologic variation of Ewing sarcoma, differing only in the degree of neuroectodermal differentiation. The Ewing sarcoma family of tumors (EFT) also includes extraskeletal Ewing sarcomas, and Askin tumors, all of which are characterized by the recurrent t(11;22)(q22;q12) chromosomal translocation. Ewing sarcoma is the second most common primary sarcoma in children, involving either bone or soft tissue, with almost 80% of affected patients younger than 20 years of age. Ewing sarcoma commonly presents as a painful mass arising in the diaphyseal or metaphyseal-diaphyseal portion of a long bone, pelvis, or ribs. Radiographically, they appear as osteolytic lesions with a characteristic multilayered periosteal reaction. Macroscopically, during a biopsy procedure, this tumor may actually be mistaken as pus, due to its often necrotic and tan-yellow, semifluid appearance. Morphologically, most EFT are composed of small round cells with round nuclei and a fine chromatin pattern, with scant clear-to-eosinophilic cytoplasm, usually containing PAS positive glycogen.

Ancillary studies

Ewing sarcoma is usually CD99 positive, with a membranous staining pattern. Markers for vimentin and nonspecific enolase are also often positive. However, the above markers are nonspecific, and newer, more specific markers, including FLI1, ERG, and EWSR1, have become available, improving the accuracy of the initial diagnosis while definitive molecular studies are pending or unavailable. The characteristic recurrent translocation t(11;22)(q22;q12) most commonly involves the EWS gene (22q12) and FLI1 genes (85% of cases), producing a chimeric protein.[8,20,51,58] The second most common combination (10%–15%) includes the fusion of EWS with the ERG gene. Other genes, such as ETS, ETV1, E1AF, FEV, and ZSG, have also been involved in the rearrangement with the EWS gene, but these are seen in less than 1% of all EFT.[22]

Prognostic implications

Molecular markers, such as TP53, telomerase expression, or CDKN2A loss, have shown prognostic significance, while the EWSR1-ETS fusion status is no longer thought to have prognostic value.[3,7,8,10,51,58,82,83] Therapeutic advances have greatly improved clinical outcomes, with most patients presenting with localized tumors being cured of disease. The presence of metastatic disease continues to be the most important prognostic factor.[10,22]

Chondrosarcoma

Chondrosarcomas are a heterogeneous group of malignant tumors, which includes the primary central, secondary central, periosteal, dedifferentiated, mesenchymal, and clear cell variants, all of which exhibit some amount of hyaline cartilage differentiation. They are the third most common primary tumor of the bone, most often arising within the pelvic bones, femur, or humerus, typically with localized pain and swelling.[3,17] Primary central chondrosarcomas are by far the most common, arise centrally within a bone, and account for 20% of all malignant bone tumors.[3,22,83]

Secondary central chondrosarcomas arise within a benign precursor, such as an enchondroma. Periosteal chondrosarcomas arise from the surface of bones, most commonly involving the long bones.[22] These chondrosarcomas have an irregular pattern of cartilage lobules that vary in size and shape that may be separated by bands of fibrosis. Myxoid changes or ossification may also be seen. Mesenchymal chondrosarcomas have a bimorphic pattern with islands of well-differentiated hyaline cartilage and areas of small round undifferentiated cells. Clear cell chondrosarcoma is a rare low-grade subtype of chondrosarcoma, composed of hyaline cartilage and bland clear cells (**Fig. 8**). Dedifferentiated chondrosarcoma accounts for approximately 10% of chondrosarcomas and contains a well-differentiated cartilaginous tumor component with an abrupt transition to a high-grade sarcoma lacking cartilaginous differentiation.[22]

Ancillary studies

Bcl-2 may be a helpful immunohistochemical marker for distinction between an osteochondroma and low-grade secondary peripheral chondrosarcoma. Isocitrate dehydrogenase genes 1 and 2 (IDH1 and IDH2) somatic mutations are seen in most chondrosarcomas.[22,97,98] In addition, RB1 pathway mutations are seen in most high-grade central chondrosarcomas.[22,97,98]

Prognostic implications

Histologic grade is the most important prognostic indicator, with low-grade tumors having the least chance of recurrence or metastasis, and a nearly 90% overall 5-year survival.[22,99] Clear cell chondrosarcomas have excellent outcomes after complete resection with clear margins, whereas dedifferentiated chondrosarcomas have the worst prognosis, with as many as 90% of patients presenting with metastatic disease within 2 years of initial diagnosis.[3,17,97–102]

Osteosarcoma

Conventional osteosarcomas are high-grade intramedullary tumors that produce any amount of osteoid (**Fig. 9**) and include the osteoblastic (80% of cases), chondroblastic, fibroblastic, and secondary variants.[22] Osteoblastic osteosarcomas have a sclerotic appearance with a predominantly osteoid matrix, which can be thick or thin and branching. Chondroblastic osteosarcomas, on the other hand, have a predominant chondroid matrix. Fibroblastic osteosarcomas produce only minimal amounts of osteoid and have high-grade spindled cell architecture. Osteosarcoma is the most common nonhematopoietic primary malignant tumor of the bone, most commonly arising within the appendicular skeleton, and affecting about 5 in every

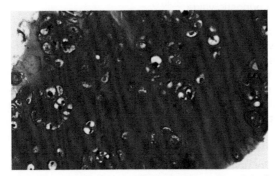

Fig. 8. Chondrosarcoma, low grade, high power (hematoxylin-eosin, original magnification ×40).

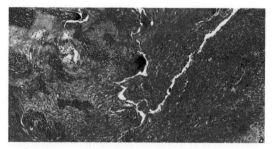

Fig. 9. Osteosarcoma, low power (hematoxylin-eosin, original magnification ×2).

million people.[22] Most cases occur in patients under the age of 25. The neoplastic cells can have one or more of many histologic appearances, including epithelioid, plasmacytoid, ovoid, multinucleated, or spindled cell morphology.[22]

Other subtypes of osteosarcoma include the telangiectatic, small cell, parosteal, periosteal, and high-grade surface osteosarcoma. Telangiectatic osteosarcoma, also previously known as malignant bone aneurysm or hemorrhagic osteosarcoma, is characterized by having large blood-filled spaces, which are usually separated by thin septa.[11,22,82] Although prognosis is thought to be similar to conventional osteosarcomas, they are much more sensitive to chemotherapy. Small cell osteosarcoma produces variable amounts of osteoid and morphologically resembles Ewing sarcoma, but lacks the t(11;22) translocation.[61] Parosteal osteosarcomas are low grade and arise on the surface of bones, most frequently involving the femur. Periosteal osteosarcomas are intermediate-grade chondroblastic osteosarcomas that also arise in the surface of bone, most commonly arising within or near the diphyseal areas of the long bones.[22]

Ancillary studies

Osteosarcomas are typically CD99 positive, and osteocalcin might be useful for highlighting osteoid, but in general immunohistochemical stains are primarily used to rule out other entities. Recurrent amplifications at 1q21 to 23 and 17p are commonly seen, and comparative genomic hybridization analysis has revealed frequent chromosomal gains, such as the gain of 8q23, seen in about half of osteosarcomas.[3,40,103] A high incidence of loss of heterozygosity has also been seen.[22,103] CDK4 with or without MDM2 is commonly amplified in aggressive osteosarcomas. Patients with hereditary retinoblastoma (RB) and Li Fraumeni syndrome have an increased risk of developing osteosarcomas. RB1 alterations have also been seen in up to 40% of sporadic osteosarcomas, whereas TP53 alterations have been seen in up to 35% of osteosarcomas. Many genetic aberrations have been found in high frequency, some of which may offer prognostic value.[22,40,42]

Prognostic implications

The overall survival, with a multidisciplinary therapeutic management approach, for osteosarcomas is about 80% to 90%.[22] Parosteal osteosarcoma carries an excellent prognosis, with a greater than 90% 5-year survival, whereas small cell osteosarcomas have slightly worse outcomes compared with conventional osteosarcomas.[22,104] Elderly patients with polyostotic Paget disease are at increased risk for developing osteosarcomas that have particularly unfavorable outcomes.[22]

Malignant Peripheral Nerve Sheath Tumor

MPNST accounts for up to 5% of all soft tissue tumors and can be found in the setting of NF1 or arising from a peripheral nerve or benign nerve sheath tumor. Individuals with NF1 have about a 50% chance developing MPNST, with a higher chance of development associated with plexiform neuromas. MPNST can be variably painful, most commonly involving a major nerve, such as the sciatic nerve, which often presents with neuropathic symptoms. Microscopically, they typically show a fascicular or whorling growth pattern of spindled cells, with alternating hypercellular and hypocellular areas and prominent, branching, HPC-like vasculature. The neoplastic cells are usually more concentrated and appear more epithelioid adjacent to the blood vessels. Up to about 15% of MPNST have heterologous elements, and the term malignant Triton tumor is used for an MPNST with skeletal muscle differentiation.[22,46,105]

Ancillary studies

Although MPNST can stain positively for S100 in up to about 50% of cases, a diffusely strong immunoreactivity is very uncommon, so other tumors within the differential diagnosis, such as melanoma, dendritic cell sarcoma, and cellular schwannoma, should be considered in that setting. Helpful histologic features include perivascular hypercellularity, tumor herniation into vascular lumens, necrosis, and expression of p75NTR, all of which are frequently associated with MPNST.[105] Glial fibrillary acidic protein (GFAP) shows positive immunoreactivity in up to 30% of MPNST.[22] Complete loss of SOX10, neurofibromin, or p16 immunoreactivity, and the presence of EGFR expression are also helpful in differentiating MPNST from a cellular schwannoma.[105] MPNSTs usually have a complex karyotype, and many have biallelic NF1 or CDK2NA gene mutations.[22]

Prognostic implications

MPNSTs with higher grade, diameter greater than 5 cm, recurrent disease, arising within the trunk region, and Triton tumors are associated with more aggressive behavior, whereas sporadic MPNSTs seem to have an overall better prognosis. Certain chromosomal arm gains and losses also seem to have prognostic significance, none of which have been found to be more associated with NF1 when compared with sporadic MPNSTs.[7,10,83]

Epithelioid Sarcoma

ESs account for up to 1% of all soft tissue sarcomas, occurring most commonly in adolescents and young adults, classically arising within acral sites with a pseudogranulomatous growth pattern. Another subtype, the "large cell" variant or proximal-type ES, usually arises within truncal regions. Histologically, the neoplastic cells may have a vaguely granulomatous growth pattern of predominantly plump epithelioid to spindled cells containing eosinophilic cytoplasm, most often with associated central or geographic necrosis.[22,106]

Ancillary studies

Most ES show positive immunoreactivity with CK 8 and 19, but are negative to focally positive for CK 5/6.[22,106] Unlike a sarcomatoid carcinoma, most ES are positive for CD34. Most also have a loss of SMARCB1 (INI1) protein expression, which likely plays an important role in the pathogenesis of these tumors.[80,107]

Prognostic implications

The overall 5-year survival for ES approaches 80%, whereas the reported 10-year overall survival is up to about 62%.[106,108–110] Metastatic disease may occur in about half of the cases, with a predilection for the lungs.[106,109,110] Unlike most sarcomas, ES is most commonly metastatic to regional lymph nodes. Factors associated with worse outcomes include tumor size of greater than 5 cm, male gender, older age, multifocality, high mitotic activity, nodal involvement, and proximal, axial, or deep soft tissue location.[22,106,110,111]

SARCOMAS WITH LOW METASTATIC POTENTIAL
Solitary Fibrous Tumor

The distinction between a SFT and an HPC has become increasingly ill-defined, so much so that the term HPC is no longer considered a separate entity for soft tissue tumors.[20,21,61] SFT (**Fig. 10**) is a mesenchymal tumor, likely fibroblastic, with the characteristic "hemangiopericytoma-like" prominent branching vascular pattern.[20-22] Most patients are middle-aged adults, with a median age of 50, and tumors can arise from any location, mostly occurring within subcutaneous tissue as a slow-growing painless mass.[3,17] Rarely, large tumors have been found to secrete hormones, leading to a paraneoplastic syndrome.[112-114] Histologic evaluation usually shows a patternless architecture with alternating hypocellular and hypercellular areas, with the classical prominent branching vasculature. Thick stromal and perivascular collagen bands are also characteristically seen. For a benign SFT, mitotic rate should be low, with less than 4 mitoses per 10 HPF. Cytologic atypia, infiltrative margins, high cellularity, and greater than 4 mitoses per HPF are features of a malignant SFT.[22]

Ancillary studies
Cytogenetic aberrations are uncommon in SFTs that are less than 10 cm in diameter. Some studies have reported near diploid or pseudodiploid karyotypes, balanced translocations, and recurrent genomic imbalances. The recurrent *NAB2-STAT6* fusion has been recently identified by integrative sequencing and has been established as the hallmark defining driver mutation of SFT.[115-120] STAT6 immunohistochemistry can also be a useful marker in the diagnosis of SFT, especially in cases with unusual morphology or location, and limited material.[115,120-122]

Prognostic implications
Only a minority of SFT behaves aggressively, with approximately 80% to 90% following a benign course.[22] SFTs that arise within the mediastinum, pelvis, and

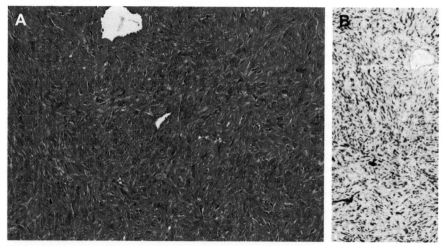

Fig. 10. Malignant SFT (*A*) (hematoxylin-eosin, original magnification ×4), showing positive nuclear immunoreactivity for STAT6 (*B*) (Original magnification ×2).

abdominal regions, and the histologically malignant SFTs are associated with more aggressive behaviors. The fusion variant *NAB2ex6-STAT6ex16/17* is associated with deep-seated extrapleural SFTs, and aggressive behavior.[121]

Inflammatory Myofibroblastic Tumor

Inflammatory myofibroblastic tumor (IMT) is a spindle cell tumor that most often arises within the soft tissue or viscera of children or young adults.[22] It is characterized by a variably cellular infiltrate of lymphocytes, eosinophils, and plasma cells, often within a myxoid or edematous background.[22]

Ancillary studies

IMT is variably positive for SMA, desmin, and focally positive for CD68.[22] Approximately one-third of cases may have keratin reactivity, and up to about 60% are ALK positive.[123,124] S100 and skeletal muscle markers are negative in these tumors.[22,124]

Prognostic implications

The likelihood of metastatic disease is usually low, with only rarely reported cases of distant metastasis. Most ALK-negative tumors are associated with an increased likelihood of metastasis; however, the round cell morphology, often associated with specific ALK fusion partners, such as RANBP2, has a greater chance of progressing to metastatic disease.[22,123–126] Aneuploidy is also a negative prognostic factor.[7,8,20,22,127]

Low-Grade Myofibroblastic Sarcoma

Low-grade myofibroblastic sarcoma, also known as myofibrosarcoma, most commonly occurs in adults with a possible predilection for the extremities or head and neck regions. They usually have fibromatosis-like features and are characterized by a diffusely infiltrative growth pattern of spindled cells, with at least focal nuclear atypia and pale to eosinophilic cytoplasm, arranged in a storiform or fascicular growth pattern.[22]

Ancillary studies

Low-grade myofibroblastic sarcomas are variably positive for smooth muscle markers and may stain positive for calponin, or sometimes with focal reactivity for CD34.[22]

Prognostic implications

Very few genetic aberrations have been reported, with overall less complex karyotypes when compared with other higher-grade sarcomas.[20,22,51,93] Although not diagnostic, gene rearrangement studies may be considered for differentiating low-grade myofibroblastic sarcoma from fibromatosis.[7,22,58] Overall, frequency of metastatic disease is very rare.[22]

Myxoinflammatory Fibroblastic Sarcoma

Myxoinflammatory fibroblastic sarcoma is characterized by large epithelioid fibroblasts within a myxoid matrix, containing prominent mixed inflammatory cells. The great majority occur in the distal extremities, especially common in the fingers, involving tenosynovial structures, usually in middle-aged individuals.[128–130] Morphologic evaluation reveals variable nuclear atypia, often with large bizarre epithelioid cells, prominent viral inclusion-like nucleoli, and sometimes with vacuolated cytoplasm.[22,128,129,131,132]

Ancillary studies

Myxoinflammatory fibroblastic sarcomas are variably positive for CD68, CD34, and SMA and may be focally positive for keratin markers.[22] They characteristically have t(1;10) breakpoints leading to the upregulation of FGF8.[22,51,58]

Prognostic implications

Myxoinflammatory fibroblastic sarcomas are considered locally aggressive tumors, with widely variable local recurrence rates reported from 20% to 70%.[22] Up to one-third of cases eventually require amputation due to repeated local recurrences.[29,130,132–134] Metastatic disease is rare, usually involving local bone or regional lymph nodes, with extremely uncommon distant metastatic disease.[83,128,129,131,132,135–137]

Dermatofibrosarcoma Protuberans

Dermatofibrosarcoma protuberans (DFSP), a low-grade fibroblastic neoplasm that usually presents in middle aged-adults, although rare, is one of the most common dermal sarcomas.[22,138] Most are sporadic, occurring in proximal extremities or trunk regions, less commonly in the head and neck or other regions, and usually present as a cutaneous plaque or nodule.[138] Histologic evaluation reveals a dense dermal proliferation of uniform spindled cells, with elongated or plump nuclei, minimal nuclear atypia, and few mitoses, arranged in a storiform pattern of growth.[22]

Ancillary studies

DFSP is usually CD34 positive and factor XIIIa negative, but may lose CD34 reactivity often with increased TP53 expression.[22,138] Gene rearrangement studies characteristically show supernumerary ring chromosomes, containing sequences from chromosomes 22 and 17, carrying the COL1A1-PDGFB (platelet-derived growth factor B-chain) fusion gene, which can be detected by FISH (preferred) or RT-PCR.[22,51] The resultant COL1A-PDGFRB fusion protein results in a functional PDGFB receptor on the cell surface that can be stimulated, driving tumor growth.[7,51,93,138–140]

Prognostic implications

Approximately 10% to 15% progress to higher-grade fibrosarcomatous DFSP, typically exhibiting fascicular architecture, which increases the metastatic potential of the tumor.[138,140,141] Tyrosine kinase inhibitors, such as imatinib mesylate, interfere with the activation of PDGFRB and are especially useful in the setting of unresectable or metastatic disease.[7,51] Molecular testing is available to help identify patients who may have clinical response.[138,139,142,143] Local recurrence rates for DFSP are lowest if wide margins can be achieved.[22,143] They very rarely metastasize unless fibrosarcomatous progression is present.[22,144–146]

Kaposi Sarcoma

Kaposi sarcoma (KS) is a locally aggressive vascular proliferation (**Fig. 11**) induced by the human herpes virus 8 (HHV8), which is also known as Kaposi sarcoma–associated herpes virus.[22,147] It characteristically presents a red-purple to brown skin patch, plaque, or nodule, usually involving the distal extremities.[3,147,148] Currently, 4 clinical forms of KS are recognized, including the classic indolent form, the endemic African form, the iatrogenic form arising in association with solid organ transplantation, and the AIDS-associated form of KS, all of which are morphologically identical.[3,147–150]

Ancillary studies

The neoplastic cells are positive for endothelial markers, including CD31, CD34, and ERG, as well as lymphatic markers such as D2-40.[151] HHV8 is nearly always positive by immunohistochemistry; however, rare cases may require PCR for confirmation.[22,148,149,152–154]

Prognostic implications

The classic KS has an indolent clinical course with only rare metastatic disease involving lymph nodes or visceral organs.[3,147] A rare form of endemic KS, the

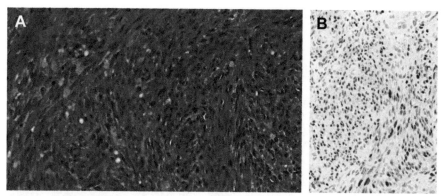

Fig. 11. KS, high power (*A*) (hematoxylin-eosin, original magnification ×20), showing the characteristic positive nuclear immunoreactivity for HHV8 (*B*) (Original magnification ×10).

lymphadenopathic variant, is rapidly progressive with a high mortality.[22] The AIDS-associated KS is overall the most aggressive form, with more widespread organ involvement, mostly involving the lungs and gastrointestinal tract.[22] The iatrogenic form is the least predictable, often improving after adjustment of immunosuppressive therapy.[3,147,151,155] New therapeutic approaches have focused on the control of HHV8 for prevention and treatment of KS. For example, antiherpes medications, such as ganciclovir, have been found to reduce the risk of KS among transplant patients, as well as in HIV-positive individuals.[147,148,155,156] In addition, targeted therapy, including inhibitors of angiogenesis, vascular endothelial growth factor, tyrosine kinase, and matrix metalloproteinases are being investigated or are under development.[147,152]

Chordoma

Chordoma is a low-grade malignant tumor showing notochordal differentiation. It is the most common primary malignancy of the sacrum; however, it more commonly arises within the base of the skull.[3,22,157] They typically present as slow-growing tumors, and morphologically are composed of epithelioid cells arranged in nests or cords with clear to eosinophilic cytoplasm (**Fig. 12**), with the so-called physaliphorous cells, which contain vacuolated cytoplasm.[22] Chordomas morphologically exhibit a lobulated appearance with tumor cells separated by fibrous septa and embedded within abundant extracellular myxoid matrix.[22] A rare variant, chondroid chordoma, contains a hyaline cartilage component, which can potentially be misdiagnosed as chondrosarcoma.[158,159]

Ancillary studies
Brachyury is a nuclear immunohistochemical marker that is specific for chordoma, and negative in chondrosarcoma.[22,158,160] Other helpful positive immunohistochemical markers for chordoma include keratin, EMA, and S-100 protein.[158,160,161] A loss of PTEN and INI-1 expression may also be useful in the diagnosis of chordoma.[158,161–165]

Prognostic implications
Dedifferentiated chordoma is a high-grade and biphasic tumor consisting of a conventional chordoma with an associated high-grade undifferentiated spindle cell sarcoma.[22,166–168] The dedifferentiated component loses expression of the above diagnostic immunohistochemical markers.[22,167–169] Imatinib may be useful for

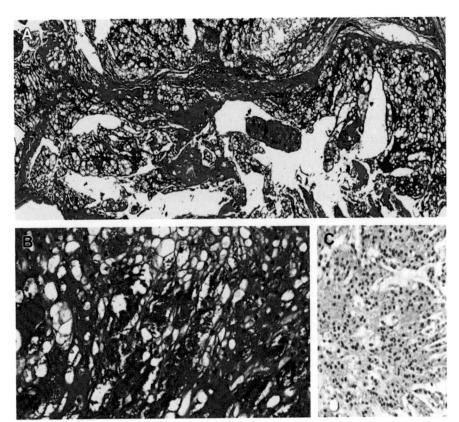

Fig. 12. Chordoma, low power (*A*) (hematoxylin-eosin, original magnification ×2) and high power (*B*) (hematoxylin-eosin, original magnification ×40), showing positive immunoreactivity for brachyury (*C*) (Original magnification ×4).

stabilization of disease or for pain reduction in locally advanced or metastatic disease if the tumor expresses platelet-derived growth factor receptor-β (PDGFR-β).[158,161,163]

Gastrointestinal Stromal Tumors

GIST is the most common mesenchymal tumor that occurs in the gastrointestinal tract and is thought to be of interstitial cell of Cajal differentiation. More than half of cases are sporadic and involve the stomach, with a clinical spectrum that ranges from benign to malignant.[170] GISTs most often have spindle cell morphology, but also frequently exhibit epithelioid cell histology. If spindle cell morphology is present, the pallisading vacuolated and sclerosing subtypes are the most common, although, with the epithelioid morphology, sclerosing, hypercellular, or discohesive histologic findings may most often be seen.[22,170]

Ancillary studies

GIST is classically strongly immunoreactive for CD117 (c-KIT). A more recent and equally specific immunomarker, DOG1, usually reacts with the approximately 5% of GISTs that are negative for CD117.[22] GISTs with spindle cell morphology are usually also positive for CD34 and rarely focally immunoreactive with smooth muscle markers, keratins, or S100.[22] GIST is characterized by activating oncogenic mutations, classically either KIT or PDGFRA.[22,51] Most GISTs harbor a mutation in KIT exon 9, KIT exon 11, or PDGFRA exon 18.[51] The few cases of GIST that are associated with the Carney triad and Carney-Stratakis syndrome typically show mutations in SDH-related genes and have a distinct morphology.[51]

Prognostic implications

Tumor size, mitotic activity, and anatomic site are currently the tumor parameters that are best used as prognostic indicators to separate patients into prognostic groups.[22,170] A Ki67 proliferative index may also be a useful tool, especially in border-line cases.[171] Mutational analysis, currently most often performed by PCR methods, is now essential for selection of therapy and for prognostic value.[51] Tyrosine kinase inhibitors, such as imatinib mesylate, have been successfully used in the treatment of GIST.[8,51,170] Recently, BRAF V600E mutations were identified in cases lacking KIT and PDGFRA mutations,[51] which may respond to BRAF therapy.[172,173] SDH-deficient GISTs have less predictable prognosis, but GISTs that arise in association with NF1 are typically multifocal with favorable outcomes.[22]

LOCALLY AGGRESSIVE SOFT TISSUE TUMORS
Atypical Lipomatous Tumor

ALT is a locally aggressive tumor with adipocytic differentiation (**Fig. 13**). This term is now preferred over the term "well-differentiated liposarcoma"; the latter has fallen out of favor due to the fact that these tumors have no metastatic potential, unless they undergo dedifferentiation.[22] Certain tumors that are deemed unresectable, usually ones located in the mediastinum or retroperitoneum, typically have locally aggressive and uncontrollably recurrent disease with a higher likelihood of eventual dedifferentiation, so the term well-differentiated liposarcoma may be justifiable in such cases.[22]

Ancillary studies

MDM2 and CDK4 testing are useful in the diagnosis of ATL and are usually negative in myxoid and pleomorphic sarcomas.[22] Gene amplification or protein overexpression of these markers can be detected by FISH or immunohistochemistry, respectively.[47,51,58]

Prognostic implications

Radiation therapy is frequently used in the management of ALT or well-differentiated liposarcoma, especially in cases with positive margins or tumors greater than 5 cm; however, there may be no significant effect on overall survival with the addition of radiation therapy, compared with surgery alone when located in the extremities.[174,175]

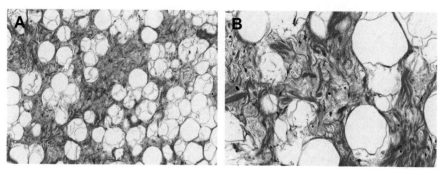

Fig. 13. Atypical lipomatous tumor, low power (*A*) (hematoxylin-eosin, original magnification ×4) and high power (*B*) (hematoxylin-eosin, original magnification ×40).

Dedifferentiation occurs in up to 10% of atypical lipomatous tumors, which then gives the tumor metastatic potential, at which point it is diagnosed as a dedifferentiated liposarcoma.[3,7,44,58,83]

Fibromatosis

Locally aggressive forms of fibromatosis include desmoid-type fibromatosis, palmar/plantar fibromatosis, and lipofibromatosis.[22] Desmoid-type fibromatosis (**Fig. 14**) typically arises within deep soft tissue and is rarer than the superficial forms.[176–179] Pathogenesis is thought to be multifactorial, with likely genetic factors.[22] Palmar and plantar fibromatosis occur more commonly in men with increasing incidence with age.[22,69] Lipofibromatosis is an exceedingly rare pediatric tumor usually arising within the hand or foot, or less commonly in the head and neck or truncal regions.[22] Each of these forms of fibromatosis has a high rate of local recurrence, but no metastatic potential.[176–178,180,181] Desmoid-type fibromatosis is a proliferation composed of uniform whorling spindled cells with infiltrative borders, often with prominent vasculature, perivascular edema, and a variable mitotic rate.[22,69,177,178,182–184]

Ancillary studies

Desmoid-type, palmar, and plantar fibromatosis usually have nuclear immunoreactivity for β–catenin and variable immunoreactivity for SMA and are usually negative for desmin, caldesmin, and S100.[22,183] Lipofibromatosis usually has a similar-appearing fibrous component with abundant mature adipose tissue, usually greater than 50% of the tumor.[22] The mutations in the gene encoding for β-catenin (CTNNB1) and APC gene mutations occur in the large majority of desmoid-type fibromatosis, resulting in the accumulation of β-catenin protein within the nucleus.[22,183] Gene rearrangement studies have shown clonal chromosomal aberrations in the minority of fibromatosis cases.[22]

Prognostic implications

Although desmoid-type fibromatosis has no metastatic potential, rare cases have been fatal due to local growth effects.[177,182,185] Unfortunately, the ability to achieve adequate margins after resection does not seem to correlate well with the rate of local recurrence, making the likelihood of recurrent disease somewhat unpredictable.[22] For palmar and plantar fibromatosis, on the other hand, the rate of local recurrence is closely related to adequacy of margins.[22] Prognostic implications of the reported gene mutations or chromosomal aberrations are currently unclear.[22,51,58,183]

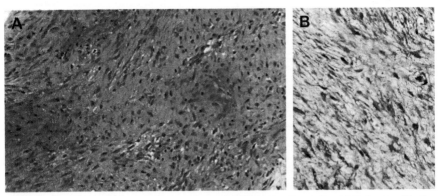

Fig. 14. Desmoid-type fibromatosis, low power (A) (hematoxylin-eosin, original magnification ×10), showing nuclear immunoreactivity for β-catenin (B) (Original magnifications ×10).

BENIGN SOFT TISSUE AND BONE TUMORS

Benign soft tissue tumors are a great deal more common than benign bone tumors and are far more common than sarcomas, with only about one out of every hundred overall soft tissue tumors found to be malignant.[22] They can be categorized based on their histologic differentiation, usually as tumors of adipocytic, cartilaginous, osteogenic, fibrogenic, fibrohistiocytic, vascular, perivascular, or neural differentiation (**Table 4**),[22] while benign bone tumors are currently most commonly classified as chondrogenic, osteogenic, fibrogenic, fibrohistiocytic, or vascular differentiation.[22] The most common benign soft tissue tumors are adipocytic, followed closely by fibrogenic tumors (**Table 5**).[20,22] A tumor should only be considered benign after ensuring that the pathologic diagnosis fits the clinical picture. This process involves gathering appropriate clinical and radiologic information, followed by adequate tissue sampling for pathologic evaluation, possibly with the aid of ancillary studies. If uncertainty persists, additional sampling or close follow-up is indicated.

GIANT CELL TUMORS
Tenosynovial Giant Cell Tumor

Tenosynovial giant cell tumors are a group of neoplastic disorders that involve synovium-lined tendon sheaths, synovial joints, and adjacent soft tissue. They are divided into localized and diffuse subtypes. The localized type is also known as nodular tenosynovitis. It presents as discrete nodules primarily affecting the tenosynovium of hands and feet (75% are in digits).[22] The nodule is grossly well circumscribed and encapsulated. The cut section shows a lobulated and tan-brown appearance. The tumor is composed of a polymorphous population of cells including osteoclast-like giant cells, larger mononuclear histiocytes, smaller mononuclear stromal cells, and macrophages that either engulf fatty content (xanthoma cells or foamy cells) or are hemosiderin-laden (pigmented). Lymphoplasmacytic infiltration is usually a minor component. Fibrous and collagenous stroma can be seen. The diffused type is also called pigmented villonodular tenosynovitis. The intra-articular lesions and the extra-articular affect the knee. The diffuse type tumors have larger and more numerous giant cells. The intra-articular lesions has typical villous pattern.

Ancillary studies
The larger mononuclear cells are positive for clusterin, while the smaller histiocytes are positive for CD68. There is also a high level of *CSF1* expression of the tumor cells resulted by the translocation of *CLO6A3* with CSF1 gene.[22]

Prognostic implications
Local type is a benign lesion with local recurrence.

Giant Cell Tumor of Bone

Giant cell tumor of bone is a benign but locally aggressive tumor. The tumor is composed of numerous characteristic giant cells that are large and osteoclast-like (**Fig. 15**). These cells are impressive morphologically; however, they are the background cells reactive to the true neoplastic cells, which are primitive mesenchymal stromal cells. The neoplastic cells are mononuclear and express receptor activator for nuclear factor -κB ligand RANKL, the master regulator of osteoclast differentiation.[22] Macrophages and osteoclasts express RANK. The interaction between the neoplastic mononuclear stromal cells and macrophages/osteoclasts by an RANKL-dependent mechanism via the stimulation of macrophage-colony stimulation factor results in neoplastic proliferation and induces osteoclast formation.[22] During this

Table 4
Common histological, immunohistochemical, and molecular findings of selected benign soft tissue tumors

Classification/ Tumor Type	Histology	Immunohistochemical	Molecular
Adipocytic			
Lipoma	Well-circumscribed, mature white adipocytes	MDM2 (−), S100 (+), leptin (+), HMGA2 (+)	MDM2 (−) HMGA2 aberrations
Lipoblastoma	Diffuse or local, lobular embryonal adipocytic cells, and fibrovascular septa	S100 (+), CD34 (+), desmin (+/−)	PLAG1
Angiolipoma	Mature adipocytes, thin capillary-sized vessels containing fibrin thrombi	S100 (+), HMGA2 (+/−)	HMGA2
Spindle cell/pleomorphic lipoma	Mature adipocytes, admixed bland spindled cells/multinucleated (often "floret-like") giant cells, thick ropelike collagen fibers, myxoid matrix	CD34 (+) spindled cells, S100 (−/+), desmin (−/+)	Losses involving 13q, 16q, 6q, 10p
Chondroid lipoma	Mature adipocytes, admixed small round lipoblasts, chondromyxoid matrix	S100 (+/−), PAS (+)	Fusion of C11of 95 (11q13) and MKL2 (16p13.3)
Hibernoma	Variable amount of polygonal, multivacuolated cells with small central nucleus, and granular cytoplasm (brown fat)	S100 (+/−), CD34 (−), desmin (−/+), UCP1 (+)	11q aberrations UCP1 expression
Cartilagenous			
Soft tissue chondroma	Lobulated mature hyaline cartilage, often hypercellular, with groups of chondrocytes	—	12q13, +5, +8, HMGA2
Fibrogenic			
Nodular fasciitis	Plump spindled fibroblasts/myofibroblasts, frequent mitoses, lacking nuclear hyperchromasia or pleomorphism, occasional osteoclast-like giant cells, tissue culture-like growth pattern	Actin (+) strong/diffuse, Desmin (−) CD68 (+) giant cells	MYH9-USP6 fusion

	Histology	IHC	Molecular/Genetics
Elastofibroma	Fibrocollagenous tissue with abnormally prominent elastic fibers	Elastin (+), tropoelastin (+)	Chromosome 1 aberrations, Xq12–22 gain
Myositis ossificans	Localized nodular fasciitis-like proliferation with osteoblasts and osteoclasts rimming irregular sheets of bone formation	Actin (+), desmin (+/–)	Limited data
Cellular angiofibroma	Uniform, spindled cells, numerous small-to-medium, thick-walled vessels, variably fibrous to edematous stroma	CD34 (+/–), actin (–/+), desmin (–/+)	AHRR-NCOA2
Gardner fibroma	Hypocellular, haphazard, thick collagen fibers	CD34 (+), nuclear β-catenin (+/–) actin (–), desmin (–)	Associated with Gardner-type FAP
Fibrohistiocytic			
Tenosynovial giant cell tumor, localized type	Lobulated, variable proportions of multinucleated giant cells and variably sized mononuclear cells with pale cytoplasm, hemosiderin deposits, and variably hyalinized stroma, arising from synovium	Clusterin (+) in larger mononuclear cells CD68 (+), CD45(+), and CD163(+) smaller cells CD68 (+), CD45 (+), tartrate-resistant acid phosphatase (+) giant cells	CSF1-COL6A3
Deep benign fibrous histiocytoma	Well-circumscribed, cellular spindled cells, storiform pattern, vesicular nuclei, many with prominent branching vascular pattern	CD34 (+), SMA (+/–)	Limited data
Neural/perineural			
Schwannoma	Majority are biphasic with compact spindled cells (Antoni A) and looser areas (Antoni B) with pallisading verocay bodies	S100 (+), collagen IV (+), laminin (+), GFAP (+/–), SOX-10 (+)	Chromosome 22 losses, NF2, SMARCB1
Neurofibroma	Loosely arranged small, spindled cells, with collagen fibers and myxoid material	S100 (focal +), GLUT1 (+), claudin-1 (+), EMA (+/–) in perineural-like cells	NF1
Perineurioma	Spindled cells with storiform growth pattern, perivascular whorls, in collagenous stroma	EMA (+), GLUT1 (+/–), claudin-1 (+/–), S100 (–), GFAP (–)	Chromosome 22 losses, NF2

(continued on next page)

Table 4
(continued)

Classification/ Tumor Type	Histology	Immunohistochemical	Molecular
Granular cell tumor	Nested to trabecular large ovoid cells with eosinophilic, granular cytoplasm, ill-defined borders. Often associated with pseudo-epitheliomatous hyperplasia of overlying epithelium	S100 (+), CD68 (+), CD63 (+), MITF (+/–), TFE (+/–), HMB45 (–), GFAP (–)	Limited data Malignant granular cell tumors may show partial loss of 5p
Smooth muscle			
Leiomyoma	Spindled cells with eosinophilic cytoplasm, cigar-shaped nuclei, arranged in fascicular growth pattern	Actin (+), desmin (+), h-caldesmon (+), S100 (–) Abdominal or inguinal tumors usually ER, PR, and WT1 (+)	Not well-described in soft tissue. Likely variable clonal chromosomal changes
Skeletal muscle			
Rhabdomyoma	Unencapsulated, lobular, large polygonal cells with abundant eosinophilic granular cytoplasm, cross-striations, or rodlike inclusions, round vesicular nuclei, and well-defined cell borders	Actin (+), desmin (+), myogenin (+)	Few reports of sonic hedgehog pathway activation
Vascular			
Hemangiomas	Multiple dilated, predominantly thin-walled, variably sized vascular channels, commonly with hemosiderin deposition, and fibrotic or myxoid stroma	WT1 (+), ERG (+), CD31 (+), CD34 (+) Epithelioid variant CK (focal +/–)	Limited data
Lymphangioma	Cystic, variably sized, lymphatic channels, lined by flattened endothelium, commonly empty or filled with proteinaceous fluid or lymphocytes	Podoplanin/D2-40 (+), PROX1 (+), CD31 (+), CD34 (+/–)	Limited data

Perivascular			
Glomus tumor	Nested small uniform, rounded cells with central round nuclei, amphophilic to eosinophilic cytoplasm, sharply defined cell borders, surrounding capillary-sized vessels	SMA (+), caldesmon (+), collagen IV (+, pericellular)	Hereditary tumor syndrome cases associated with GLMN or NF1
Myopericytoma	Nodular or lobular, uniform oval spindled myoid cells, with multilayered, concentric perivascular growth. Neoplastic cells with plump, spindled nuclei and eosinophilic cytoplasm	Perivascular cells SMA (+), caldesmon (+), Neoplastic cells desmin (focal +/−), CD34 (focal +/−)	ACTB-GLI1 fusion
Angioleiomyoma	Spindled cells with eosinophilic cytoplasm, cigar-shaped nuclei, arranged in fascicular pattern with intervening vascular channels	Actin (+), calponin (+), caldesmon (+/−)	Variable, most commonly with 22q11.2 loss or Xq gain
Uncertain differentiation			
Acral fibromyxoma	Spindled to stellate-shaped fibroblasts within collagenous or myxoid stroma, loose fascicular to storiform patterns, usually with numerous vessels and mast cells	CD34 (+), EMA (+/−)	GNAS (−)
Intramuscular myxoma	Spindled to stellate-shaped fibroblasts within abundant, often vacuolated, myxoid stroma, and sparse small vessels	CD34 (+/−), desmin (+/−), actin (+/−)	GNAS
Deep angiomyxoma	Spindled to stellate myoid cells, with loose myxoedematous to collagenous stroma	ER/PR (+/−), CD34 (+/−), actin (+/−), desmin (+/−), HMGA2 (+/−)	12q13–15, HMGA2

Data from Refs.[22,23,51,54,58,93,103,186–189]

Table 5
Common histologic, immunohistochemical, and molecular findings of selected benign bone tumors

Classification/Tumor Type	Histology	Immunohistochemical	Molecular
Chondrogenic			
Osteochondroma	Perichondrium, cartilage, and bone layers. Continuous cortical and medullary bone with stalk	—	EXT1 or EXT2 Negative for IDH1 or IDH2 mutations
Chondromas	Encondroma: Hypocellular, avascular, with prominent hyaline cartilage matrix Periosteal chondroma: Similar, but beneath periosteum, occasional with mild nuclear pleomorphism	—	IDH mutations
Chondromyxoid fibroma	Peripherally, spindled cells with fibrous stroma. Centrally, stellate and chondrocyte-like cells with chondromyxoid stroma	—	Chromosome 6 aberrations
Osteogenic			
Osteoma	Compact, spongious, or mixed lamellar bone, with osteoblastic remodeling, in a well-vascularized, moderately cellular, fibrous stroma	—	Limited data
Osteoid osteoma	Small (<2 cm) tumor with central (nidus) of osteoblastic activity, producing osteoid and often bone	—	Rare reports of clonal chromosomal aberrations
Osteoblastoma	Similar to osteoid osteoma, except >2 cm and richly vascular	—	Variable reported, limited data
Fibrohistiocytic			
Nonossifying fibroma	Large proliferation of bland spindled fibroblasts, with storiform growth pattern, extending into medullary cavities	—	Limited data

(continued on next page)

Table 5 (continued)			
Classification/Tumor Type	**Histology**	**Immunohistochemical**	**Molecular**
Benign fibrous histiocytoma	Identical histologic findings as nonossifying fibroma, but different clinical and radiologic presentation (smaller, usually involving nonmetaphyseal long bones or pelvis)	—	Limited data
Notochordal			
Benign notochordal cell tumor	Well-defined tumor with vacuolated cells, small centrally or peripherally located round or oval nuclei, and no nuclear atypia. Lacks the lobular architecture, fibrous bands, and myxoid matrix seen in chordoma	S100 (+), EMA (+), keratin (+), brachyury (+)	Limited data
Undefined neoplastic nature			
Aneurysmal bone cyst	Well-circumscribed, cystic spaces filled with blood, separated by cellular fibrous septa containing bland fibroblasts, scattered multinucleated osteoclast-like cells and woven bone rimmed by osteoblasts, often mitotically active	—	USP6 fusion with CDH11, TRAP150, ZNF9, OMD, or COLA1

Data from Fletcher CDM, World Health Organization, International Agency for Research on Cancer. WHO classification of tumours of soft tissue and bone. World Health Organization classification of tumours. 4th edition. Lyon (France): IARC Press; 2013. p. 468; and Letson GD, Muro-Cacho CA. Genetic and molecular abnormalities in tumors of the bone and soft tissues. Cancer Control 2001;8(3):239–51.

process, tumor-associated macrophage-like osteoclast precursors, which are also mononuclear cells, are recruited by tumoral stromal cells to participate in osteoclast differentiation and activation. Because osteoclast formation is the major consequence of GCTB, inhibition of osteoclast formation and activity is the key therapeutic approach. For example, bisphosphonate inhibits osteoclast-mediated resorption of bone/osteolysis and anti-RANKL antibody targets the RANKL-dependent mechanism of GCTB formation.[186,190–193]

Osteoprotegerin (OPG) is a soluble decoy receptor that is produced by osteoblasts to inhibit osteoclast differentiation through its binding to RANKL, which prevents

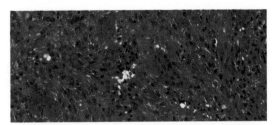

Fig. 15. Giant cell tumor of bone, high power (hematoxylin-eosin, original magnification ×40).

RANK binding. OPG expression reflects a protective mechanism of the skeleton to compensate increased bone resorption. Bone remodeling is mainly controlled by the balance of RANKL/OPG. Osteoprotegerin ligand (OPGL), also named receptor activator of RANKL, is also expressed in the stromalike tumor cells of GCTB. The ratio of OPGL/OPG by tumor cells may contribute to the degree of osteogenesis and bone resorption.[194]

Grossly, the tumor is red-brown with hemorrhage. Yellow areas reflect lipid-laden macrophage-rich areas. Histologically, the tumor is composed of numerous giant cells with multinucleation and scattered mononuclear cells that are round or spindle shaped. Lipid-laden or hemosiderin-laden macrophages are also present. The tumor is mainly solid and may contain cystic areas. Secondary aneurysmal bone cyst component is seen in 10% of GCTB.[22] The tumor may be mitotically active; however, a benign giant cell tumor typically does not have atypical mitosis or significant nuclear atypia. The latter is associated with a malignant transformation of GCTB. One diagnostic pitfall is to avoid misdiagnosing an osteosarcoma when a pathologic fracture is in association with a malignant giant cell tumor.

Ancillary studies
Giant cell tumor of soft tissue is positive for CD68, with some mononuclear cells showing SMA positivity.[190,191,195,196] A ligand for RANKL is also expressed by the mononuclear cells and is important for osteoclastic recruitment.[190,197,198]

Prognostic implications
Local recurrence rates of up to 12% have been reported with only rare cases of metastatic disease reported.[196,197,199–202] Although complete resection improves local recurrence rates, prognostic factors are otherwise currently unknown.[22,190,202]

Giant Cell Tumor of Soft Tissue

Giant cell tumor of soft tissue is clinically and histologically similar to giant cell tumor of bone. It most often presents in middle-aged adults, usually as a superficial painless extremity soft tissue tumor, less often affecting the trunk or head and neck regions.[22] Morphologic evaluation shows a multinodular proliferation of cellular nodules containing mononuclear and multinuclear osteoclast-like giant cells, often with frequent mitoses, within a richly vascular stroma.[22] About half of these tumors present with metaplastic bone formation, and other common histologic features include cystic changes, stromal fibrosis, stromal hemorrhage, and foamy macrophages.[22,190]

SUMMARY

Recent advances in immunohistochemical markers, cytogenetics, and molecular pathology techniques summarized here have improved the diagnosis and management of sarcomas. The most recent version of the WHO classification of soft tissue and bone tumors better defines pathological diagnostic criteria, allowing for more reproducible diagnoses. Ongoing improvements in our understanding of the molecular characteristics of tumors will undoubtedly continue to shed light on the factors that influence the pathogenesis of soft tissue and bone tumors and optimize the management of sarcomas.

REFERENCES

1. Dufresne A, Blay JY, Cassier P, et al. Recommendations for diagnostic and therapeutic management of soft tissue sarcoma. Bull Cancer 2009;96(9):909–15 [in French].
2. Amankwah EK, Conley AP, Reed DR. Epidemiology and therapies for metastatic sarcoma. Clin Epidemiol 2013;5:147–62.
3. Burningham Z, Hashibe M, Spector L, et al. The epidemiology of sarcoma. Clin Sarcoma Res 2012;2(1):14.
4. Moley JF, Brother MB, Wells SA, et al. Low frequency of ras gene mutations in neuroblastomas, pheochromocytomas, and medullary thyroid cancers. Cancer Res 1991;51(6):1596–9.
5. Gibson TN, Hanchard B, Waugh N, et al. A fifty-year review of soft tissue sarcomas in Jamaica: 1958-2007. West Indian Med J 2012;61(7):692–7.
6. Gronchi A, Miceli R, Allard MA, et al. Personalizing the approach to retroperitoneal soft tissue sarcoma: histology-specific patterns of failure and postrelapse outcome after primary extended resection. Ann Surg Oncol 2015;22(5): 1447–54.
7. Demicco EG. Sarcoma diagnosis in the age of molecular pathology. Adv Anat Pathol 2013;20(4):264–74.
8. Al-Zaid T, Somaiah N, Lazar AJ. Targeted therapies for sarcomas: new roles for the pathologist. Histopathology 2014;64(1):119–33.
9. Fletcher JA. Molecular biology and cytogenetics of soft tissue sarcomas: relevance for targeted therapies. Cancer Treat Res 2004;120:99–116.
10. Taylor BS, Barretina J, Maki RG, et al. Advances in sarcoma genomics and new therapeutic targets. Nat Rev Cancer 2011;11(8):541–57.
11. Ligier K, Maynou C, Leroy X, et al. Improvement of the initial management of sarcomas after the dissemination of evidence-based guidelines depends on the primary sarcoma location: a population-based study. BMC Cancer 2015;15:218.
12. Goldbraich E, Waks Z, Farkash A, et al. Understanding deviations from clinical practice guidelines in adult soft tissue sarcoma. Stud Health Technol Inform 2015;216:280–4.
13. Nijhuis PH, Schaapveld M, Otter R, et al. Soft tissue sarcoma–compliance with guidelines. Cancer 2001;91(11):2186–95.
14. Bagaria SP, Ashman JB, Daugherty LC, et al. Compliance with national comprehensive cancer network guidelines in the use of radiation therapy for extremity and superficial trunk soft tissue sarcoma in the United States. J Surg Oncol 2014;109(7):633–8.
15. Demetri GD, Baker LH, Beech D, et al. Soft tissue sarcoma clinical practice guidelines in oncology. J Natl Compr Canc Netw 2005;3(2):158–94.

16. Perrier L, Buja A, Mastrangelo G, et al. Clinicians' adherence versus non adherence to practice guidelines in the management of patients with sarcoma: a cost-effectiveness assessment in two European regions. BMC Health Serv Res 2012; 12:82.

17. Honore C, Méeus P, Stoeckle E, et al. Soft tissue sarcoma in France in 2015: epidemiology, classification and organization of clinical care. J Visc Surg 2015;152(4):223–30.

18. von Mehren M, Randall RL, Benjamin RS, et al. Soft tissue sarcoma, version 2.2014. J Natl Compr Canc Netw 2014;12(4):473–83.

19. Doyle LA. Sarcoma classification: an update based on the 2013 World Health Organization classification of tumors of soft tissue and bone. Cancer 2014; 120(12):1763–74.

20. Fletcher CD. The evolving classification of soft tissue tumours—an update based on the new 2013 WHO classification. Histopathology 2014;64(1):2–11.

21. Jo VY, Fletcher CD. WHO classification of soft tissue tumours: an update based on the 2013 (4th) edition. Pathology 2014;46(2):95–104.

22. Fletcher CDM, World Health Organization and International Agency for Research on Cancer. WHO classification of tumours of soft tissue and bone. World Health Organization classification of tumours. 4th edition. Lyon (France): IARC Press; 2013. p. 468.

23. Fletcher CD. Recently characterized soft tissue tumors that bring biologic insight. Mod Pathol 2014;27(Suppl 1):S98–112.

24. Zambo I, Vesely K. WHO classification of tumours of soft tissue and bone 2013: the main changes compared to the 3rd edition. Cesk Patol 2014;50(2):64–70 [in Czech].

25. Costa J, Wesley RA, Glatstein E, et al. The grading of soft tissue sarcomas. Results of a clinicohistopathologic correlation in a series of 163 cases. Cancer 1984;53(3):530–41.

26. Golouh R, Bračko M. What is current practice in soft tissue sarcoma grading? Radiol Oncol 2001;35(1):47–52.

27. Coindre JM, Trojani M, Contesso G, et al. Reproducibility of a histopathologic grading system for adult soft tissue sarcoma. Cancer 1986;58(2):306–9.

28. Deyrup AT, Weiss SW. Grading of soft tissue sarcomas: the challenge of providing precise information in an imprecise world. Histopathology 2006; 48(1):42–50.

29. Damjanov I, Fan F. Cancer grading manual. 2nd edition. New York: Springer; 2013. p. 220, xi.

30. Gustafson P, Akerman M, Alvegård TA, et al. Prognostic information in soft tissue sarcoma using tumour size, vascular invasion and microscopic tumour necrosis-the SIN-system. Eur J Cancer 2003;39(11):1568–76.

31. Recommendations for the reporting of soft tissue sarcomas. Association of Directors of Anatomic and Surgical Pathology. Mod Pathol 1998;11(12):1257–61.

32. Guillou L, Coindre JM, Bonichon F, et al. Comparative study of the National Cancer Institute and French Federation of Cancer Centers Sarcoma Group grading systems in a population of 410 adult patients with soft tissue sarcoma. J Clin Oncol 1997;15(1):350–62.

33. Kilpatrick SE. Histologic prognostication in soft tissue sarcomas: grading versus subtyping or both? A comprehensive review of the literature with proposed practical guidelines. Ann Diagn Pathol 1999;3(1):48–61.

34. Coindre JM, Terrier P, Bui NB, et al. Prognostic factors in adult patients with locally controlled soft tissue sarcoma. A study of 546 patients from the French Federation of Cancer Centers Sarcoma Group. J Clin Oncol 1996;14(3):869–77.

35. Hashimoto H, Daimaru Y, Takeshita S, et al. Prognostic significance of histologic parameters of soft tissue sarcomas. Cancer 1992;70(12):2816–22.

36. Edge SB, American Joint Committee on Cancer. AJCC cancer staging manual. 7th edition. New York: Springer; 2010. p. 648, xiv.

37. Inwards CY, Unni KK. Classification and grading of bone sarcomas. Hematol Oncol Clin North Am 1995;9(3):545–69.

38. Folpe AL, Inwards CY. Bone and soft tissue pathology. Philadelphia: Saunders/Elsevier; 2010.

39. Sobin L, Gospodarowicz M, Ch W, editors. UICC TNM classification of malignant tumours. 7th edition. New York: Wiley-Liss; 2009.

40. Egas-Bejar D, Anderson PM, Agarwal R, et al. Theranostic profiling for actionable aberrations in advanced high risk osteosarcoma with aggressive biology reveals high molecular diversity: the human fingerprint hypothesis. Oncoscience 2014;1(2):167–79.

41. Warenius HM, Seabra L, Kyritsi L, et al. Theranostic proteomic profiling of cyclins, cyclin dependent kinases and Ras in human cancer cell lines is dependent on p53 mutational status. Int J Oncol 2008;32(4):895–907.

42. Ahmed N, Fessi H, Elaissari A. Theranostic applications of nanoparticles in cancer. Drug Discov Today 2012;17(17–18):928–34.

43. Aleixo PB, Hartmann AA, Menezes IC, et al. Can MDM2 and CDK4 make the diagnosis of well differentiated/dedifferentiated liposarcoma? An immunohistochemical study on 129 soft tissue tumours. J Clin Pathol 2009;62(12):1127–35.

44. Ghadimi MP, Al-Zaid T, Madewell J, et al. Diagnosis, management, and outcome of patients with dedifferentiated liposarcoma systemic metastasis. Ann Surg Oncol 2011;18(13):3762–70.

45. Fritchie KJ, Goldblum JR, Tubbs RR, et al. The expanded histologic spectrum of myxoid liposarcoma with an emphasis on newly described patterns: implications for diagnosis on small biopsy specimens. Am J Clin Pathol 2012;137(2):229–39.

46. Iwasaki H, Nabeshima K, Nishio J, et al. Pathology of soft-tissue tumors: daily diagnosis, molecular cytogenetics and experimental approach. Pathol Int 2009;59(8):501–21.

47. Matthyssens LE, Creytens D, Ceelen WP. Retroperitoneal liposarcoma: current insights in diagnosis and treatment. Front Surg 2015;2:4.

48. Pedeutour F, Suijkerbuijk RF, Forus A, et al. Complex composition and co-amplification of SAS and MDM2 in ring and giant rod marker chromosomes in well-differentiated liposarcoma. Genes Chromosomes Cancer 1994;10(2):85–94.

49. Creytens D, van Gorp J, Ferdinande L, et al. Array-based comparative genomic hybridization analysis of a pleomorphic myxoid liposarcoma. J Clin Pathol 2014;67(9):834–5.

50. Narendra S, Valente A, Tull J, et al. DDIT3 gene break-apart as a molecular marker for diagnosis of myxoid liposarcoma–assay validation and clinical experience. Diagn Mol Pathol 2011;20(4):218–24.

51. Henderson-Jackson EB, Bui MM. Molecular pathology of soft-tissue neoplasms and its role in clinical practice. Cancer Control 2015;22(2):186–92.

52. Marino-Enriquez A, Hornick JL, Dal Cin P, et al. Dedifferentiated liposarcoma and pleomorphic liposarcoma: a comparative study of cytomorphology and

MDM2/CDK4 expression on fine-needle aspiration. Cancer Cytopathol 2014; 122(2):128–37.

53. Gustafson P, Rydholm A, Willén H, et al. Liposarcoma: a population-based epidemiologic and prognostic study of features of 43 patients, including tumor DNA content. Int J Cancer 1993;55(4):541–6.

54. van de Rijn M, Fletcher JA. Genetics of soft tissue tumors. Annu Rev Pathol 2006;1:435–66.

55. Oda Y, Yamamoto H, Takahira T, et al. Frequent alteration of p16(INK4a)/ p14(ARF) and p53 pathways in the round cell component of myxoid/round cell liposarcoma: p53 gene alterations and reduced p14(ARF) expression both correlate with poor prognosis. J Pathol 2005;207(4):410–21.

56. Wang L, Ren W, Zhou X, et al. Pleomorphic liposarcoma: a clinicopathological, immunohistochemical and molecular cytogenetic study of 32 additional cases. Pathol Int 2013;63(11):523–31.

57. Garcia JJ, Folpe AL. The impact of advances in molecular genetic pathology on the classification, diagnosis and treatment of selected soft tissue tumors of the head and neck. Head Neck Pathol 2010;4(1):70–6.

58. Hemmings C. Morphology, molecular genetics and multidisciplinary management: soft tissue pathology in 2014 and beyond. Pathology 2014;46(2):93–4.

59. Lo CH, Cheng SN, Lin KT, et al. Successful treatment of infantile fibrosarcoma spinal metastasis by chemotherapy and stereotactic hypofractionated radiotherapy. J Korean Neurosurg Soc 2013;54(6):528–31.

60. Gallego S, Pericas N, Barber I, et al. Infantile fibrosarcoma of the retroperitoneum: a site of unfavorable prognosis? Pediatr Hematol Oncol 2011;28(5): 451–3.

61. Fletcher CDM, Bridge JA, Hoagendoorn PCW, et al. WHO classification of tumours of soft tissue and bone. In: Bosman FT, Jaffe ES, Lakhani SR, et al, editors. World Health Organization classification of tumours. 4th edition. Lyon (France): International Agency for Reasearch on Cancer; 2013.

62. Sadri N, Barroeta J, Pack SD, et al. Malignant round cell tumor of bone with EWSR1-NFATC2 gene fusion. Virchows Arch 2014;465(2):233–9.

63. Yamaguchi S, Yamazaki Y, Ishikawa Y, et al. EWSR1 is fused to POU5F1 in a bone tumor with translocation t(6;22)(p21;q12). Genes Chromosomes Cancer 2005;43(2):217–22.

64. Doyle LA, Fletcher CD, Hornick JL. Nuclear expression of CAMTA1 distinguishes epithelioid hemangioendothelioma from histologic mimics. Am J Surg Pathol 2016;40(1):94–102.

65. Deyrup AT, Tighiouart M, Montag AG, et al. Epithelioid hemangioendothelioma of soft tissue: a proposal for risk stratification based on 49 cases. Am J Surg Pathol 2008;32(6):924–7.

66. Barison A, Pastormerlo LE, Mirizzi G, et al. Leiomyosarcoma of the inferior vena cava in a patient with Budd-Chiari syndrome. Rev Port Cardiol 2014;33(12): 807–9.

67. Chia-Hsin L. Education and imaging. Hepatobiliary and pancreatic: Budd-Chiari syndrome secondary to leiomyosarcoma of the inferior vena cava. J Gastroenterol Hepatol 2010;25(1):218.

68. Kelly KJ, Yoon SS, Kuk D, et al. Comparison of perioperative radiation therapy and surgery versus surgery alone in 204 patients with primary retroperitoneal sarcoma: a retrospective 2-institution study. Ann Surg 2015;262(1):156–62.

69. von Mehren M, Benjamin RS, Bui MM, et al. Soft tissue sarcoma, version 2.2012: featured updates to the NCCN guidelines. J Natl Compr Canc Netw 2012;10(8): 951–60.
70. Maekawa A, Kohashi K, Setsu N, et al. Expression of Forkhead Box M1 in soft tissue leiomyosarcoma: clinicopathological and in vitro study using a newly established cell line. Cancer Sci 2016;107(1):95–102.
71. Rosenberg AE. WHO classification of soft tissue and bone, fourth edition: summary and commentary. Curr Opin Oncol 2013;25(5):571–3.
72. Fletcher CD. The evolving classification of soft tissue tumours: an update based on the new WHO classification. Histopathology 2006;48(1):3–12.
73. Tailor IK, Motabi I, Alshehry N, et al. Alveolar rhabdomyosarcoma masquerading as Burkitt's lymphoma in bone marrow. Hematol Oncol Stem Cell Ther 2015;8(1): 38–9.
74. Win KT, Lee MY, Tan TD, et al. Nasopharyngeal alveolar rhabdomyosarcoma expressing CD56: a mimicker of extranodal natural killer/T-cell lymphoma. Int J Clin Exp Pathol 2014;7(1):451–5.
75. Ganesan P, Thulkar S, Rajan A, et al. Solid variant of alveolar rhabdomyosarcoma mimicking non-Hodgkin lymphoma: case report and review of literature. J Pediatr Hematol Oncol 2008;30(10):772–4.
76. Tsai SC, Reale LD, Flomenberg N, et al. Alveolar rhabdomyosarcoma mimicking a lymphoma at presentation. J Clin Oncol 2006;24(24):4031–2.
77. Miller RW. Contrasting epidemiology of childhood osteosarcoma, Ewing's tumor, and rhabdomyosarcoma. Natl Cancer Inst Monogr 1981;(56):9–15.
78. Sultan I, Qaddoumi I, Yaser S, et al. Comparing adult and pediatric rhabdomyosarcoma in the surveillance, epidemiology and end results program, 1973 to 2005: an analysis of 2,600 patients. J Clin Oncol 2009;27(20):3391–7.
79. Busam KJ, Fletcher CD. The clinical role of molecular genetics in soft tissue tumor pathology. Cancer Metastasis Rev 1997;16(1–2):207–27.
80. Oda Y, Tsuneyoshi M. Recent advances in the molecular pathology of soft tissue sarcoma: implications for diagnosis, patient prognosis, and molecular target therapy in the future. Cancer Sci 2009;100(2):200–8.
81. La Starza R, Nofrini V, Pierini T, et al. Molecular cytogenetics detect an unbalanced t(2;13)(q36;q14) and PAX3-FOXO1 fusion in rhabdomyosarcoma with mixed embryonal/alveolar features. Pediatr Blood Cancer 2015;62(12):2238–41.
82. Demicco EG, Lazar AJ. Clinicopathologic considerations: how can we fine tune our approach to sarcoma? Semin Oncol 2011;38(Suppl 3):S3–18.
83. Husain N, Verma N. Current concepts in pathology of soft tissue sarcoma. Indian J Surg Oncol 2011;2(4):302–8.
84. Todd R, Lunec J. Molecular pathology and potential therapeutic targets in soft-tissue sarcoma. Expert Rev Anticancer Ther 2008;8(6):939–48.
85. Rubin BP, Goldblum JR. Pathology of soft tissue sarcoma. J Natl Compr Canc Netw 2007;5(4):411–8.
86. Slominski A, Wortsman J, Carlson A, et al. Molecular pathology of soft tissue and bone tumors. A review. Arch Pathol Lab Med 1999;123(12):1246–59.
87. Kubo T, Shimose S, Fujimori J, et al. Prognostic value of PAX3/7-FOXO1 fusion status in alveolar rhabdomyosarcoma: systematic review and meta-analysis. Crit Rev Oncol Hematol 2015;96(1):46–53.
88. Kosemehmetoglu K, Vrana JA, Folpe AL. TLE1 expression is not specific for synovial sarcoma: a whole section study of 163 soft tissue and bone neoplasms. Mod Pathol 2009;22(7):872–8.

89. Blackett J. Difficulties in diagnosing soft-tissue sarcomas: a case of synovial sarcoma of the foot. N Z Med J 2011;124(1346):83–7.

90. He R, Patel RM, Alkan S, et al. Immunostaining for SYT protein discriminates synovial sarcoma from other soft tissue tumors: analysis of 146 cases. Mod Pathol 2007;20(5):522–8.

91. Garcia Del Muro X, de Alava E, Artigas V, et al. Clinical practice guidelines for the diagnosis and treatment of patients with soft tissue sarcoma by the Spanish group for research in sarcomas (GEIS). Cancer Chemother Pharmacol 2016; 77(1):133–46.

92. Coindre JM. Grading of soft tissue sarcomas: review and update. Arch Pathol Lab Med 2006;130(10):1448–53.

93. Dei Tos AP. A current perspective on the role for molecular studies in soft tissue tumor pathology. Semin Diagn Pathol 2013;30(4):375–81.

94. Tang Y, Song H, Bao Y, et al. Multimodal treatment of abdominal and pelvic desmoplastic small round cell tumor with relative good prognosis. Int J Surg 2015; 16(Pt A):49–54.

95. Palomeque Jimenez A, Pérez Cabrera B, González Puga C, et al. Desmoplastic small-round-cell tumor of the peritoneum: an uncommon entity with poor prognosis. Gastroenterol Hepatol 2015;38(6):383–5 [in Spanish].

96. Casey DL, Wexler LH, LaQuaglia MP, et al. Favorable outcomes after whole abdominopelvic radiation therapy for pediatric and young adult sarcoma. Pediatr Blood Cancer 2014;61(9):1565–9.

97. Roos E, van Coevorden F, Verhoef C, et al. Prognosis of primary and recurrent chondrosarcoma of the rib. Ann Surg Oncol 2016;23(3):811–7.

98. Rozeman LB, Hogendoorn PC, Bovee JV. Diagnosis and prognosis of chondrosarcoma of bone. Expert Rev Mol Diagn 2002;2(5):461–72.

99. Verdegaal SH, Bovée JV, Pansuriya TC, et al. Incidence, predictive factors, and prognosis of chondrosarcoma in patients with Ollier disease and Maffucci syndrome: an international multicenter study of 161 patients. Oncologist 2011; 16(12):1771–9.

100. Lu N, Lin T, Wang L, et al. Association of SOX4 regulated by tumor suppressor miR-30a with poor prognosis in low-grade chondrosarcoma. Tumour Biol 2015; 36(5):3843–52.

101. Tsukamoto S, Honoki K, Kido A, et al. Chemotherapy improved prognosis of mesenchymal chondrosarcoma with rare metastasis to the pancreas. Case Rep Oncol Med 2014;2014:249757.

102. Jin Z, Han YX, Han XR. Loss of RUNX3 expression may contribute to poor prognosis in patients with chondrosarcoma. J Mol Histol 2013;44(6):645–52.

103. Letson GD, Muro-Cacho CA. Genetic and molecular abnormalities in tumors of the bone and soft tissues. Cancer Control 2001;8(3):239–51.

104. Pappo AS, Vassal G, Crowley JJ, et al. A phase 2 trial of R1507, a monoclonal antibody to the insulin-like growth factor-1 receptor (IGF-1R), in patients with recurrent or refractory rhabdomyosarcoma, osteosarcoma, synovial sarcoma, and other soft tissue sarcomas: results of a Sarcoma Alliance for Research Through Collaboration study. Cancer 2014;120(16):2448–56.

105. Pekmezci M, Reuss DE, Hirbe AC, et al. Morphologic and immunohistochemical features of malignant peripheral nerve sheath tumors and cellular schwannomas. Mod Pathol 2015;28(2):187–200.

106. Sobanko JF, Meijer L, Nigra TP. Epithelioid sarcoma: a review and update. J Clin Aesthet Dermatol 2009;2(5):49–54.

107. Sonobe H, Ohtsuki Y, Sugimoto T, et al. Involvement of 8q, 22q, and monosomy 21 in an epithelioid sarcoma. Cancer Genet Cytogenet 1997;96(2):178–80.
108. Iavazzo C, Gkegkes ID, Vrachnis N. Dilemmas in the management of patients with vulval epithelioid sarcoma: a literature review. Eur J Obstet Gynecol Reprod Biol 2014;176:1–4.
109. Ong AC, Lim TY, Tan TC, et al. Proximal epithelioid sarcoma of the vulva: a case report and review of current medical literature. J Obstet Gynaecol Res 2012;38(7):1032–5.
110. Halling AC, Wollan PC, Pritchard DJ, et al. Epithelioid sarcoma: a clinicopathologic review of 55 cases. Mayo Clin Proc 1996;71(7):636–42.
111. Feely MG, Fidler ME, Nelson M, et al. Cytogenetic findings in a case of epithelioid sarcoma and a review of the literature. Cancer Genet Cytogenet 2000;119(2):155–7.
112. Khowaja A, Johnson-Rabbett B, Bantle J, et al. Hypoglycemia mediated by paraneoplastic production of insulin like growth factor-2 from a malignant renal solitary fibrous tumor—clinical case and literature review. BMC Endocr Disord 2014;14:49.
113. Mohammedi K, Abi Khalil C, Olivier S, et al. Paraneoplastic hypoglycemia in a patient with a malignant solitary fibrous tumor. Endocrinol Diabetes Metab Case Rep 2014;2014:140026.
114. Tominaga N, Kawarasaki C, Kanemoto K, et al. Recurrent solitary fibrous tumor of the pleura with malignant transformation and non-islet cell tumor-induced hypoglycemia due to paraneoplastic overexpression and secretion of high-molecular-weight insulin-like growth factor II. Intern Med 2012;51(23):3267–72.
115. Tanaka K, Kishimoto T, Ohtsuka M, et al. Importance of NAB2-STAT6 fusion in the diagnosis of pancreatic solitary fibrous tumor with hamartoma-like features: a case report and review of the literature. Case Rep Pathol 2015;2015:149606.
116. Tai HC, Chuang IC, Chen TC, et al. NAB2-STAT6 fusion types account for clinicopathological variations in solitary fibrous tumors. Mod Pathol 2015;28(10):1324–35.
117. Nakada S, Minato H, Takegami T, et al. NAB2-STAT6 fusion gene analysis in two cases of meningeal solitary fibrous tumor/hemangiopericytoma with late distant metastases. Brain Tumor Pathol 2015;32(4):268–74.
118. Koelsche C, Schweizer L, Renner M, et al. Nuclear relocation of STAT6 reliably predicts NAB2-STAT6 fusion for the diagnosis of solitary fibrous tumour. Histopathology 2014;65(5):613–22.
119. Chmielecki J, Crago AM, Rosenberg M, et al. Whole-exome sequencing identifies a recurrent NAB2-STAT6 fusion in solitary fibrous tumors. Nat Genet 2013;45(2):131–2.
120. Robinson DR, Wu YM, Kalyana-Sundaram S, et al. Identification of recurrent NAB2-STAT6 gene fusions in solitary fibrous tumor by integrative sequencing. Nat Genet 2013;45(2):180–5.
121. Barthelmess S, Geddert H, Boltze C, et al. Solitary fibrous tumors/hemangiopericytomas with different variants of the NAB2-STAT6 gene fusion are characterized by specific histomorphology and distinct clinicopathological features. Am J Pathol 2014;184(4):1209–18.
122. NAB2-STAT6 fusions are a hallmark of solitary fibrous tumors. Cancer Discov 2013;3(3):OF18.
123. Zhou J, Jiang G, Zhang D, et al. Epithelioid inflammatory myofibroblastic sarcoma with recurrence after extensive resection: significant clinicopathologic

characteristics of a rare aggressive soft tissue neoplasm. Int J Clin Exp Pathol 2015;8(5):5803–7.

124. Sigel JE, Smith TA, Reith JD, et al. Immunohistochemical analysis of anaplastic lymphoma kinase expression in deep soft tissue calcifying fibrous pseudotumor: evidence of a late sclerosing stage of inflammatory myofibroblastic tumor? Ann Diagn Pathol 2001;5(1):10–4.

125. Masciocchi C, Lanni G, Conti L, et al. Soft-tissue inflammatory myofibroblastic tumors (IMTs) of the limbs: potential and limits of diagnostic imaging. Skeletal Radiol 2012;41(6):643–9.

126. Donner LR, Trompler RA, White RR 4th. Progression of inflammatory myofibroblastic tumor (inflammatory pseudotumor) of soft tissue into sarcoma after several recurrences. Hum Pathol 1996;27(10):1095–8.

127. Karanian M, Coindre JM. Fourth edition of WHO classification tumours of soft tissue. Ann Pathol 2015;35(1):71–85 [in French].

128. Lombardi R, Jovine E, Zanini N, et al. A case of lung metastasis in myxoinflammatory fibroblastic sarcoma: analytical review of one hundred and thirty eight cases. Int Orthop 2013;37(12):2429–36.

129. Alaggio R, Coffin CM, Dall'igna P, et al. Myxoinflammatory fibroblastic sarcoma: report of a case and review of the literature. Pediatr Dev Pathol 2012;15(3): 254–8.

130. Lang JE, Dodd L, Martinez S, et al. Case reports: acral myxoinflammatory fibroblastic sarcoma: a report of five cases and literature review. Clin Orthop Relat Res 2006;445:254–60.

131. Togral G, Arikan M, Aktas E, et al. Giant myxoinflammatory fibroblastic sarcoma with bone invasion: a very rare clinical entity and literature review. Chin J Cancer 2014;33(8):406–10.

132. Silver AG, Baynosa RC, Mahabir RC, et al. Acral myxoinflammatory fibroblastic sarcoma: a case report and literature review. Can J Plast Surg 2013;21(2):92–4.

133. Xiang H, Shi XL, Li QX, et al. Myxoinflammatory fibroblastic sarcoma: a clinicopathologic study of 6 cases with review of literature. Zhonghua Bing Li Xue Za Zhi 2011;40(2):94–8 [in Chinese].

134. Baumhoer D, Glatz K, Schulten HJ, et al. Myxoinflammatory fibroblastic sarcoma: investigations by comparative genomic hybridization of two cases and review of the literature. Virchows Arch 2007;451(5):923–8.

135. Bishop AJ, Zagars GK, Demicco EG, et al. Soft tissue solitary fibrous tumor: combined surgery and radiation therapy results in excellent local control. Am J Clin Oncol 2015. [Epub ahead of print].

136. DeVito N, Henderson E, Han G, et al. Clinical characteristics and outcomes for solitary fibrous tumor (SFT): a single center experience. PLoS One 2015;10(10): e0140362.

137. Lahon B, Mercier O, Fadel E, et al. Solitary fibrous tumor of the pleura: outcomes of 157 complete resections in a single center. Ann Thorac Surg 2012;94(2): 394–400.

138. Stacchiotti S, Pedeutour F, Negri T, et al. Dermatofibrosarcoma protuberans-derived fibrosarcoma: clinical history, biological profile and sensitivity to imatinib. Int J Cancer 2011;129(7):1761–72.

139. Stacchiotti S, Pantaleo MA, Negri T, et al. Efficacy and biological activity of imatinib in metastatic dermatofibrosarcoma protuberans (DFSP). Clin Cancer Res 2016;22(4):837–46.

140. Saeki H, Hoashi T, Tada Y, et al. Analysis of gene mutations in three cases of dermatofibrosarcoma protuberans (DFSP): ordinary DFSP, DFSP with

fibrosarcomatous lesion (DFSP-FS) and lung metastasis of DFSP-FS. J Dermatol Sci 2003;33(3):161–7.

141. Belyaeva EA, Elenitsas R, Roth R, et al. Dermatofibrosarcoma protuberans (DFSP) with fibrosarcomatous changes in a patient with psoriasis treated with adalimumab. JAAD Case Rep 2015;1(5):272–3.

142. Hong JY, Liu X, Mao M, et al. Genetic aberrations in imatinib-resistant dermatofibrosarcoma protuberans revealed by whole genome sequencing. PLoS One 2013;8(7):e69752.

143. Rutkowski P, Dębiec-Rychter M, Nowecki Z, et al. Treatment of advanced dermatofibrosarcoma protuberans with imatinib mesylate with or without surgical resection. J Eur Acad Dermatol Venereol 2011;25(3):264–70.

144. Wang C, Luo Z, Chen J, et al. Target therapy of unresectable or metastatic dermatofibrosarcoma protuberans with imatinib mesylate: an analysis on 22 Chinese patients. Medicine (Baltimore) 2015;94(17):e773.

145. Premalata CS, Rama Rao C, Padma M, et al. Myxoinflammatory fibroblastic sarcoma–report of a rare case at an unusual site with review of the literature. Int J Dermatol 2008;47(1):68–71.

146. Ortiz AE, Wu JJ, Linden KG. Letter: clear margins after the use of imatinib mesylate prior to resection of extensive dermatofibrosarcoma protuberans. Dermatol Surg 2008;34(8):1151.

147. Fatahzadeh M. Kaposi sarcoma: review and medical management update. Oral Surg Oral Med Oral Pathol Oral Radiol 2012;113(1):2–16.

148. Feller L, Lemmer J, Wood NH, et al. HIV-associated oral Kaposi sarcoma and HHV-8: a review. J Int Acad Periodontol 2007;9(4):129–36.

149. Eaton C, Dorer R, Aboulafia DM. Human herpesvirus-8 infection associated with kaposi sarcoma, multicentric Castleman's disease, and plasmablastic microlymphoma in a man with AIDS: a case report with review of pathophysiologic processes. Patholog Res Int 2010;2011:647518.

150. Feller L, Anagnostopoulos C, Wood NH, et al. Human immunodeficiency virus-associated Kaposi sarcoma as an immune reconstitution inflammatory syndrome: a literature review and case report. J Periodontol 2008;79(2):362–8.

151. Rosado FG, Itani DM, Coffin CM, et al. Utility of immunohistochemical staining with FLI1, D2-40, CD31, and CD34 in the diagnosis of acquired immunodeficiency syndrome-related and non-acquired immunodeficiency syndrome-related Kaposi sarcoma. Arch Pathol Lab Med 2012;136(3):301–4.

152. Cao W, Vyboh K, Routy B, et al. Imatinib for highly chemoresistant Kaposi sarcoma in a patient with long-term HIV control: a case report and literature review. Curr Oncol 2015;22(5):e395–9.

153. Marti N, Monteagudo C, Pinazo I, et al. Negative herpesvirus-8 immunoreactivity does not exclude a diagnosis of Kaposi sarcoma. Br J Dermatol 2011;164(1):209–11.

154. Patel RM, Goldblum JR, Hsi ED. Immunohistochemical detection of human herpes virus-8 latent nuclear antigen-1 is useful in the diagnosis of Kaposi sarcoma. Mod Pathol 2004;17(4):456–60.

155. Xiao J, Selvaggi SM, Leith CP, et al. Kaposi sarcoma herpesvirus/human herpesvirus-8-negative effusion-based lymphoma: report of 3 cases and review of the literature. Cancer Cytopathol 2013;121(11):661–9.

156. Casper C, Wald A. The use of antiviral drugs in the prevention and treatment of Kaposi sarcoma, multicentric Castleman disease and primary effusion lymphoma. Curr Top Microbiol Immunol 2007;312:289–307.

157. Housari G, González M, Calero P, et al. Sacral chordoma: management of a rare disease in a tertiary hospital. Clin Transl Oncol 2013;15(4):327–30.
158. Walcott BP, Nahed BV, Mohyeldin A, et al. Chordoma: current concepts, management, and future directions. Lancet Oncol 2012;13(2):e69–76.
159. Mika K, Fuminari K, Hitoshi T, et al. Endoscopic management of a lower clival chondroid chordoma: case report. Turk Neurosurg 2012;22(1):123–6.
160. Kayani B, Hanna SA, Sewell MD, et al. A review of the surgical management of sacral chordoma. Eur J Surg Oncol 2014;40(11):1412–20.
161. Ferraresi V, Nuzzo C, Zoccali C, et al. Chordoma: clinical characteristics, management and prognosis of a case series of 25 patients. BMC Cancer 2010;10:22.
162. Ozger H, Eralp L, Sungur M, et al. Surgical management of sacral chordoma. Acta Orthop Belg 2010;76(2):243–53.
163. Lee DH, Zhang Y, Kassam AB, et al. Combined PDGFR and HDAC inhibition overcomes PTEN disruption in chordoma. PLoS One 2015;10(8):e0134426.
164. Choy E, MacConaill LE, Cote GM, et al. Genotyping cancer-associated genes in chordoma identifies mutations in oncogenes and areas of chromosomal loss involving CDKN2A, PTEN, and SMARCB1. PLoS One 2014;9(7):e101283.
165. Chen K, Mo J, Zhou M, et al. Expression of PTEN and mTOR in sacral chordoma and association with poor prognosis. Med Oncol 2014;31(4):886.
166. Chou WC, Hung YS, Lu CH, et al. De novo dedifferentiated chordoma of the sacrum: a case report and review of the literature. Chang Gung Med J 2009; 32(3):330–5.
167. Masood Q, Bilal M, Tariq A, et al. Dedifferentiated chordoma with a sarcomatous component: an overlooked diagnosis. J Ayub Med Coll Abbottabad 2009;21(1): 164–5.
168. Sahasrabudhe NS, Jadhav MV, Holla VV. Dedifferentiated chordoma–a case report. Indian J Pathol Microbiol 2002;45(3):353–4.
169. Kim SC, Cho W, Chang UK, et al. Two cases of dedifferentiated chordoma in the sacrum. Korean J Spine 2015;12(3):230–4.
170. Borgaonkar V, Deshpande S, Borgaonkar V, et al. Gastrointestinal stromal tumor—single-center experience with review of the literature. Indian J Surg 2015;77(Suppl 2):678–81.
171. Pyo JS, Kang G, Sohn JH. Ki-67 labeling index can be used as a prognostic marker in gastrointestinal stromal tumor: a systematic review and meta-analysis. Int J Biol Markers 2016;31(2):e204–10.
172. Falchook GS, Trent JC, Heinrich MC, et al. BRAF mutant gastrointestinal stromal tumor: first report of regression with BRAF inhibitor dabrafenib (GSK2118436) and whole exomic sequencing for analysis of acquired resistance. Oncotarget 2013;4(2):310–5.
173. Matin RN, Gonzalez D, Thompson L, et al. KIT and BRAF mutational status in a patient with a synchronous lentigo maligna melanoma and a gastrointestinal stromal tumor. Am J Clin Dermatol 2012;13(1):64–5.
174. Baldini EH, Raut C. Radiation therapy for extremity soft tissue sarcoma: in the absence of a clear survival benefit, why do we give it? Ann Surg Oncol 2014; 21(8):2463–5.
175. Lazarides AL, Eward WC, Speicher PJ, et al. The use of radiation therapy in well-differentiated soft tissue sarcoma of the extremities: an NCDB review. Sarcoma 2015;2015:186581.
176. Kasper B, Baumgarten C, Bonvalot S, et al. Management of sporadic desmoid-type fibromatosis: a European consensus approach based on patients' and

professionals' expertise—a sarcoma patients EuroNet and European Organisation for research and treatment of cancer/soft tissue and bone sarcoma group initiative. Eur J Cancer 2015;51(2):127–36.

177. Mori T, Yamada T, Ohba Y, et al. A case of desmoid-type fibromatosis arising after thoracotomy for lung cancer with a review of the English and Japanese literature. Ann Thorac Cardiovasc Surg 2014;20(Suppl):465–9.

178. La Greca G, Santangelo A, Primo S, et al. Clinical and diagnostic problems of desmoid-type fibromatosis of the mesentery: case report and review of the literature. Ann Ital Chir 2014;85.

179. Oudot C, Orbach D, Minard-Colin V, et al. Desmoid fibromatosis in pediatric patients: management based on a retrospective analysis of 59 patients and a review of the literature. Sarcoma 2012;2012:475202.

180. Schmoyer CJ, Brereton HD, Blomain EW. Contralateral recurrence of aggressive fibromatosis in a young woman: a case report and review of the literature. Oncol Lett 2015;10(1):325–8.

181. Veith NT, Tschernig T, Histing T, et al. Plantar fibromatosis–topical review. Foot Ankle Int 2013;34(12):1742–6.

182. Yoon GW, Kim JD, Chung SH. The analysis of treatment of aggressive fibromatosis using oral methotrexate chemotherapy. Clin Orthop Surg 2014;6(4): 439–42.

183. Ghanem M, Heinisch A, Heyde CE, et al. Diagnosis and treatment of extraabdominal desmoid fibromatosis. GMS Interdiscip Plast Reconstr Surg DGPW 2014; 3:Doc01.

184. Coindre JM. New WHO classification of tumours of soft tissue and bone. Ann Pathol 2012;32(5 Suppl):S115–6 [in French].

185. Kucuk L, Keçeci B, Sabah D, et al. Aggressive fibromatosis: evaluation of prognostic factors and outcomes of surgical treatment. Acta Orthop Traumatol Turc 2014;48(1):55–60.

186. Nishio J. Updates on the cytogenetics and molecular cytogenetics of benign and intermediate soft tissue tumors. Oncol Lett 2013;5(1):12–8.

187. Jo VY, Fletcher CD. Myoepithelial neoplasms of soft tissue: an updated review of the clinicopathologic, immunophenotypic, and genetic features. Head Neck Pathol 2015;9(1):32–8.

188. Papachristou DJ, Palekar A, Surti U, et al. Malignant granular cell tumor of the ulnar nerve with novel cytogenetic and molecular genetic findings. Cancer Genet Cytogenet 2009;191(1):46–50.

189. Sandberg AA. Updates on the cytogenetics and molecular genetics of bone and soft tissue tumors: leiomyoma. Cancer Genet Cytogenet 2005;158(1):1–26.

190. Bresler SC, Wanat KA, Elenitsas R. Giant cell tumor of soft tissue. Cutis 2014; 93(6):278, 286–8.

191. Kumar S, Carter LF. Giant cell tumor of soft tissue of hand: simple but rare diagnosis, which is often missed. Clin Pract 2011;1(3):e54.

192. Morgan T, Atkins GJ, Trivett MK, et al. Molecular profiling of giant cell tumor of bone and the osteoclastic localization of ligand for receptor activator of nuclear factor kappaB. Am J Pathol 2005;167(1):117–28.

193. Rao UN, Goodman M, Chung WW, et al. Molecular analysis of primary and recurrent giant cell tumors of bone. Cancer Genet Cytogenet 2005;158(2): 126–36.

194. Huang L, Xu J, Wood DJ, et al. Gene expression of osteoprotegerin ligand, osteoprotegerin, and receptor activator of NF-kappaB in giant cell tumor of bone:

possible involvement in tumor cell-induced osteoclast-like cell formation. Am J Pathol 2000;156(3):761–7.

195. Garcia-Bennett J, Olivé CS, Rivas A, et al. Soft tissue solitary fibrous tumor. Imaging findings in a series of nine cases. Skeletal Radiol 2012;41(11):1427–33.

196. Asotra S, Sharma S. Giant cell tumor of soft tissue: cytological diagnosis of a case. J Cytol 2009;26(1):33–5.

197. Icihikawa K, Tanino R. Soft tissue giant cell tumor of low malignant potential. Tokai J Exp Clin Med 2004;29(3):91–5.

198. Roux S, Amazit L, Meduri G, et al. RANK (receptor activator of nuclear factor kappa B) and RANK ligand are expressed in giant cell tumors of bone. Am J Clin Pathol 2002;117(2):210–6.

199. Jain D, Arava S, Mishra B, et al. Soft tissue giant cell tumor of low malignant potential of mediastinum: a rare case report. Int J Surg Pathol 2015;23(1):71–4.

200. Guo H, Garcia RA, Perle MA, et al. Giant cell tumor of soft tissue with pulmonary metastases: pathologic and cytogenetic study. Pediatr Dev Pathol 2005;8(6): 718–24.

201. Kim NR, Han J. Primary giant cell tumor of soft tissue. Report of a case with fine needle aspiration cytologic and histologic findings. Acta Cytol 2003;47(6): 1103–6.

202. Holst VA, Elenitsas R. Primary giant cell tumor of soft tissue. J Cutan Pathol 2001;28(9):492–5.

Radiologic Approach to Bone and Soft Tissue Sarcomas

Jamie T. Caracciolo, MD, MBA[a,b,c],*, G. Douglas Letson, MD[b,c,d,e]

KEYWORDS

- Imaging • Radiology • Diagnostic evaluation • Bone lesion • Soft tissue mass
- Sarcoma

KEY POINTS

- Diagnostic imaging plays an important role in the evaluation and treatment planning of patients with musculoskeletal tumors.
- Following a thorough history and physical examination, imaging examinations may be requested to evaluate a palpable abnormality; soft tissue mass; or clinical symptoms, such as pain and swelling.
- In some cases, the clinical presentation including patient age, symptomatology, and past medical history may suggest a specific diagnosis, although in most cases the clinical examination is nonspecific.
- Whether detected incidentally or in the setting of clinical symptoms, musculoskeletal neoplasms can often be accurately characterized utilizing appropriate imaging examinations.

Diagnostic imaging is a critical component of a multidisciplinary approach to the diagnosis and treatment of musculoskeletal neoplasms. Following a thorough history and physical examination, imaging examinations may be requested to evaluate a palpable abnormality; soft tissue mass; or clinical symptoms, such as pain and swelling. In some cases, the clinical presentation including patient age, symptomatology, and past medical history may suggest a specific diagnosis, although in most cases the clinical examination is nonspecific. With greater accessibility to and use of advanced imaging modalities, musculoskeletal tumors may be identified incidentally on studies

[a] Musculoskeletal Imaging, Department of Diagnostic Imaging, Moffitt Cancer Center, 12902 Magnolia Drive, WCB-RAD MD/OPI, Tampa, FL 33612, USA; [b] Department of Radiology, University of South Florida Morsani College of Medicine, 12901 Bruce B Downs Blvd, Tampa, FL 33612, USA; [c] Department of Orthopedics/Sports Medicine, University of South Florida Morsani College of Medicine, 12901 Bruce B Downs Blvd, Tampa, FL 33612, USA; [d] Moffitt Cancer Center, Tampa, FL, USA; [e] Department of Surgery, University of South Florida Morsani College of Medicine, 12901 Bruce B Downs Blvd, Tampa, FL 33612, USA
* Corresponding author. Musculoskeletal Imaging, Department of Diagnostic Imaging, Moffitt Cancer Center, 12902 Magnolia Drive, WCB-RAD MD/OPI, Tampa, FL 33612.
E-mail address: Jamie.caracciolo@moffitt.org

Surg Clin N Am 96 (2016) 963–976
http://dx.doi.org/10.1016/j.suc.2016.05.007
0039-6109/16/$ – see front matter © 2016 Elsevier Inc. All rights reserved.
surgical.theclinics.com

performed for other reasons. In any of these scenarios, the initial objective of diagnostic imaging is confirmation of the presence of a musculoskeletal neoplasm versus an alternative explanation of symptoms, such as traumatic injury or infection. When a mass is present, initial characterization of the tumor as benign or malignant is based on features, such as size, margins, enhancement pattern, and internal homogeneity versus heterogeneity. After the initial assessment of benignity versus malignancy, further evaluation may provide for a more specific diagnosis based on tumor characteristics, such as anatomic location, morphology, pattern of growth, and intrinsic tumor composition. Ideally, a subspecialized multidisciplinary review of the clinical history, diagnostic imaging, and histopathologic findings at a tertiary cancer referral center would direct optimal patient treatment planning.[1–4]

This article discusses several important concepts in musculoskeletal tumor imaging and presents relevant imaging features of several common musculoskeletal neoplasms. A complete and thorough review of musculoskeletal tumor imaging is beyond the scope of this review, with numerous textbooks dedicated to the subject. In this article, we discuss the following:

- Imaging modalities most often used in the evaluation of musculoskeletal tumors including the advantages and disadvantages of each modality
- Our approach to the diagnostic evaluation of a newly suspected musculoskeletal neoplasm including determination of risk of malignancy
- An assessment of internal tumor composition allowing for a specific preoperative histopathologic diagnosis including features of several common soft tissue sarcomas
- Findings relevant to tumor staging and preoperative planning including response to neoadjuvant therapy
- Postoperative surveillance plans for local tumor recurrence following limb-salvage procedures

IMAGING MODALITIES

Several different diagnostic imaging examinations may be used in the initial evaluation of a suspected musculoskeletal neoplasm.[5–10] Each modality presents unique advantages and disadvantages as shown in **Table 1**. However, in most cases complementary information is provided by each study. For example, MRI provides greater soft tissue contrast than computed tomography (CT) and therefore often allows for better definition of internal tumor soft tissue composition/intrinsic elements of the tumor, whereas CT better demonstrates tumor mineralization than MRI. In another example, CT better depicts cortical bone involvement including pathologic fractures, whereas MRI better demonstrates medullary edema and bone marrow lesions including skip metastases not uncommonly seen in patients with primary bone tumors, such as osteosarcoma.

EVALUATION OF A NEWLY SUSPECTED MUSCULOSKELETAL TUMOR

Although a thorough clinical history and physical examination are important in the initial evaluation of a patient with a possible musculoskeletal neoplasm, symptomatology and physical findings are often nonspecific with significant overlap among presentations of neoplastic and nonneoplastic causes of musculoskeletal complaints.[11] Even when findings suggest the presence of a tumor, physical examination is often limited in differentiating benign and malignant neoplasms. As such, most patients with musculoskeletal symptoms are referred for diagnostic imaging. When imaging

Table 1
A comparison of imaging modalities commonly used in musculoskeletal tumors

Modality	Advantages	Disadvantages	Indications/Usefulness
Diagnostic radiography, orthogonal roentgenogram	• Diagnostic • Accessible • Inexpensive • Critical in evaluating bone tumors • Demonstrates tumor mineralization and adipocytic tumors	• Ionizing radiation • Limited evaluation of nonadipocytic soft tissue tumors	• Evaluation of bone tumor margin, matrix, and periosteal reaction • Soft tissue tumor density and internal mineralization
CT	• Accessible • Rapid acquisition/short scan time • Contiguous imaging of large anatomic regions • Greater spatial and temporal resolution than MRI	• Ionizing radiation • Less soft tissue contrast resolution compared with MRI	• Evaluate tumor matrix • Involvement of cortical bone including pathologic fractures • Tumor staging including chest CT for pulmonary metastases • CT-guided biopsy
MRI	• Greater soft tissue contrast resolution than CT • No ionizing radiation • Direct multiplanar imaging	• Small confined space; claustrophobia • Cost • Contraindications to MRI	• Evaluation of internal tumor composition • Local extent of disease including neurovascular involvement • Bone marrow involvement, skip metastases
Ultrasound	• Real-time imaging • Assess solid versus cystic mass and tumor vascularity (Doppler)	Limited ability to differentiate soft tissue masses	Ultrasound-guided biopsy
PET	Tumor/tissue viability, assessment of metabolic activity	• Ionizing radiation • Reimbursement in sarcomas	• May help differentiate benign and malignant tumors (ie, neurogenic tumors) • Evaluate tumor response to neoadjuvant therapy
Whole-body bone scan	Assessment of the entire skeletal system in a single examination	Ionizing radiation	Assessment of skeletal metastases and osteomyelitis

Abbreviation: CT, computed tomography.

is indicated, initial evaluation begins with orthogonal radiographs of the affected area, which may be followed by cross-sectional imaging, such as CT or MRI as shown in **Fig. 1**.

Step 1: Determination of Risk of Malignancy

The first and foremost role of imaging in the setting of a musculoskeletal neoplasm should be confirmation of the presence of a tumor and an assessment of tumor characteristics, which help predict benignity versus malignancy. After establishing the risk of malignancy, a further assessment of imaging findings providing for a more specific diagnosis is performed. With patient counseling based on the potential risk of malignancy, patients may be appropriately informed on treatment options, which may include surveillance, biopsy, or surgery. For example, consider a young patient with a geographic well-defined metadiaphyseal lytic lesion with circumferential marginal sclerosis. These findings suggest a low likelihood of malignancy and conservative observation may be preferred to biopsy. In cases of soft tissue tumors, the surgical

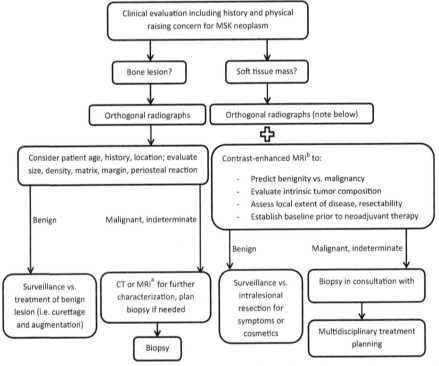

Fig. 1. Flowchart demonstrating our approach to the initial evaluation of a suspected musculoskeletal neoplasm. [a] See text for discussion of CT versus MRI. [b] MRI protocol for MSK neoplasm includes multiplanar imaging (axial, sagittal, and coronal) of the entire compartment obtaining T1-weighted imaging, a fluid-sensitive sequence (T2-weighted imaging or short tau inversion recovery [STIR]), a fat-suppressed sequence (STIR or chemically selective fat saturation technique), diffusion-weighted imaging, and fat-suppressed T1-weighted intravenous contrast-enhanced imaging. In practice, radiographs may not be considered before MRI in cases of suspected soft tissue tumors. However, whether obtained before or following MRI, radiographs are often useful in correlation with findings seen at MRI, particularly areas of mineralization. MSK, musculoskeletal.

approach to percutaneous biopsy or resection differs based on the likelihood of malignancy. Here, we discuss imaging features of musculoskeletal neoplasms that help predict benignity versus malignancy.

Bone lesions

In cases of bone tumors, diagnostic orthogonal radiography (ie, anteroposterior and lateral) allows an assessment of radiographic density (osteolytic vs osteoblastic), size, location, margination, internal matrix, and periosteal reaction. Additionally, radiographs may demonstrate the presence of a pathologic fracture or an associated extraosseous soft tissue mass. These features allow prediction of tumor aggressiveness, growth rate, and risk of malignancy. In 1980, Lodwick and colleagues[12] first demonstrated a correlation between tumor margination and rate of growth. Subsequent contributions of Madewell and colleagues[13] established three distinct types of osteolysis. Since their early works on this subject, a useful grading system to describe lytic bone lesions has been incorporated into clinical practice such that radiographic grade is commonly used to predict risk of malignancy.

In many cases, the radiographic appearance of a bone lesion alone provides sufficient information regarding biologic activity and risk of malignancy.[14] More specifically, lesion margination, or zone of transition, described as narrow or wide, correlates with rate of growth. This important radiographic feature forms the basis of the current widely used grading system of lytic bone lesions. Lytic lesions are described as geographic (grade I) or nongeographic (grade II or III). Grade I lesions are further classified as IA, IB, or IC. Geographic lesions demonstrate a clear delineation between involved and uninvolved bone, and the margins of the lesion are generally described as well-defined with a sclerotic rim (IA), well-defined without a sclerotic rim (IB), or ill-defined with a wide zone of transition (IC). Grade II and III lesions are nongeographic moth-eaten and permeative bone lesions with an indistinct transition between normal and pathologic bone. Increasing grade correlates with increased rate of growth such that grade IA lesions are largely benign and IB lesions are indeterminate with a moderate risk of malignancy, whereas grade IC and higher lesions are considered malignant until proven otherwise. Our ongoing research hopes to expand the existing classification system to include lytic lesions with changing margination and radiographically occult bone lesions.

Although margination and grade assignment of a bone lesion may be most important in predicting risk of malignancy, other radiographic features provide information on tumor aggressiveness and histopathology.[15–22] The presence or absence of periosteal reaction or an extraosseous soft tissue mass should be evaluated on bone radiographs. Periosteal reaction may be described as smooth, solid, or continuous most often in benign etiologies or irregular, lamellated, interrupted, or spiculated in malignant diseases. Cortical disruption with an extraosseous soft tissue mass is highly suggestive of a malignant bone tumor. Meanwhile, such findings as radiographic density (lytic or sclerotic) and the pattern of matrix mineralization (osteoid, chondroid, or ground glass) may point to a specific histologic diagnosis. Patient age and site of disease (long bone vs flat bone; central vs eccentric; epiphyseal vs metadiaphyseal) also contribute to the construction of a differential diagnosis (**Figs. 2** and **3**).

Soft tissue masses

When evaluating a soft tissue mass, the objective should first be differentiation of benign from malignant lesions, as in cases of newly diagnosed bone lesions. Even for experienced musculoskeletal radiologists, this can be more difficult than for bone lesions because there is significant overlap in the imaging appearance of benign

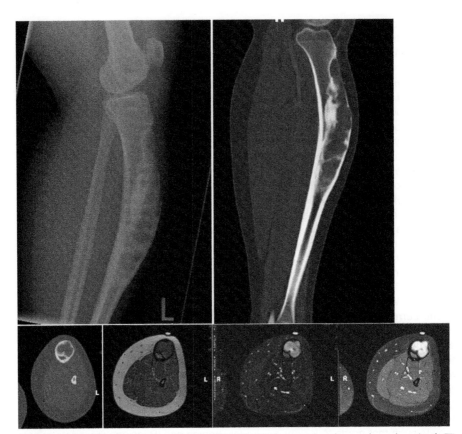

Fig. 2. Benign bone lesion in a 15-year-old girl. (*Top*) Lateral radiograph and sagittal CT reconstruction of the left tibia demonstrate a well-defined, geographic, cortically based, diaphyseal mixed lytic and sclerotic lesion along the anterior tibia with marginal sclerosis and areas of dense osteoid mineralization. (*Bottom*) Axial CT, T1-weighted, STIR, and contrast-enhanced MRIs demonstrate a lytic lesion with fibrous matrix involving the anterior tibial cortex with circumferential sclerosis, which encroaches on but does not invade the medullary cavity. Biopsy-confirmed osteofibrous dysplasia.

and malignant tumors, particularly when small and superficial. However, certain imaging features are helpful when evaluating a soft tissue mass and predicting whether it is more likely to be benign or malignant.

In cases of soft tissue tumors, initial diagnostic radiography can provide valuable information regarding tumor density (ie, adipocytic tumors), mineralization with a soft tissue mass (ie, synovial sarcoma and liposarcoma), involvement of the underlying bone, and nonneoplastic processes that mineralize (ie, myositis ossificans).[23,24] However, most soft tissue masses are referred for cross-sectional imaging. In the absence of any contraindication, for reasons discussed previously, we typically perform multiplanar, multiweighted, and contrast-enhanced MRI of the entire compartment (joint-to-joint coverage) suspected to be involved by a musculoskeletal tumor. Several imaging features help differentiate benign from malignant neoplasms.[25–29] Benign lesions tend to be small, homogeneous, and superficial to the investing fascia when arising in the extremities, whereas soft tissue masses that are large (>4 cm), heterogeneous, and deep-seated are more worrisome for malignancy

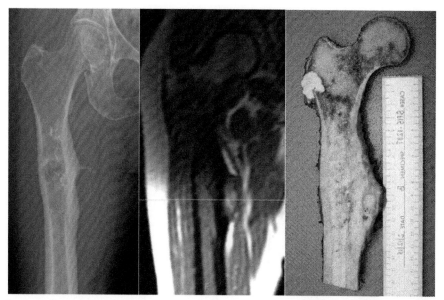

Fig. 3. Malignant bone lesion in a 56-year-old man. Anteroposterior radiograph of the proximal right femur demonstrates a geographic, but poorly marginated lytic medullary lesion with chondroid mineralization, moderate endosteal scalloping with medial cortical thickening, and elevation of the periosteum suggesting an extraosseous soft tissue mass. Coronal T1-weighted MRI demonstrates extent of medullary cavity involvement and confirms a medial extraosseous mass. Gross pathology specimen correlated with MRI-confirmed chondrosarcoma.

(**Figs. 4** and **5**). Malignant tumors often demonstrate enhancement with areas of internal necrosis and hemorrhage contributing to tumor heterogeneity. Although cystic lesions, such as ganglia, and fluid collections, such as postoperative seromas, do not enhance or show thin smooth peripheral rim enhancement, most benign and malignant solid neoplasms demonstrate intravenous contrast enhancement. However, benign masses are more likely to demonstrate mild patchy or uniform homogeneous enhancement than malignant tumors, which often demonstrate internal areas of nonenhancing necrosis and/or hemorrhage. Associated findings, such as a hypointense pseudocapsule and hyperintense peritumoral edema (reactive zone) on T2-weighted or short tau inversion recovery (STIR) imaging, are more commonly seen in soft tissue sarcomas than benign soft tissue masses. Finally, regional lymphadenopathy (albeit less common in sarcoma than other primary cancers) and satellite nodules or distant sites of disease concerning for metastases may be present with malignant soft tissue tumors.

Step 2: Assessment of Tumor Composition to Predict a Specific Histopathologic Diagnosis

Following an assessment of tumor aggressiveness, a specific histopathologic diagnosis or concise differential diagnosis can be presented for most musculoskeletal neoplasms by evaluating the internal matrix or intrinsic composition of a mass. Demographic information, such as age and gender, site of disease, and pattern of growth, also contributes to the construction of a differential diagnosis. The internal matrix of a bone lesion is best evaluated at radiography or CT and points to cell lineage

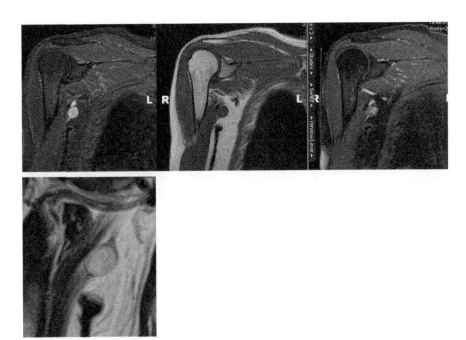

Fig. 4. Benign soft tissue mass. (*Top*) Coronal STIR, T1-weighted, and contrast-enhanced MRIs demonstrate a small, superficial, well-defined, and smoothly marginated soft tissue nodule with mild intravenous contrast enhancement, features typical of benign soft tissue neoplasms. (*Bottom*) After assessing risk of malignancy, further evaluation of internal tumor composition and identification of any pathognomonic findings, such as a "string sign" in this example of a benign peripheral nerve sheath tumor, allows for a specific diagnosis.

(ie, osteoid, chondroid, or fibrohistiocytic), whereas MRI better demonstrates internal soft tissue elements within a soft tissue mass (ie, lipomatous, myxomatous, or fibrous). Imaging features of common components and associated findings of osseous and soft tissue neoplasms are presented in **Table 2**.

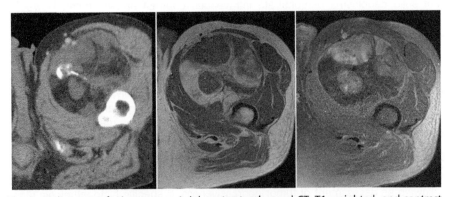

Fig. 5. Malignant soft tissue mass. Axial contrast-enhanced CT, T1-weighted, and contrast-enhanced MRIs demonstrate a large, heterogeneous, deep-seated soft tissue mass in the anterior proximal thigh, features typical of malignant soft tissue neoplasms. Further inspection of the internal composition of the mass demonstrates intrinsic fat indicating a lipomatous neoplasm with areas of mineralization and nonadipocytic soft tissue elements consistent with dedifferentiated liposarcoma.

Table 2
Imaging findings of common components of musculoskeletal neoplasms

Tissue Composition	Radiography or CT	MRI
Bone tumors		
Osteoid matrix	Dense, sclerotic, amorphous, cloud-like mineralization	Dark signal intensity on T1- and T2-weighted imaging
Chondroid matrix	Punctate, stippled, linear, or rings and arcs mineralization; lucent lesion with lobular pattern of growth and endosteal scalloping	Bright signal intensity on T2-weighted imaging with peripheral and internal septal pattern of enhancement
Fibrohistiocytic matrix	Radiolucent ground glass appearance without evidence of mineralization	Variable with somewhat whorled appearance, often with areas of dark T2-weighted signal
Soft tissue masses		
Lipomatous tissue	Radiolucent; low density on CT with negative Hounsfield units similar to subcutaneous fat	Bright signal intensity on T1- and T2-weighted imaging; signal drop out with fat suppression techniques
Myxomatous tissue	Hypodense on CT with similar attenuation to fluid	Markedly bright signal on T2-weighted imaging similar to fluid, but with intravenous contrast enhancement
Fibrous tissue	Similar density to skeletal muscle on CT	Dark signal intensity on T1- and T2-weighted imaging with variable enhancement; often infiltrative pattern of growth
Hemorrhage[a]	Hyperdense on CT	Hyperintense signal on T1-weighted, heterogeneous; hemosiderin appears dark with "blooming" susceptibility artifact on gradient echo imaging caused by iron
Necrosis	Hypodense on CT without enhancement	Bright T2-weighted signal intensity without enhancement
Pseudocapsule	Difficult to delineate on CT	Dark rim of signal intensity on T2-weighted imaging
Peritumoral edema	Hypodense, but difficult to delineate on CT	Infiltrative-appearing, bright signal intensity on T2-weighted imaging surrounding a mass

[a] Appearance of hemorrhage depends on acuity/chronicity of blood products.

The initial evaluation of a soft tissue mass should begin with orthogonal radiographs. Radiography is most helpful in cases of adipocytic and mineralizing neoplasms.[24] Fatty tumors, such as lipomas, atypical lipomatous tumors, and liposarcomas, demonstrate radiolucency relative to skeletal muscle, whereas most other soft tissue masses demonstrate density similar to muscle and are not well defined on radiographs. Some tumors and nonneoplastic lesions demonstrate patterns of mineralization specific to the diagnosis. For example, long-standing adipocytic tumors can demonstrate metaplastic, mature-appearing bone formation. Soft tissue hemangiomas commonly present with numerous rounded and lamellated phleboliths. Synovial sarcoma often demonstrates irregular dystrophic mineralization. Myositis ossificans demonstrates a typical pattern of peripheral mineralization allowing for diagnosis despite a nonspecific mass-like appearance on cross-sectional, which may mimic a soft tissue sarcoma.

Following radiography, cross-sectional imaging is often performed to further characterize musculoskeletal neoplasms with the goal of providing a specific preoperative histopathologic diagnosis.[30] CT and MRI provide different but complementary information. CT has the advantage of better depiction of tumor matrix mineralization and cortical bone involvement, such as depth of endosteal scalloping seen in cartilaginous bone tumors. Although fat within an adipocytic neoplasm is well demonstrated by both CT and MRI, greater soft tissue contrast afforded by MRI often allows for differentiation of other intrinsic elements, such as myxomatous or fibrous components, which may allow for a more specific preoperative diagnosis. The selection of CT or MRI for tumor characterization largely depends on the clinical question to be answered. However, in most cases, MRI provides greater soft tissue contrast and definition of internal tumor composition, internal necrosis, hemorrhage, and associated findings common to soft tissue sarcomas, such as a pseudocapsule and peritumoral edema.

When evaluating a soft tissue mass on cross-sectional imaging, we first attempt to determine whether the mass contains any intrinsic fat given the incidence of benign and malignant lipomatous neoplasms among most patient populations. The presence of internal fat within a mass typically indicates an adipocytic neoplasm.[31,32] Fat appears hypodense on CT and hyperintense on T1- and T2-weighted MRI similar to subcutaneous tissues with evidence of signal suppression on chemically selective fat-suppressed imaging or STIR. Adipocytic tumors tend to demonstrate a somewhat lobulated pattern of growth. Simple lipomas are comprised entirely of fat without any internal nodularity or thickened septations, although smooth thin (<2 mm) bands may be seen. The presence of internal fat stranding ("dirty fat") or nodularity on STIR or contrast-enhanced imaging may indicate atypical lipomatous tumor or well-differentiated liposarcoma. Continuing along the spectrum of adipocytic neoplasms, the presence of nonadipocytic soft tissue elements within a fatty mass indicates liposarcoma. This may include myxomatous tissue seen as markedly T2-weighted hyperintense and enhancing areas on MRI in cases of myxoid liposarcoma.[33] The hallmark of dedifferentiated liposarcoma is the presence of nonadipocytic enhancing soft tissue elements.[32] Pleomorphic liposarcoma typically presents as an indeterminate heterogeneous mass, which may not demonstrate any obvious macroscopic fat on CT or MRI.[32]

When intrinsic fat is not identified at cross-sectional imaging within an aggressive-appearing soft tissue mass, we then consider nonadipocytic soft tissue sarcomas, such as undifferentiated high-grade pleomorphic sarcoma (UPS) and leiomyosarcoma (LMS) among other sarcomas depending on additional factors, such as patient age and site of disease. UPS, formerly referred to as malignant fibrous histiocytoma, typically presents as a large, heterogeneous enhancing mass with extensive internal hemorrhage and necrosis, a pseudocapsule, and peritumoral edema.[34] UPS is the most common soft tissue sarcoma among elderly patients. LMS tends to appear as a mostly solid, avidly enhancing hypervascular soft tissue mass with less necrosis than typical of UPS commonly arising from a large blood vessel, such as the interior vena cava, pulmonary artery, or peripheral vessel, such as the femoral vein.[35] LMS often grows into the lumen of the vessel of origin and may result in thrombosis. LMS also may arise from smooth muscle cells of the retroperitoneum, genitourinary or gastrointestinal tract, or hair pillars of the skin and should be considered in cases of small, superficial, solid enhancing soft tissue masses, features more common among benign lesions.

Several other soft tissue sarcomas demonstrate characteristic imaging features warranting mention. Rhabdomyosarcoma has a predilection for the head and neck in pediatric patients.[36] Synovial sarcoma also tends to occur in the adolescent and young adult patient population in a periarticular location with a propensity for internal hemorrhage, mineralization, regional lymph node metastases, and osseous invasion.[37] Benign and malignant fibrous neoplasms, such as fibromatosis, myxofibrosarcoma, and adult fibrosarcoma, typically demonstrate intrinsic fibrous elements appearing hypointense on T1- and T2-weighted MRI with variable enhancement often arising along fascial planes with a characteristic "fascial tail."[38] Myxofibrosarcoma is often microscopically infiltrative with higher rates of local tumor recurrence than other soft tissue sarcomas. Angiosarcoma is often an infiltrative vascular neoplasm with a propensity for the scalp and breast.

TUMOR STAGING, RESPONSE TO NEOADJUVANT THERAPY, AND POSTOPERATIVE SURVEILLANCE

Tumor staging in the setting of a musculoskeletal neoplasm includes an assessment of local extent of disease and an evaluation of distant metastatic disease.[39] Because most soft tissue sarcomas tend to respect compartmental boundaries, imaging of the primary site of disease should include the entire compartment to visualize the entirety of the mass and detect any intracompartmental skip metastases, more common in bone tumors, such as osteosarcoma, but occasionally seen in soft tissue sarcomas. Local extent of disease directs treatment planning and attention must be directed to identify neurovascular involvement and contiguous bone involvement via direct extension. Lymph node metastases are uncommon in most soft tissue sarcomas, although several types more commonly spread to locoregional lymph nodes including synovial sarcoma, epithelioid sarcoma, clear cell sarcoma, and angiosarcoma. Pulmonary metastases are the most common site of distant disease and we recommend unenhanced chest CT for this reason, although some argue that chest radiographs are sufficient to identify significant pulmonary nodules. Whole-body bone scan and PET/CT are not routinely performed in our practice in the initial staging of soft tissue sarcomas. Of note, experience has shown that myxoid liposarcomas have a propensity for retroperitoneal and paraspinal soft tissue metastases and therefore contrast-enhanced CT of the chest, abdomen, and pelvis is typically performed in these patients.

Neoadjuvant chemotherapy and/or radiation therapy is often used in patients with large tumors at increased risk for local recurrence or to improve the likelihood of a margin-negative surgical resection. Response to neoadjuvant chemotherapy also yields prognostic information in cases of osteosarcoma. Restaging examinations are commonly performed following neoadjuvant therapy immediately before surgery. Several imaging findings identified on MRI are consistent to assess response to therapy.[40,41] An overall decrease in tumor size or tumor volume indicates a positive response. In some cases of neurovascular abutment or partial encasement, the tumor may retract from the neurovascular bundle providing for a surgical plane between the tumor and the bundle. Alternatively, a tumor may increase in size following treatment, while the amount of viable enhancing neoplastic tissue decreases. In these cases, enlargement is caused by tumor necrosis and hemorrhage in response to therapy. Diffusion-weighted MRI has more recently shown the ability to identify changes in apparent diffusion coefficients in response to therapy.[42] Densely packed tumor cells exhibit limited diffusivity of water molecules in the interstitial space, which manifests as areas of restricted diffusion on diffusion-weighted MRI. Cell death in response to therapy creates increased interstitial space allowing for increased mobility of interstitial water molecules via brownian motion. Increased movement of water results in a quantifiable change in diffusivity depicted on diffusion-weighted images as higher apparent diffusion coefficients values.

Given risk of local tumor recurrence, patients with surgically resected soft tissue sarcomas should undergo postoperative surveillance imaging of the operative bed. The frequency of surveillance imaging depends on the patient's risk of local recurrence determined by tumor size, grade, histology, and margin status following surgery. Early recurrence typically presents as a small enhancing soft tissue nodule within the operative field. Recurrent disease usually demonstrates similar signal characteristics to the primary tumor and therefore comparison with preoperative and postoperative baseline examinations is imperative.[40] Knowledge of the surgical procedure including reconstruction technique and soft tissue changes following adjuvant radiation therapy aids interpretation of postoperative scans. Radiation-induced soft tissue changes are usually infiltrative and geographic with demarcated borders conforming to the radiation field. Patchy, ill-defined bone marrow edema may indicate radiation-induced osteitis. Postoperative seromas are common and demonstrate internal fluid signal intensity with thin rim enhancement without mural nodularity. Hematomas may be heterogeneous on MRI with increased T1-weighted signal, variable T2-weighted signal, and often a peripheral hypointense rim caused by mural hemosiderin deposition.

Following clinical assessment of a newly suspected musculoskeletal neoplasm, diagnostic imaging plays an important role in initial tumor characterization, tumor staging, treatment planning, evaluation of response to therapy, and postoperative surveillance. We have presented our diagnostic algorithm for the initial work-up of primary bone and soft tissue tumors. We have also reviewed the advantages and disadvantages of different imaging modalities and the complementary information each provides, discussed pertinent imaging features that help predict the likelihood of benignity versus malignancy, and highlighted intrinsic imaging characteristics defining internal tumor composition that allow for specific preoperative histopathologic diagnoses. Despite dramatic improvements in imaging technologies, expertise in image interpretation, improved understanding of tumor biology, and advancements in neoadjvant/adjuvant therapies and limb-salvage surgical options, musculoskeletal sarcomas remain exceedingly rare in comparison with visceral carcinomas and hematologic malignancies and continue to carry a significant risk of disease-related morbidity and mortality. For these and other reasons, we advocate a multidisciplinary approach to the diagnosis and treatment of musculoskeletal neoplasms preferably at a local or regional tertiary care center with specialized physician and ancillary services in the management of these tumors.

REFERENCES

1. Lehnhardt M, Daigeler A, Hauser J, et al. The value of expert second opinion in diagnosis of soft tissue sarcomas. J Surg Oncol 2008;97(1):40–3.

2. Blay JY, Sleijfer S, Schoffski P, et al. International expert opinion on patient-tailored management of soft tissue sarcomas. Eur J Cancer 2014;50(4):679–89.
3. Gutierrez JC, Perez E, Moffat FL, et al. Should soft tissue sarcomas be treated at high-volume centers? An analysis of 4205 patients. Ann Surg 2007;245(6):952–8.
4. Klein MJ. Radiographic correlation in orthopedic pathology. Adv Anat Pathol 2005;12(4):155–79.
5. Robinson E, Bleakney RR, Ferguson PC, et al. Oncodiagnosis panel: 2007 multidisciplinary management of soft tissue sarcoma. Radiographics 2008;28: 2069–86.
6. Aga P, Singh R, Parihar A, et al. Imaging spectrum in soft tissue sarcomas. Indian J Surg Oncol 2011;2(4):271–9.
7. Amini B, Jessop AC, Ganeshan DM, et al. Contemporary imaging of soft tissue sarcomas. J Surg Oncol 2015;111:496–503.
8. Knapp EL, Kransdorf MJ, Letson GD. Diagnostic imaging update: soft tissue sarcomas. Cancer Control 2005;12(1):22–6.
9. Varma DG. Optimal radiologic imaging of soft tissue sarcomas. Semin Surg Oncol 1999;17(1):2–10.
10. Gilbert NF, Cannon CP, Lin PP, et al. Soft-tissue sarcoma. J Am Acad Orthop Surg 2009;17(1):40–7.
11. Stacy GS, Dixon LB. Pitfalls in MR image interpretation prompting referrals to an orthopedic oncology clinic. Radiographics 2007;27:805–28.
12. Lodwick GS, Wilson AJ, Farrell C, et al. Determining growth rates of focal lesions of bone from radiographs. Radiology 1980;134(3):577–83.
13. Madewell JE, Ragsdale BD, Sweet DE. Radiologic and pathologic analysis of solitary bone lesions. Part I: internal margins. Radiol Clin North Am 1981;19(4): 715–48.
14. Domb BG, Tyler W, Ellis S, et al. Radiographic evaluation of pathological bone lesions: current spectrum of disease and approach to diagnosis. J Bone Joint Surg Am 2004;86:84–90.
15. Miller TT. Bone tumors and tumorlike conditions: analysis with conventional radiography. Radiology 2008;246(3):662–74.
16. Ragsdale BD, Madewell JE, Sweet DE. Radiologic and pathologic analysis of solitary bone lesions. Part II: periosteal reactions. Radiol Clin North Am 1981;19(4): 749–83.
17. Greenfield GB, Warren DL, Clark RA. MR imaging of periosteal and cortical changes of bone. Radiographics 1991;11(4):611–23.
18. Moser RP, Madewell JE. An approach to primary bone tumors. Radiol Clin North Am 1987;25(6):1049–93.
19. Kricun ME. Radiographic evaluation of solitary bone lesions. Orthop Clin North Am 1983;14(1):39–64.
20. Weber KL. Evaluation of the adult patient (aged >40years) with a destructive bone lesion. J Am Acad Orthop Surg 2010;18(3):169–79.
21. Priolo F, Cerase A. The current role of radiography in the assessment of skeletal tumors and tumor-like lesions. Eur J Radiol 1998;27:S77–85.
22. Pommersheim WJ, Chew FS. Imaging, diagnosis, and staging of bone tumors: a primer. Semin Roentgenol 2004;39(3):361–72.
23. Kransdorf MJ, Jelinek JS, Moser RP. Imaging of soft tissue tumors. Radiol Clin North Am 1993;31(2):359–72.
24. Kransdorf MJ, Murphey MD. Radiologic evaluation of soft-tissue masses: a current perspective. AJR Am J Roentgenol 2000;175:575–87.

25. Kransdorf MJ, Murphey MD. Imaging of soft tissue tumors. 2nd edition. Philadelphia: Lippincott Williams & Wilkins; 2006.

26. Wu JS, Hochman MG. Soft-tissue tumors and tumorlike lesions: a systematic imaging approach. Radiology 2009;253(2):297–316.

27. Ma LD, Frassica FJ, Scott WW, et al. Differentiation of benign and malignant musculoskeletal tumors: potential pitfalls with MR imaging. Radiographics 1995;15: 349–66.

28. Vilanova JC, Woertler K, Narvaez JA, et al. Soft-tissue tumors update: MR imaging features according to the WHO classification. Eur Radiol 2007;17(1):125–38.

29. Simon MA, Finn HA. Diagnostic strategy for bone and soft-tissue tumors. J Bone Joint Surg Am 1993;75(4):622–31.

30. Murphey MD. World Health Organization classification of bone and soft tissue tumors: modifications and implications for radiologists. Semin Musculoskelet Radiol 2007;11(3):201–14.

31. Murphey MD, Carroll JF, Flemming DJ, et al. Benign musculoskeletal lipomatous lesions. Radiographics 2004;24(5):1433–66.

32. Murphey MD, Arcara LK, Fanburg-Smith J. Imaging of musculoskeletal liposarcoma with radiologic-pathologic correlation. Radiographics 2005;25(5):1371–95.

33. Petscavage-Thomas JM, Walker EA, Logie CI, et al. Soft-tissue myxomatous lesions: review of salient imaging features with pathologic comparison. Radiographics 2014;34(4):964–80.

34. Murphey MD, Gross TM, Rosenthal HG. Musculoskeletal malignant fibrous histiocytoma: radiologic-pathologic correlation. Radiographics 1994;14:807–26.

35. Cortecero JM, Guirau Rubio MD, Roma AP. Leiomyosarcoma of the inferior vena cava. Radiographics 2015;35:616–20.

36. Razek AA, Huang BY. Soft tissue tumors of the head and neck: imaging-based review of the WHO classification. Radiographics 2011;31(7):1923–54.

37. Murphey MD, Gibson MS, Jennings BT, et al. Imaging of synovial sarcoma with radiologic-pathologic correlation. Radiographics 2006;26:1543–65.

38. Murphey MD, Ruble CM, Tyszko SM, et al. Musculoskeletal fibromatoses: radiologic-pathologic correlation. Radiographics 2009;29(7):2143–83.

39. Tzeng CW, Smith JK, Heslin MJ. Soft tissue sarcoma: preoperative and postoperative imaging for staging. Surg Oncol Clin N Am 2007;16(2):389–402.

40. Garner HW, Kransdorf MJ, Bancroft LW, et al. Benign and malignant soft-tissue tumors: posttreatment MR imaging. Radiographics 2009;29:119–34.

41. Tirkes T, Hollar M, Tann M, et al. Response criteria in oncologic imaging: review of traditional and new criteria. Radiographics 2013;33:1323–41.

42. Subhawong TK, Jacobs MA, Fayad LM. Diffusion-weighted MR imaging for characterizing musculoskeletal lesions. Radiographics 2014;34:1163–77.

Multimodality Management of Soft Tissue Tumors in the Extremity

Aimee M. Crago, MD, PhD[a,b,*], Ann Y. Lee, MD[a]

KEYWORDS

- Soft tissue sarcoma • Extremity sarcoma • Limbs • Resection • Radiotherapy

KEY POINTS

- Work-up for an extremity mass suspicious for a soft tissue sarcoma includes cross-sectional imaging with an MRI and a core biopsy done in line with the planned incision.
- The standard for treatment of extremity soft tissue sarcomas is limb-sparing surgery with a margin of 1 to 2 cm. Overlying fascial layers (ie, muscular fascia, femoral sheath, periosteum) are often barriers to tumor extension and are acceptable margins when major neurovascular or bony structures are in close proximity.
- Rates of local and distant recurrence vary by histologic subtype. These differences inform surgical margins and the use of chemotherapy and radiation.
- Radiation therapy is used to decrease rates of local recurrence in high-risk tumors. Neoadjuvant (vs adjuvant) radiation can minimize side effects to nearby joints and normal tissues, but is associated with increased rates of wound complications and has equivalent rates of local control.
- Use of adjuvant chemotherapy is controversial. Neoadjuvant chemotherapy should be routinely prescribed for high-risk, chemosensitive subtypes (ie, Ewing sarcoma and rhabdomyosarcoma). It can be selectively prescribed for moderately chemosensitive subtypes based on other risk factors, such as size.

INTRODUCTION

Soft tissue sarcoma (STS) is a term referring to approximately 100 different subtypes of cancer.[1] These diseases are rare, and as a group are diagnosed in only approximately 12,000 patients in the United States each year.[2] Although STS is identified in

---

Disclosures: The authors have no disclosures to report.
This work was supported by the Memorial Sloan Kettering Cancer Center Core Grant (P30 CA008748) and the Kristen Ann Carr Fund.
[a] Sarcoma Disease Management Team, Department of Surgery, Memorial Sloan Kettering Cancer Center, 1275 York Avenue, H1220, New York, NY 10065, USA; [b] Department of Surgery, Weill Cornell Medical College, 1300 York Avenue, New York, NY 10065, USA
* Corresponding author. Gastric and Mixed Tumor Service, Department of Surgery, 1275 York Avenue, H1220, New York, NY 10065.
E-mail address: cragoa@mskcc.org

Surg Clin N Am 96 (2016) 977–992
http://dx.doi.org/10.1016/j.suc.2016.05.001
0039-6109/16/$ – see front matter © 2016 Elsevier Inc. All rights reserved.

surgical.theclinics.com

any site within the body, 40% are located in the extremities, and multimodality treatment is used to manage patients with localized disease.[3] What combination of surgery, radiation, and systemic treatment is best for a particular patient depends on histologic subtype, which is diagnosed using a combination of cross-sectional imaging, microscopy, and molecular diagnostics. The most common histologies in the extremity are liposarcoma, undifferentiated pleomorphic sarcoma, myxofibrosarcoma, and synovial sarcoma (**Fig. 1**). Each carries a different risk for distant metastases and local recurrence; for example, dermatofibrosarcoma protuberans (DFSP) carries a higher long-term risk of local recurrence than leiomyosarcoma, but its risk of metastasis is much lower. We present an algorithm for diagnosis and treatment of STS, highlighting modifications that should be made based on the biologic behavior of specific histologic subtypes.

CLINICAL PRESENTATION AND DIAGNOSIS

Most patients eventually diagnosed with an STS present with a painless mass. More than 90% of painless masses are benign lesions, such as lipomas. Therefore, sarcomas are sometimes initially diagnosed as lipomas, resulting in a delay in the correct diagnosis. In general, lipomas tend to be softer, be in a subcutaneous location, have a history of prolonged stability, and be uniformly mobile with no overlying skin changes.

In contrast, STS may be firm, deep, enlarging over time, multifocal, and associated with neovascularization of the overlying skin. Radicular pain or swelling in the distal extremity related to underlying neurovascular involvement may reflect locally advanced disease. A history of nearby trauma may be reported by the patient, but it is unclear that trauma can initiate STS development. More likely, trauma brings attention to a preexisting mass.

IMAGING THE PRIMARY TUMOR

Work-up of an extremity mass begins with cross-sectional imaging for all but the smallest superficial lesions (<2–3 cm), which can be managed with an excisional

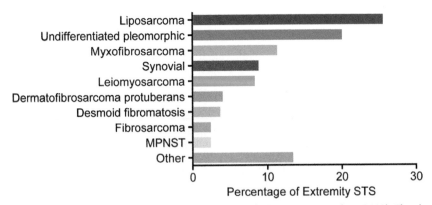

Fig. 1. Histologic distribution of primary extremity soft tissue sarcomas (n = 3103). The data are derived from all surgically resected soft tissue sarcomas followed prospectively at Memorial Sloan-Kettering Cancer Center between 1980 and 2014. Tumors previously designated as malignant fibrous histiocytoma are denoted as undifferentiated pleomorphic sarcoma. Histologic subtypes that represented ≤2% of all cases are grouped as other. MPNST, malignant peripheral nerve sheath tumor.

biopsy. MRI with contrast is the preferred study modality, because it provides detailed anatomic information necessary for surgical planning. MRI allows the vascular structures to be easily delineated, and T1 images allow the clinician to trace branches of major peripheral nerves. Computed tomography (CT) is beneficial only when bony involvement is expected and complex reconstruction may be necessary during surgical resection of the tumor. The MRI appearance can also be predictive of histologic subtype (**Fig. 2**). For example, myxoid lesions are associated with high T2 signal, even in the absence of gadolinium contrast. This is the case for myxofibrosarcoma, which often has enhancing tails extending from the multifocal, nodular components of the lesion, highlighting its infiltrative nature.[4] Collagenous regions are low in signal on T1 and T2 imaging, so a persistent low signal in regions of the tumor may indicate a desmoid-type fibromatosis or a collagenous fibroma. However, in none of these instances is the diagnosis pathognomonic, and pretreatment biopsy is recommended.

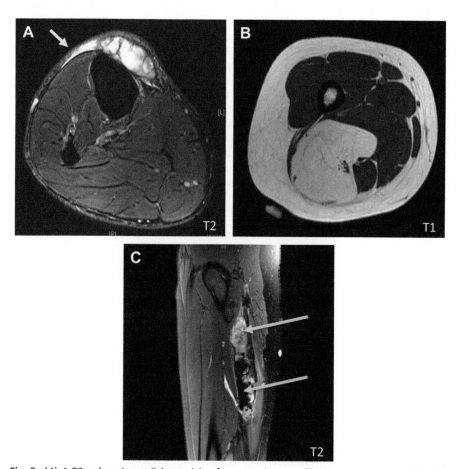

Fig. 2. (*A*) A T2-enhancing tail (*arrow*) is often seen in myxofibrosarcoma, representing its infiltrative borders. (*B*) A lipomatous mass in the posterior thigh compartment with multiple septations consistent with an atypical lipomatous tumor. (*C*) Desmoids are mixed intensity on T2-weighted imaging, with high-T2 areas representing cellular components (*orange arrow*) and low-T2 areas representing collagenous components (*green arrow*).

There is only one STS type for which imaging is considered diagnostic (and only when reviewed by an experienced radiologist). This type is atypical lipomatous neoplasm/well-differentiated liposarcoma/dedifferentiated liposarcoma, and has a signal profile almost identical to subcutaneous fat, but with enhancing septae and, if a dedifferentiated component is present, with solid nodules.[5,6]

BIOPSY TECHNIQUES

When imaging is not pathognomonic, biopsy is necessary before treatment is planned. Historically, this was performed by incisional biopsy. However, subsequent studies have shown that core biopsy of STS is accurate not only in demonstrating the presence of malignancy, but also in determining grade (in 88% of cases) and histologic subtype (in 75% of cases).[7] Core biopsy often provides enough tissue for immunohistochemistry and cytogenetic studies, which can be of significant benefit in diagnosis. Characteristic genomic alterations for common histologic subtypes of extremity sarcoma and their associated diagnostic tests are presented in **Table 1**. Although fine-needle aspiration has been examined as a means of obtaining biopsy of soft tissue lesions at the time of presentation, its utility is limited by the rarity of specialists trained both in cytology and STS histology and the limited amount of tissue obtained from such specimens. Fine-needle aspiration may be appropriate for initial diagnosis of malignant tumor or confirmation of a recurrence, but it is often inadequate for histologic subtyping. Regardless of the type of biopsy performed, care should be made to orient the incision or core needle in such a way that the biopsy tract is completely excised at the time of eventual surgery. For incisional or excisional biopsy, this means orienting the incision longitudinally along the extremity. This greatly facilitates closure of the incision at the time of re-excision. If the incisional biopsy is oriented transversely, removing the incision with requisite margin during the definitive resection often leaves a defect requiring skin graft.

Table 1
Characteristic genomic alterations and diagnostic testing for different extremity histologic subtypes

Histologic Subtype	Genomic Alteration	Diagnostic Testing
Atypical lipomatous tumor and dedifferentiated liposarcoma	12q13–15 amplification	FISH or IHC for *CDK4* or *MDM2*
Desmoid fibromatosis	*CTNNB1* mutation or APC loss	IHC for nuclear β-catenin
Epithelioid sarcoma	*SMARCB1* deletion	IHC for SMARCB1
Myxoid and round cell liposarcomas	*FUS-DDIT3* fusion or *EWSR1-DDIT3* fusion	FISH or PCR for *FUS-DDIT3* or *EWSR1-DDIT3*
Synovial sarcoma	*SYT-SSX1*, *SYT-SSX2*, or *SYT-SSX3* fusion	PCR for *SYT-SSX1-3*
Ewing sarcoma	*EWSR1-FLI1* fusion	PCR for *EWSR1-FLI1*
Dermatofibrosarcoma protuberans	*COL1A1-PDGRB* fusion	PCR for *COL1A1-PDGFB*
Solitary fibrous tumor	*NAB2-STAT6* fusion	IHC for STAT6

Abbreviations: FISH, fluorescence in situ hybridization; IHC, immunohistochemistry; PCR, polymerase chain reaction.

STAGING AND EXTENT OF DISEASE WORK-UP

American Joint Committee on Cancer (AJCC) staging (**Table 2**) takes into account tumor size and depth (T), nodal metastases (N), distant metastases (M), and histologic grade (G). Unlike carcinomas, STSs rarely metastasize to regional lymph nodes. The histologic subtypes with the highest rates of lymph node metastasis are angiosarcoma, epithelioid sarcoma, and embryonal rhabdomyosarcoma. The more common route of metastasis is direct hematogenous spread. Most STSs metastasize preferentially to the lung, and National Comprehensive Cancer Network staging guidelines

Table 2
AJCC staging for soft tissue sarcoma

Primary tumor (T)	
TX	Primary tumor cannot be assessed
T0	No evidence of primary tumor
T1	Tumor ≤5 cm in greatest dimension
T1a	Superficial tumor (not involving underlying fascia)
T1b	Deep tumor (involving or deep to fascia)
T2	Tumor >5 cm in greatest dimension
T2a	Superficial tumor
T2b	Deep tumor

Regional lymph nodes (N)	
NX	Regional lymph nodes cannot be assessed
N0	No regional lymph node metastasis
N1	Regional lymph node metastasis

Distant metastases (M)	
M0	No distant metastasis
M1	Distant metastasis

Histologic grade (G)	
GX	Grade cannot be assessed
G1	Grade 1
G2	Grade 2
G3	Grade 3

Stage	T	N	M	G
Stage IA	T1a	N0	M0	G1, GX
	T1b	N0	M0	G1, GX
Stage IB	T2a	N0	M0	G1, GX
	T2b	N0	M0	G1, GX
Stage IIA	T1a	N0	M0	G2, G3
	T1b	N0	M0	G2, G3
Stage IIB	T2a	N0	M0	G2
	T2b	N0	M0	G2
Stage III	T2a	N0	M0	G3
	T2b	N0	M0	G3
	Any T	N1	M0	Any G
Stage IV	Any T	Any N	M1	Any G

generally recommend chest radiograph or CT scan to rule out distant disease. In general, the use of chest imaging can be tailored to the metastatic risk associated with a given lesion. This risk can be estimated based on AJCC staging or, more accurately, based on prognostic nomograms, many of which are subtype-specific.[8–10] For example, atypical lipomatous tumors do not metastasize. In general, low-grade STSs rarely spread; local recurrence is more common and staging can be completed with preoperative chest radiograph. Large, high-grade undifferentiated pleomorphic sarcoma or leiomyosarcoma have rates of disease-specific death that may approach 50%, and distant metastases are common, so chest CT is reasonable as a means of determining extent of disease for these high-risk patients. Special consideration is given to myxoid/round cell liposarcoma, which has a unique pattern of spread with a propensity for metastasis to soft tissue fat pads and the spine. CT of the chest, abdomen, and pelvis is generally performed in high-risk patients, and MRI of the total spine can be considered.[11,12] PET scan is not clearly warranted for routine extent of disease work-up in STS; many histologic subtypes are not fluorodeoxyglucose-sensitive, and PET is less sensitive than CT for identifying subcentimeter pulmonary nodules.

SURGICAL APPROACH

Benign soft tissue tumors can often be observed, and tumors of a few types, such as nodular fasciitis, may spontaneously regress. However, for intermediate and malignant subtypes of soft tissue tumors, surgery has been considered the gold standard of treatment. Historically, STS of the extremity was treated with amputation. However, in a randomized clinical trial of 43 patients who received adjuvant chemotherapy and underwent limb-sparing surgery followed by radiation or amputation (2:1 randomization), only 15% of patients undergoing limb-sparing experienced local recurrences, and the two treatment groups did not differ in 5-year disease-specific or overall survival.[13] For this reason, limb-sparing procedures are now the standard for treatment of extremity STS. Initially, this was performed by resecting the entire involved muscle, but the current standard for most STS histologies is resection of a 1-cm margin. For superficial lesions, the underlying muscular fascia is removed with the specimen. Similarly, for intramuscular tumors, the fascial barrier between muscle bodies or compartments can provide an adequate barrier and should be resected with the specimen. The key principles of surgery for extremity sarcomas are summarized in **Box 1**.

In the extremity, extent of resection can sometimes be limited by adjacent neurovascular bundles. Generally, the STS is resected away from a neurovascular bundle

---

Box 1
Principles of surgery in extremity soft tissue sarcoma

- Core biopsy should be done in line with the planned surgical incision and then excised at the time of definitive resection.
- Plan for 1-cm margin except for the infiltrative subtypes (myxofibrosarcoma and DFSP), which require a 2-cm margin.
- Superficial sarcomas should be excised with the underlying fascia. For deep/intramuscular tumors, the fascia between muscle bodies or compartments provides a good barrier to tumor extension and should be resected with the specimen.
- Skeletonize vessels and motor nerves unless encased by high-grade sarcoma. Low-grade tumors can be bivalved around critical structures to minimize morbidity.

with the overlying fascial layer (eg, femoral sheath) or the perineurium so as to optimize margins. Encasement of a major neurovascular structure by a low-grade STS is generally managed by bivalving the tumor to minimize morbidity. Encasement by a high-grade lesion may necessitate resection of a major neurovascular structure. Arterial reconstruction can be planned when the artery is involved; venous reconstruction is generally unsuccessful and is often deferred. If the patient develops venous congestion, compression and elevation are prescribed to minimize morbidity as alternative routes of venous drainage develop.

Patients should be carefully counseled regarding expected results of a nerve resection. Sciatic or peroneal resection is generally well tolerated, but results in foot drop and requires ankle bracing. Interruption of the tibial branches of the sciatic causes paresthesias on the plantar aspect of the foot, and patients should be instructed to monitor their feet routinely for trauma that may occur secondary to an insensate foot.[14] Femoral nerve injury results in instability of the knee and may necessitate bracing, particularly in older patients, and patients are at increased risk of fracture in the long term.[15] Resection of one of the three major nerves in the upper extremity generally allows some retention of function, but may necessitate bracing of the limb, result in significant paresthesias, or limit opposition. Advanced maneuvers, such as tendon transfers, are considered in collaboration with a hand specialist.

Special consideration should be given to tumors associated with high rates of local recurrence, mainly myxofibrosarcoma, DFSP, and desmoid-type fibromatosis.[16–18] Both myxofibrosarcoma and DFSP have microscopic components that extend outward from the visible tumor. In the context of myxofibrosarcoma, these may be visible on MRI as enhancing tails (see **Fig. 2**A), and 2-cm margins should be planned circumferentially around the dominant nodules and these tails. In the context of DFSP, a reasonable margin is 2 cm around visible disease. In a retrospective analysis of 206 DFSPs, approximately 85% of surgeries planned with 1- to 2-cm margins resulted in complete microscopic resection.[19] Both DFSP with fibrosarcomatous degeneration and myxofibrosarcoma may invade through fascial margins, so these planes should not be considered as adequate alternatives to the full width of the margin as they can be in most tumor histologies.

Desmoid-type fibromatosis was historically treated like a low-grade fibrosarcoma and managed with aggressive surgical extirpation. However, surgery is currently being used less aggressively for all but the smallest extremity desmoids that can be removed with wide margins, for three reasons. First, related metastases have never been identified for desmoids. Second, extremity desmoids have high rates of local recurrence (>50%–60% in some series),[20–22] and repeated surgeries or amputation cause significant morbidity. Finally, over time, many desmoids remain stable in size or regress.[23] Observation is a reasonable alternative, or in the context of symptoms, systemic therapy can be considered. Traditional agents (ie, doxorubicin or vincristine/methotrexate combinations) and targeted therapies (ie, sorafenib and notch inhibitors) show responses and alleviate symptoms in clinical trials, so they are being used increasingly in management of patients with high-risk desmoids.[24–26] Aggressive surgery is less and less frequently considered for some other histologic subtypes for which, as for desmoids, rates of local or regional recurrence are high even after complete microscopic resection, progression follows an indolent course, and surgery is associated with significant morbidity. These include multifocal epithelioid hemangioendothelioma in a single extremity and tenosynovial giant cell tumors, which can be infiltrative lesions affecting entire muscle compartments and may be responsive to tyrosine kinase inhibitors.

Lymph node metastases occur in less than 5% of STS so that routine sentinel lymph node biopsy or nodal dissection is not performed. When clinically positive nodes are present, prognosis is poor, however. In these instances, radical lymphadenectomy for isolated regional nodal recurrence is associated with improved survival. The histologic subtypes most frequently associated with lymph node metastases are angiosarcoma, rhabdomyosarcoma, clear cell, and epithelioid sarcoma where rates of nodal metastases are approximately 25%.[27–29] In these histologies, it has been proposed that sentinel lymph node biopsy may be of prognostic or therapeutic benefit. However, the role of sentinel lymph node biopsy is unclear because prospective studies have only demonstrated a 5% to 7% rate of occult lymph node metastases in patients with these higher risk subtypes and no survival advantage has been observed in patients undergoing the procedure.[30,31] The small number of patients in these studies makes it difficult to draw any definitive conclusions, but most benefit obtained from sentinel node biopsy is likely related to improved prognostication as opposed to true therapeutic benefit, and we do not routinely recommend the procedure even in high-risk histologies.

CLINICAL OUTCOMES

Rates of local and distant recurrence differ by histologic subtype. For extremity STS, distant metastases are the primary cause of sarcoma-specific death. This is in contrast to retroperitoneal sarcomas, where local recurrence can cause significant morbidity and even disease-specific death. The local recurrence–free survival and distant recurrence–free survival of the six most common subtypes of extremity STS are shown in **Fig. 3**. Highlighted by these survival curves is the high rate of local recurrence for myxofibrosarcoma, high rate of early distant recurrence of undifferentiated pleomorphic sarcoma, and particularly low rate of distant recurrence for DFSP. Even within the group of liposarcomas there are differences, with pleomorphic liposarcomas and round cell liposarcomas having a notably higher risk of distant recurrence. These differences in local and distant recurrence help inform patient management and follow-up. General risk factors for sarcoma-related death are size greater than 5 cm, age greater than 50 years, deep location, high grade, and incomplete gross resection.

MULTIMODALITY TREATMENT

Adjuvant radiation and chemotherapy are considered in conjunction with surgery to prevent local or distant recurrence. Although adjuvant and neoadjuvant radiation

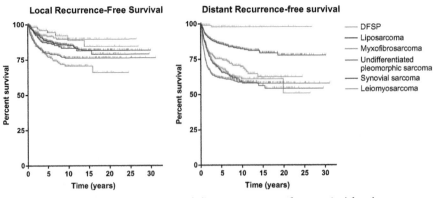

Fig. 3. Local recurrence-free survival and distant recurrence-free survival for the most common subtypes of extremity sarcoma (n = 2498).

have relatively clear indications, the role of adjuvant chemotherapy is controversial, with wide differences in treatment strategies used even across highly specialized sarcoma centers.

Adjuvant and Neoadjuvant Radiation

The role of local radiation to prevent local recurrence has been defined in a range of clinical trials and prospective studies. Adjuvant radiation was used in conjunction with limb-sparing surgery in the National Institutes of Health–led trial defining amputation as unnecessary in routine management of STS. A second randomized trial, again led by investigators at the National Institutes of Health, examined whether adjuvant radiation affects patient outcomes. Ninety-one patients were randomized to undergo adjuvant radiation versus observation after their surgery. Local recurrence rates were lower in patients receiving adjuvant radiation than in those on observation and overall survival did not significantly differ. Similar findings were recorded in subsets of patients with low-grade and high-grade tumors, and these results were durable when reanalyzed with a median follow-up of 18 years.[32,33] Analogous findings were observed when patients were randomized to receive brachytherapy versus no further therapy after limb-sparing surgery; specifically, lower rates of local recurrence were observed in patients receiving radiation than in those treated with surgery alone. In this context, however, the observed benefit was restricted to patients with high-grade lesions. Again, radiation was not associated with better overall or disease-specific survival.[34]

Because adjuvant radiation has not been shown to improve rates of overall survival, the risks associated with radiation should be considered before recommending the treatment of a given patient. Radiation can result in postoperative wound complications, radiation-associated fracture, fibrosis in nearby joints, neuritis, and secondary sarcomas. For this reason, when the baseline risk of local recurrence is small or a local recurrence could be easily salvaged with secondary surgeries, adjuvant radiation is not advised. A prospective study of patients with T1 STS treated with surgery alone showed that forgoing radiation seemed to be safe in most cases. At a median follow-up of 75 months, 5-year local recurrence rates after R0 resection (n = 74) were only 8%.[35] In low-risk lesions, such as these, most clinicians would defer the use of radiation unless local recurrence would be salvageable only with a morbid procedure. Previous studies have identified age greater than 50,[36,37] microscopically positive margins,[36–41] high grade,[39–42] deep location,[37,40] and recurrent tumors[36,37] as risk factors for local recurrence. Many of these factors, and atypical lipomatous tumor histology (a positive prognostic factor), have been integrated into a nomogram that estimates a patient's risk of local recurrence after surgery alone and can therefore be used to predict whether the patient is likely to benefit from adjuvant treatment.[41]

Radiation is administered in either the adjuvant or the neoadjuvant setting; to determine which is appropriate for the individual patient, the clinician should carefully consider the risks and benefits of each regimen (**Box 2**). These risks and benefits were defined in a randomized trial of 94 patients reported by O'Sullivan and colleagues.[43] Participants received either 50 Gy preoperatively with a 5-Gy postoperative boost to the tumor bed or 66 Gy administered postoperatively. At a median follow-up of 3.3 years, the two groups had equivalent rates of local recurrence. However, significant wound complications (defined as requiring operative intervention, prolonged packing, or invasive procedures to minimize complications) were more frequent in those who received neoadjuvant radiation than in those who received their treatment in the adjuvant setting (35% vs 17%; $P = .01$). This difference was exclusively related

---

Box 2
Advantages of neoadjuvant versus adjuvant radiation therapy

Neoadjuvant

Decreased joint toxicity

Decreased field size and radiation dose

Decreased surgical field

Avoid radiating complex reconstruction

Adjuvant

Fewer wound complications

---

to high rates of wound complications in the thigh (affecting 45% of patients with tumors resected from the upper leg).

Despite its association with wound complications in the thigh, neoadjuvant radiation can have significant benefit compared with adjuvant radiation. Standard delivery of radiation involves radiating a field that extends 1.5 cm radially and 4 cm proximally and distally from the site of the tumor or surgical bed.[43] Because the tumor is resected with a margin of normal tissue where possible, a larger volume of normal tissue must be included in the radiation field if radiation is given to the surgical bed as opposed to the tumor in situ. In addition, adjuvant radiation is generally given to doses of 66 Gy as opposed to preoperative doses that are maximally 55 Gy. Neoadjuvant radiation is, therefore, theoretically able to minimize risks of radiation-associated side effects, such as neuritis. Long-term follow-up of patients in the O'Sullivan and colleagues[43] study has demonstrated concrete reductions in joint fibrosis, which was noted in 31% of patients who received neoadjuvant radiation and 48% of patients who received adjuvant radiation ($P = .07$). In addition, patients receiving neoadjuvant treatment tended to have less edema (15% vs 23%) and less joint stiffness (18% vs 23%).[44] Implementation of newer modes of radiation delivery, such as image-guided intensity-modulated radiotherapy (IMRT) or proton beam therapy, may minimize nonspecific injury to normal margins and minimize side effects further. IMRT is similar to conventional radiation therapy for minimizing local recurrence, and in an initial IMRT series postoperative edema was 11% and joint fibrosis was 5.6%, frequencies lower than in historical control subjects. No joint fractures were reported.[45]

Given the increased availability of modalities, such as IMRT and proton beam therapy, most institutions now routinely use neoadjuvant radiation therapy for patients at high risk of local recurrence. In our own case, because of the persistent increase in wound complications related to neoadjuvant treatment and the increased need for complex wound closures that may complicate reresection in the event of local recurrence, we prescribe neoadjuvant radiation selectively. It is prescribed for tumors near a joint, preferentially in the upper extremity and in instances where locally advanced disease may necessitate extensive resection. For tumors in the upper thigh, where wound complications are highest, we tend to resect first and treat with radiation in the adjuvant setting. Radiation should not be prescribed in the neoadjuvant setting if preoperative biopsy is inconclusive regarding grade and/or histology, because radiation would constitute overtreatment if the tumor is low risk or benign.

Adjuvant and Neoadjuvant Chemotherapy

Recommendations regarding the prescription of adjuvant chemotherapy in patients with STS of the extremity vary greatly, even among high-volume specialty centers.

This variability comes from the range of results in randomized clinical trials and the limitations associated with these trials in general. Early trials examined small cohorts of patients undergoing surgery (with or without radiation), who were randomized to undergo adjuvant systemic treatment versus observation. In an early study, 88 patients with FNCLCC grade II or III STS were randomized to systemic therapy (epirubicin with or without ifosfamide) versus no systemic therapy. Although the systemic therapy group had significantly better recurrence-free survival (44% vs 69% at 5 years; $P = .01$), no difference in overall survival was identified.[46] Several subsequent studies, generally randomizing patients to observation versus doxorubicin/ifosfamide-based regimens, had similar outcomes with no consistent evidence that systemic regimens improve overall or disease-specific survival.

The most recent of these randomized trial reports was an European Organization for Research and Treatment of Cancer (EORTC)-sponsored trial (EORTC 62931).[36] Patients with grade II or III STS (n = 351) were randomized to either five cycles of doxorubicin and ifosfamide or to no chemotherapy following treatment of local disease. In this trial, no difference was observed between the two groups in either relapse-free survival or overall survival. As part of the study, however, the investigators performed a meta-analysis of data presented in previously reported clinical trials and their own data for a combined 1071 patients receiving adjuvant chemotherapy and 1074 observed following treatment of local disease. Although 46.5% of patients who did not receive adjuvant chemotherapy died during follow-up, only 41.4% of patients in adjuvant arms died (hazard ratio, 0.86; $P = .02$), suggesting an absolute risk reduction of approximately 5% associated with adjuvant chemotherapy. Although the paucity of survival benefit has led many groups to argue against the routine use of adjuvant chemotherapy, the meta-analysis result, combined with the limitations of published trials (specifically the heterogeneity of tumor types eligible for entrance), has led others to argue that at least a subset of patients may have more substantial benefit from treatment than that observed in the cohort as a whole.[47]

The argument in favor of chemotherapy for subsets of patients with sarcoma has been further bolstered by subset analysis of the patient cohort enrolled on EORTC 62931. In ad hoc analyses, the patients whose outcomes tended to be most improved in the adjuvant chemotherapy arm were those patients with tumors that were grade III, located in the limb (vs trunk or central site), and greater than or equal to 10 cm in diameter. These subset analyses did not reach statistical significance, but results leave open the possibility that these clinical characteristics may define cohorts who would receive the most benefit from adjuvant chemotherapy.[47] Retrospective series have given further credence to this hypothesis, particularly those examining patients with single histologic subtype of STS with known sensitivity to chemotherapy. An example is a review of 255 patients treated for localized synovial sarcoma. Data for patients who did not receive adjuvant chemotherapy were used to contract a nomogram based on tumor size and site, among other variables. Patients treated with adjuvant chemotherapy, however, had significantly better 3-year disease-specific survival than predicted by the nomogram.[9] Another study suggested that improved outcomes in patients with pleomorphic or round cell liposarcoma are associated with receipt of adjuvant ifosfamide-based chemotherapy.[48]

In general, our own practice has been to consider neoadjuvant chemotherapy for high-risk patients. The neoadjuvant setting allows for observation of the tumor in situ and for early discontinuation of the treatment if there is no evidence of response. An additional criterion for chemotherapy is the relative chemosensitivity of the STS subtype (**Table 3**). For example, patients with rhabdomyosarcoma and Ewing sarcoma have risks of sarcoma-specific death that can be more than 50%, and these

Table 3
Risk of distant metastases and chemosensitivity for high-grade extremity sarcomas

		Chemosensitivity		
		Low	Moderate	High
Risk of distant metastases	Low	Dedifferentiated liposarcoma	Myxofibrosarcoma	
	Moderate		Undifferentiated pleomorphic sarcoma Leiomyosarcoma	
	High		Round cell liposarcoma Pleomorphic liposarcoma Angiosarcoma Synovial sarcoma	Ewing sarcoma Rhabdomyosarcoma

tumors are sensitive to chemotherapy; therefore, in our practice, all of these patients receive neoadjuvant systemic therapy. Moderately chemosensitive histologies are treated with chemotherapy when a high-risk tumor is more than 5 cm in size (eg, synovial sarcoma), a moderate-risk tumor is more than 8 cm (eg, undifferentiated pleomorphic sarcoma), and a low-risk tumor is more than 10 cm (eg, myxofibrosarcoma). Chemoresistant histologies, such as dedifferentiated liposarcoma ,are not treated with neoadjuvant chemotherapy.

ISOLATED LIMB PERFUSION

Limb-sparing surgery is the standard of care for extremity sarcoma; however, resection of some extremity sarcomas requires an amputation because of involvement of major neurovascular bundles or multifocality. Isolated limb perfusion has been used in patients that would otherwise require an amputation in an attempt to convert them to a limb-sparing operation. Isolated limb perfusion with melphalan alone had limited success[49]; however combination treatment with tumor necrosis factor-α has been shown to have clinical response and limb salvage rates of 70% to 80%.[50–55] This finding has not significantly altered therapeutic paradigms in the United States, however, because tumor necrosis factor-α is not available in North American centers.

FOLLOW-UP

After resection and adjuvant therapy for localized STS, the National Comprehensive Cancer Network guidelines generally recommend follow-up every 3 to 6 months for 2 to 3 years and every 6 to 12 months thereafter, depending on stage. Patients with tumors of higher metastatic risk generally undergo chest radiograph or chest CT. In practice, low-grade tumors and small, high-grade tumors may have minimal risk of distant metastases and are initially followed every 6 to 12 months. More frequent surveillance is undertaken for patients with large, high-grade tumors identified in the deep compartments of the extremity. Care should be taken for certain histologies to ensure that screening examinations are tailored to the unique patterns of spread. For example, round cell liposarcoma has a propensity to metastasize to fat pads, so after resection, CT of the abdomen and pelvis may be considered in addition to chest scans. Local recurrence can generally be detected by physical examination, although MRI is considered for deep lesions and those with infiltrative histologies, such as myxofibrosarcoma that may not be palpable early.

SUMMARY

Work-up of a mass suspicious for STS starts with a detailed history and physical, followed by cross-sectional imaging (MRI preferred) and a well-planned core needle biopsy for pathologic diagnosis. Rates of local recurrence, distant metastasis (typically to lungs), and sarcoma-specific survival vary significantly among different histologic subtypes, and these differences help inform multimodality treatment planning.

The standard of care for extremity sarcoma is limb-sparing surgery with a margin of 1 to 2 cm (depending on histology), with fascial boundaries providing an acceptable margin to limit morbidity of the resection when major neurovascular or bony structures are in close proximity. Radiation therapy should be considered for tumors with a high risk of local recurrence. The timing of radiation is best determined by weighing the increased risk of wound complications from neoadjuvant radiation against the increased risk of side effects to surrounding tissues and joints from adjuvant radiation. The use of adjuvant chemotherapy is controversial; however, there are relative indications for neoadjuvant chemotherapy for chemosensitive subtypes with moderate or high risk of distant metastases. Currently there are approximately 100 histologic subtypes of STS with variable biology, and these nuances in the therapeutic algorithm highlight the importance of patients being evaluated and managed by a multidisciplinary team with experience and expertise in sarcoma.

ACKNOWLEDGMENTS

The authors thank Janet Novak for editorial assistance.

REFERENCES

1. Fletcher CDM, Bridge JA, Hogendoorn PCW, et al. WHO classification of tumours of soft tissue and bone. 4th edition. Lyon (France): IARC; 2013.
2. Siegel RL, Miller KD, Jemal A. Cancer statistics, 2015. CA Cancer J Clin 2015; 65(1):5–29.
3. Brennan MF, Antonescu CR, Moraco N, et al. Lessons learned from the study of 10,000 patients with soft tissue sarcoma. Ann Surg 2014;260(3):416–21 [discussion: 421–2].
4. Lefkowitz RA, Landa J, Hwang S, et al. Myxofibrosarcoma: prevalence and diagnostic value of the "tail sign" on magnetic resonance imaging. Skeletal Radiol 2013;42(6):809–18.
5. Jelinek JS, Kransdorf MJ, Shmookler BM, et al. Liposarcoma of the extremities: MR and CT findings in the histologic subtypes. Radiology 1993;186(2):455–9.
6. Murphey MD, Arcara LK, Fanburg-Smith J. From the archives of the AFIP: imaging of musculoskeletal liposarcoma with radiologic-pathologic correlation. Radiographics 2005;25(5):1371–95.
7. Heslin MJ, Lewis JJ, Woodruff JM, et al. Core needle biopsy for diagnosis of extremity soft tissue sarcoma. Ann Surg Oncol 1997;4(5):425–31.
8. Eilber FC, Brennan MF, Eilber FR, et al. Validation of the postoperative nomogram for 12-year sarcoma-specific mortality. Cancer 2004;101(10):2270–5.
9. Canter RJ, Qin LX, Maki RG, et al. A synovial sarcoma-specific preoperative nomogram supports a survival benefit to ifosfamide-based chemotherapy and improves risk stratification for patients. Clin Cancer Res 2008;14(24):8191–7.
10. Dalal KM, Kattan MW, Antonescu CR, et al. Subtype specific prognostic nomogram for patients with primary liposarcoma of the retroperitoneum, extremity, or trunk. Ann Surg 2006;244(3):381–91.

11. Hoffman A, Ghadimi MP, Demicco EG, et al. Localized and metastatic myxoid/round cell liposarcoma: clinical and molecular observations. Cancer 2013; 119(10):1868–77.

12. Schwab JH, Boland PJ, Antonescu C, et al. Spinal metastases from myxoid liposarcoma warrant screening with magnetic resonance imaging. Cancer 2007; 110(8):1815–22.

13. Rosenberg SA, Tepper J, Glatstein E, et al. The treatment of soft-tissue sarcomas of the extremities: prospective randomized evaluations of (1) limb-sparing surgery plus radiation therapy compared with amputation and (2) the role of adjuvant chemotherapy. Ann Surg 1982;196(3):305–15.

14. Brooks AD, Gold JS, Graham D, et al. Resection of the sciatic, peroneal, or tibial nerves: assessment of functional status. Ann Surg Oncol 2002;9(1):41–7.

15. Jones KB, Ferguson PC, Deheshi B, et al. Complete femoral nerve resection with soft tissue sarcoma: functional outcomes. Ann Surg Oncol 2010;17(2):401–6.

16. Mentzel T, Calonje E, Wadden C, et al. Myxofibrosarcoma. Clinicopathologic analysis of 75 cases with emphasis on the low-grade variant. Am J Surg Pathol 1996;20(4):391–405.

17. Huang HY, Lal P, Qin J, et al. Low-grade myxofibrosarcoma: a clinicopathologic analysis of 49 cases treated at a single institution with simultaneous assessment of the efficacy of 3-tier and 4-tier grading systems. Hum Pathol 2004;35(5): 612–21.

18. Fields RC, Hameed M, Qin LX, et al. Dermatofibrosarcoma protuberans (DFSP): predictors of recurrence and the use of systemic therapy. Ann Surg Oncol 2011; 18(2):328–36.

19. Farma JM, Ammori JB, Zager JS, et al. Dermatofibrosarcoma protuberans: how wide should we resect? Ann Surg Oncol 2010;17(8):2112–8.

20. Crago AM, Denton B, Salas S, et al. A prognostic nomogram for prediction of recurrence in desmoid fibromatosis. Ann Surg 2013;258(2):347–53.

21. Merchant NB, Lewis JJ, Woodruff JM, et al. Extremity and trunk desmoid tumors: a multifactorial analysis of outcome. Cancer 1999;86(10):2045–52.

22. Salas S, Dufresne A, Bui B, et al. Prognostic factors influencing progression-free survival determined from a series of sporadic desmoid tumors: a wait-and-see policy according to tumor presentation. J Clin Oncol 2011;29(26):3553–8.

23. Fiore M, Rimareix F, Mariani L, et al. Desmoid-type fibromatosis: a front-line conservative approach to select patients for surgical treatment. Ann Surg Oncol 2009;16(9):2587–93.

24. de Camargo VP, Keohan ML, D'Adamo DR, et al. Clinical outcomes of systemic therapy for patients with deep fibromatosis (desmoid tumor). Cancer 2010; 116(9):2258–65.

25. Gounder MM, Lefkowitz RA, Keohan ML, et al. Activity of sorafenib against desmoid tumor/deep fibromatosis. Clin Cancer Res 2011;17(12):4082–90.

26. Messersmith WA, Shapiro GI, Cleary JM, et al. A phase I, dose-finding study in patients with advanced solid malignancies of the oral gamma-secretase inhibitor PF-03084014. Clin Cancer Res 2015;21(1):60–7.

27. Fong Y, Coit DG, Woodruff JM, et al. Lymph node metastasis from soft tissue sarcoma in adults. Analysis of data from a prospective database of 1772 sarcoma patients. Ann Surg 1993;217(1):72–7.

28. Riad S, Griffin AM, Liberman B, et al. Lymph node metastasis in soft tissue sarcoma in an extremity. Clin Orthop Relat Res 2004;(426):129–34.

29. Behranwala KA, A'Hern R, Omar AM, et al. Prognosis of lymph node metastasis in soft tissue sarcoma. Ann Surg Oncol 2004;11(7):714–9.

30. Maduekwe UN, Hornicek FJ, Springfield DS, et al. Role of sentinel lymph node biopsy in the staging of synovial, epithelioid, and clear cell sarcomas. Ann Surg Oncol 2009;16(5):1356–63.
31. Andreou D, Boldt H, Werner M, et al. Sentinel node biopsy in soft tissue sarcoma subtypes with a high propensity for regional lymphatic spread: results of a large prospective trial. Ann Oncol 2013;24(5):1400–5.
32. Yang JC, Chang AE, Baker AR, et al. Randomized prospective study of the benefit of adjuvant radiation therapy in the treatment of soft tissue sarcomas of the extremity. J Clin Oncol 1998;16(1):197–203.
33. Beane JD, Yang JC, White D, et al. Efficacy of adjuvant radiation therapy in the treatment of soft tissue sarcoma of the extremity: 20-year follow-up of a randomized prospective trial. Ann Surg Oncol 2014;21(8):2484–9.
34. Pisters PW, Harrison LB, Leung DH, et al. Long-term results of a prospective randomized trial of adjuvant brachytherapy in soft tissue sarcoma. J Clin Oncol 1996;14(3):859–68.
35. Pisters PW, Pollock RE, Lewis VO, et al. Long-term results of prospective trial of surgery alone with selective use of radiation for patients with T1 extremity and trunk soft tissue sarcomas. Ann Surg 2007;246(4):675–81 [discussion: 681–2].
36. Pisters PW, Leung DH, Woodruff J, et al. Analysis of prognostic factors in 1,041 patients with localized soft tissue sarcomas of the extremities. J Clin Oncol 1996;14(5):1679–89.
37. Gronchi A, Casali PG, Mariani L, et al. Status of surgical margins and prognosis in adult soft tissue sarcomas of the extremities: a series of patients treated at a single institution. J Clin Oncol 2005;23(1):96–104.
38. Stojadinovic A, Leung DH, Hoos A, et al. Analysis of the prognostic significance of microscopic margins in 2,084 localized primary adult soft tissue sarcomas. Ann Surg 2002;235(3):424–34.
39. Trovik CS, Bauer HC, Alvegard TA, et al. Surgical margins, local recurrence and metastasis in soft tissue sarcomas: 559 surgically-treated patients from the Scandinavian Sarcoma Group Register. Eur J Cancer 2000;36(6):710–6.
40. Coindre JM, Terrier P, Bui NB, et al. Prognostic factors in adult patients with locally controlled soft tissue sarcoma. A study of 546 patients from the French Federation of Cancer Centers Sarcoma Group. J Clin Oncol 1996;14(3):869–77.
41. Cahlon O, Brennan MF, Jia X, et al. A postoperative nomogram for local recurrence risk in extremity soft tissue sarcomas after limb-sparing surgery without adjuvant radiation. Ann Surg 2012;255(2):343–7.
42. Fabrizio PL, Stafford SL, Pritchard DJ. Extremity soft-tissue sarcomas selectively treated with surgery alone. Int J Radiat Oncol Biol Phys 2000;48(1):227–32.
43. O'Sullivan B, Davis AM, Turcotte R, et al. Preoperative versus postoperative radiotherapy in soft-tissue sarcoma of the limbs: a randomised trial. Lancet 2002;359(9325):2235–41.
44. Davis AM, O'Sullivan B, Turcotte R, et al. Late radiation morbidity following randomization to preoperative versus postoperative radiotherapy in extremity soft tissue sarcoma. Radiother Oncol 2005;75(1):48–53.
45. O'Sullivan B, Griffin AM, Dickie CI, et al. Phase 2 study of preoperative image-guided intensity-modulated radiation therapy to reduce wound and combined modality morbidities in lower extremity soft tissue sarcoma. Cancer 2013; 119(10):1878–84.
46. Petrioli R, Coratti A, Correale P, et al. Adjuvant epirubicin with or without ifosfamide for adult soft-tissue sarcoma. Am J Clin Oncol 2002;25(5):468–73.

47. Woll PJ, Reichardt P, Le Cesne A, et al. Adjuvant chemotherapy with doxorubicin, ifosfamide, and lenograstim for resected soft-tissue sarcoma (EORTC 62931): a multicentre randomised controlled trial. Lancet Oncol 2012;13(10):1045–54.

48. Eilber FC, Eilber FR, Eckardt J, et al. The impact of chemotherapy on the survival of patients with high-grade primary extremity liposarcoma. Ann Surg 2004; 240(4):686–95 [discussion: 695–7].

49. Krementz ET, Carter RD, Sutherland CM, et al. Chemotherapy of sarcomas of the limbs by regional perfusion. Ann Surg 1977;185(5):555–64.

50. Eggermont AM, Schraffordt Koops H, Lienard D, et al. Isolated limb perfusion with high-dose tumor necrosis factor-alpha in combination with interferon-gamma and melphalan for nonresectable extremity soft tissue sarcomas: a multicenter trial. J Clin Oncol 1996;14(10):2653–65.

51. Eggermont AM, Schraffordt Koops H, Klausner JM, et al. Isolated limb perfusion with tumor necrosis factor and melphalan for limb salvage in 186 patients with locally advanced soft tissue extremity sarcomas. The cumulative multicenter European experience. Ann Surg 1996;224(6):756–64 [discussion: 764–5].

52. Deroose JP, Eggermont AM, van Geel AN, et al. Long-term results of tumor necrosis factor alpha- and melphalan-based isolated limb perfusion in locally advanced extremity soft tissue sarcomas. J Clin Oncol 2011;29(30):4036–44.

53. Rastrelli M, Campana LG, Valpione S, et al. Hyperthermic isolated limb perfusion in locally advanced limb soft tissue sarcoma: a 24-year single-centre experience. Int J Hyperthermia 2016;32(2):165–72.

54. Bhangu A, Broom L, Nepogodiev D, et al. Outcomes of isolated limb perfusion in the treatment of extremity soft tissue sarcoma: a systematic review. Eur J Surg Oncol 2013;39(4):311–9.

55. Bonvalot S, Laplanche A, Lejeune F, et al. Limb salvage with isolated perfusion for soft tissue sarcoma: could less TNF-alpha be better? Ann Oncol 2005;16(7): 1061–8.

Retroperitoneal Sarcomas

Andrea S. Porpiglia, MD, MS[a], Sanjay S. Reddy, MD[b],
Jeffrey M. Farma, MD[b],*

KEYWORDS

- Retroperitoneal sarcoma • Retroperitoneal liposarcoma • Radiation
- Chemotherapy • Surgery

KEY POINTS

- Retroperitoneal sarcomas are a rare disease, and 5-year survival rates vary from 12% to 70%.
- Although surgery represents the mainstay of treatment, the emphasis is on extended resections to achieve negative margins.
- In the main, patients eventually succumb to metastatic disease, so, in order to treat these patients better, there needs to be better adoption of multimodality therapies both in the neoadjuvant and adjuvant settings.
- Because this disease is rare, multi-institutional collaborations are the only way advances can be made.

INTRODUCTION

Retroperitoneal sarcomas are rare tumors and make up a small subset of all sarcomas; approximately 15%. They tend to grow and can be sizable, and thus patients can present with very large tumors. Most patients present with an abdominal mass and abdominal pain, although most symptoms are nonspecific. The most common subtypes are liposarcoma and leiomyosarcoma. Clinicians should also consider other primary retroperitoneal tumors, including lymphomas, germ cell tumors, and testicular cancer, as a differential diagnosis. The role for surgery in the treatment of retroperitoneal sarcomas remains the gold standard compared with other modalities of therapy. Chemotherapy has limited efficacy, and radiation can be limited by toxicity to adjacent intra-abdominal structures.[1,2] The challenge is often that multivisceral resections are needed to clear disease. The authors advocate patients should be managed at a center specializing in a multimodality treatment, given poor survival rates caused by difficulty with resectability and high recurrence rates.[3]

Disclosures: None.
[a] Crozer Keystone Health Network, Department of Surgery, 2100 Keystone Ave, Drexell Hill, PA 19026, USA; [b] Fox Chase Cancer Center, Department of Surgery, 333 Cottman Ave, Philadelphia, PA 19111, USA
* Corresponding author.
E-mail address: jeffrey.farma@fccc.edu

Surg Clin N Am 96 (2016) 993–1001
http://dx.doi.org/10.1016/j.suc.2016.05.009
0039-6109/16/$ – see front matter © 2016 Elsevier Inc. All rights reserved.

Most patients present with an abdominal mass, early satiety, increase in abdominal girth, or abdominal pain.[4] Evaluation should include a complete history and physical examination with abdominal imaging (either computed tomography [CT] or MRI) to determine the extent of disease. Chest imaging should be included to complete staging. Approximately 11% of patients present with metastatic disease.[1,4] Staging of retroperitoneal sarcomas is based on the American Joint Committee on Cancer staging system. The authors generally advocate preoperative core biopsy of the lesion. If imaging is consistent with a large lipoma versus well-differentiated liposarcoma, we generally defer biopsy and plan for surgical resection (**Figs. 1** and **2**). Gene expression analysis is being used by pathologists to help distinguish liposarcoma subtypes; murine double minute-2 (MDM2) is overexpressed in liposarcomas.[5] Preoperative biopsy allows for discussion and consideration for a clinical trial or for neoadjuvant therapy. Patients with retroperitoneal sarcomas should be discussed at a multidisciplinary sarcoma tumor board.

SURGERY

Surgery is the mainstay of treatment of retroperitoneal sarcomas and is the only potentially curative treatment. As for many different types of cancers, the ability to remove tumors with negative margins is one of the most important prognostic factors relating to survival. Singer and colleagues[6] confirmed that incomplete resections and contiguous organ resections were independent prognostic factors for survival. Unique histologic subtype also played a role in prognosis. Dedifferentiated histologic subtypes and the need for contiguous organ resection were associated with an increased risk for local and distant recurrence.[6] The practice of multivisceral resections in order to obtain negative margins is imbedded in surgical teachings; however, what extent of surgical resection is considered too much?

Complete resection is the most important prognostic factor for prolonged survival. There is noted to be a high rate of recurrence up to 48% of patients and complete excision occurs less than 70% of the time.[7,8] Multivisceral en bloc resection may be necessary in up to 83% of patients in order to achieve negative margins.[9] The kidney, colon, adrenal, pancreas, bladder, and spleen are the most common organs resected.[1,10]

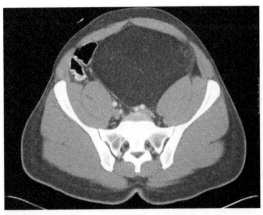

Fig. 1. CT of the abdomen showing a well-differentiated retroperitoneal liposarcoma.

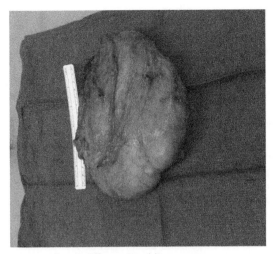

Fig. 2. Resected specimen of well-differentiated liposarcoma.

Bonvalot and colleagues[11] described 3 tiers of surgical resection for primary retroperitoneal sarcomas. Complete compartmental resections were used in those patients who had resections of uninvolved contiguous organs so that a rim of normal tissue was removed to ensure wide excision. A simple complete resection was used where the tumor was shelled out. The third classification included procedures in which contiguously involved organs were removed because of invasion. Patients undergoing complete compartmental resections had a 3.29-fold lower rate of abdominal recurrence compared with simple resection alone.[11] This finding is directly correlated with obtaining a negative margin of resection. Bremjit and colleagues[12] performed a retrospective review of a large single-institutional database. Forty-five percent of patients underwent a margin-negative resection, and 44% had a microscopic margin-positive resection. Tumor grade and margin status were predictors of progression-free and overall survival.[12] Another large experience was published by Erzen and colleagues,[13] in which 155 patients underwent surgery, and survival rates were considerably higher in those who underwent a margin-negative resection. The current trend in surgical management of these retroperitoneal sarcomas is not only to remove the tumors but to ensure that the extent of resection creates negative margins, even if this means that an extended resection is needed. Given the location of retroperitoneal sarcomas, reliable assessment of microscopic margins can be challenging. Gronchi and colleagues[14] expounded on the idea of the complete compartmental resections proposed by Bonvalot and colleagues.[11] Simple resections were performed early in their experience, and, more recently, the liberal en bloc resection of surrounding tissues and organs was performed. Results showed greater local control in the more aggressive extended resections, with a 28% 5-year local recurrence rate versus 48% when a less aggressive operation was done.[14] Ultimately the fate of many of these patients is the same, because overall survival is affected by development of metastatic disease. Whether or not adequate systemic treatments are available is disputed among experts; however, Miura and colleagues[15] recently reviewed the National Cancer Database and, in 8653 patients with surgically resected retroperitoneal sarcomas, the use of chemotherapy in the neoadjuvant or adjuvant setting did not confer a survival benefit.

RADIATION THERAPY

Radiation therapy has been shown to be one of the significant prognostic factors that contribute to a decrease in local recurrence.[7] However, radiation therapy is challenging in treating retroperitoneal sarcomas because they are often adjacent to radiosensitive structures and require large fields.[16] Radiation therapy has been described preoperatively, intraoperatively, and postoperatively.

Preoperative Radiation Therapy

An advantage to preoperative radiation therapy is in decreasing the size of the tumor, allowing it to be amenable to surgical resection. Another advantage is improvement of the negative margins obtained.[17] Pawlik and colleagues[18] reported on 2 prospective trials evaluating the use of preoperative radiation therapy in intermediate-grade to high-grade retroperitoneal sarcomas. The University of Toronto evaluated patients in whom preoperative radiation was used and a select group of patients received a radiation boost with brachytherapy. MD Anderson Cancer Center was the other site, and their patients received low-dose doxorubicin with concurrent external beam irradiation. The patients received intraoperative radiation therapy in a select number of cases. Seventy-nine percent of patients who started with preoperative radiation underwent surgical resection and 95% of those had an R1 or R0 resection. Fifty-two percent of the patients who completed neoadjuvant radiation and had surgical resection developed recurrent disease (31% local failure, 15% with distant failure, 6% in both). The time to recurrence was 17.2 months, with 2-year and 5-year local recurrence-free survival of 79% and 60%.

Another retrospective review from Bremjit and colleagues[12] showed no benefit in overall survival or progression-free survival in those patients who received preoperative radiation. Furthermore, there have been no prospective randomized trials evaluating the role of preoperative radiation therapy. The American College of Surgeons Oncology Group tried to perform a randomized trial evaluating the role of preoperative therapy but it closed early because of poor accrual. There is a phase III randomized controlled trial being conducted by the European Organisation for Research and Treatment of Cancer, comparing preoperative radiation therapy plus surgery versus surgery alone for patients with retroperitoneal sarcomas.[19] The trial is still accruing so it will be years before the results are available.

Postoperative Radiation Therapy

There are several retrospective series and multiple single-institutional studies evaluating the use of postoperative radiation therapy. Postoperative radiation therapy has been shown to be effective in local control. However, high doses result in significant toxicities.[3] The University of Florida described their experience with postoperative radiation therapy. More than half the patients received preoperative radiation therapy. Forty-seven percent developed local recurrence compared with only 16% in the patients treated with preoperative radiation. The study also reported a greater local control in the patients who had negative surgical margins, despite the sequence of radiation treatment. The 5-year overall survival was also higher in those with negative margins: 69% compared with 12% in those with positive margins.[20] The University of Michigan retrospectively reviewed their experience of preoperative and postoperative radiation therapy.[21] The patients with postoperative radiation therapy had an increased rate of local recurrence compared with those who received preoperative radiation therapy. However, there was no statistically significant difference in toxicity.

There has been more discussion of aggressive up-front surgery to decrease local recurrence. In a French study, Le Pechoux and colleagues[22] reviewed their experience of patients with primary retroperitoneal sarcomas who underwent frontline aggressive surgery alone or who received adjuvant radiation therapy. There were 56 patients who had surgery alone versus 42 patients who had surgery plus adjuvant radiation therapy. The patients who received adjuvant radiation therapy were more likely to have an R1 or R2 resection ($P = .03$) and more likely to have received neoadjuvant therapy ($P \leq .0001$). They found improved local recurrence-free survival rates with postoperative radiation therapy (hazard ratio [HR], 0.43; 95% confidence interval [CI], 0.20–0.88; $P = .02$). Local relapse rates at 5 years were 22% for surgery plus adjuvant radiation and 36% for the surgery-only group, and these were not statistically significant. The study showed only a small benefit of adjuvant radiation therapy in local recurrence-free survival, but no difference in local relapse rates.

There have been several Surveillance, Epidemiology, and End Result (SEER) database analyses focusing on the use of radiation therapy in the treatment of retroperitoneal sarcomas. Choi and colleagues[23] analyzed 558 patients with retroperitoneal sarcomas who underwent surgical resection alone and 204 patients who underwent surgery plus radiation. The results showed no reduced hazard of death with radiation therapy and, with propensity score matching, no difference in disease-specific or overall survival with the use of radiation therapy. Radiation therapy included external beam radiation, radioactive implants, and combination of beam and radioactive implants. In addition, the study included patients receiving preoperative radiation, postoperative radiation, intraoperative radiation, and a combination. Tseng and colleagues[24] used the SEER database to evaluate the benefit of adjuvant radiation therapy in 1535 patients and found no difference in overall survival and disease-specific survival between those who received adjuvant radiation therapy and those who did not. However, there was improved survival with the malignant fibrous histiocytoma (MFH) histologic subtype. Bates and colleagues[25] performed a SEER database review and again noted an overall survival benefit with adjuvant radiation therapy in patients with MFH. Other reviews of SEER databases have noted limited survival benefit with adjuvant radiation therapy.[26,27]

Postoperative radiation therapy can be considered in patients with close or positive surgical margins or high-grade disease. However, further prospective studies need to be performed to better delineate the role of radiation therapy in retroperitoneal sarcomas. At our institution, we recommend preoperative radiation therapy for high-grade or dedifferentiated retroperitoneal sarcomas.

Intraoperative Radiation Therapy

Intraoperative radiation therapy has been described in conjunction with either preoperative or postoperative radiation therapy. Sindelar and colleagues[28] performed a prospective randomized trial by comparing intraoperative radiotherapy in combination with postoperative external beam radiation with postoperative external beam radiation alone. The study was small, with only 35 patients. However, there was improved locoregional control with those who received intraoperative radiotherapy, but similar median survival. Single-institution series have shown improved 5-year local control rates of 59% to 62%.[29,30]

However, there are no large randomized controlled trials comparing preoperative, intraoperative, and postoperative radiation therapy. Decisions on the use of radiation therapy should be made in a multidisciplinary setting.

CHEMOTHERAPY

There are some data on the use of chemotherapy in the treatment of retroperitoneal sarcomas. Because there are no prospective data, Miura and colleagues[15] conducted a retrospective cohort study using the National Cancer Data Base. From 1998 to 2011 there were 8653 patients with retroperitoneal sarcomas who underwent surgical resection and only 17.6% received chemotherapy. Ten percent received neoadjuvant chemotherapy, 32% received adjuvant chemotherapy, and 1% received both. A propensity-matched cohort noted that those who received chemotherapy had worse overall survival than those who had surgery alone (40 months vs 52.4 months; $P = .002$). The investigators were unable to show any survival benefit in patients with high-grade tumors, R1/R2 resections, or tumor size greater than 10 cm.

A meta-analysis of 18 trials evaluating the use of adjuvant chemotherapy in patients with localized resectable retroperitoneal sarcomas showed a benefit with adjuvant chemotherapy.[31] Doxorubicin-based chemotherapy reduced overall recurrence (0.69; 95% CI, 0.56–0.86; $P = .0008$). However, there was no benefit of adjuvant doxorubicin-based chemotherapy on overall survival. There was a survival benefit noted with doxorubicin combined with ifosfamide (HR, 0.56; 95% CI; 0.36–0.85; $P = .01$). The meta-analysis showed a small benefit of adjuvant chemotherapy. However, there are limitations with a meta-analysis and there are no prospective randomized trials. Adjuvant therapy should be discussed in a multidisciplinary setting.

RECURRENCE

Despite adequate surgical resection, chemotherapy, and radiation, the risks for recurrence locally or distant remains high. Patients presenting with this rare disease often inquire what these aggressive treatments will mean for them in the long term. The group from Memorial Sloan Kettering established a nomogram to assist in answering these questions. Bagaria and colleagues[32] performed a retrospective review of the SEER registry, and entered data from 9237 patients into this nomogram. The results confirmed a better predictive ability than the current American Joint Committee on Cancer system; however, there remains room for improvement on prognostication.[32] The rarity and diverse histologic subtypes of this disease make it difficult to predict outcomes. Despite this, histologic subtype remains one of the most important independent predictors of recurrence and survival.[6,33,34]

SURVEILLANCE

In general, patients should be followed with imaging every 3 to 6 months for the first 2 to 3 years, then every 6 months for the next 2 years, then annually. Patients who are found to have locally recurrent disease should be discussed in a multidisciplinary fashion with a strong consideration for radiation if they have not had this before, and if surgically resectable should consider resection of the recurrence. If the patient has already received radiation therapy, a consideration should be made for intraoperative radiation therapy or brachytherapy catheters in the hope of decreasing the chance of recurrence.

SUMMARY

Retroperitoneal sarcoma is a rare disease, and 5-year survival rates vary from 12% to 70%.[35,36] Although surgery represents the mainstay of treatment, the emphasis is on extended resections to achieve negative margins. Patients eventually succumb to metastatic disease, so, in order to treat this subset of patients better, there needs to be better adoption of multimodality therapies in both the neoadjuvant and adjuvant settings and enrollment into clinical trials. Because this disease is rare, multi-institutional collaborations are the only way advances can be made.

REFERENCES

1. Lewis JJ, Leung D, Woodruff JM, et al. Retroperitoneal soft-tissue sarcoma: analysis of 500 patients treated and followed at a single institution. Ann Surg 1998; 228(3):355–65.
2. Lewis JJ, Benedetti F. Adjuvant therapy for soft tissue sarcomas. Surg Oncol Clin N Am 1997;6(4):847–62.
3. Tzeng CW, Fiveash JB, Popple RA, et al. Preoperative radiation therapy with selective dose escalation to the margin at risk for retroperitoneal sarcoma. Cancer 2006;107(2):371–9.
4. Hueman MT, Herman JM, Ahuja N. Management of retroperitoneal sarcomas. Surg Clin North Am 2008;88(3):583–97, vii.
5. Singer S, Socci ND, Ambrosini G, et al. Gene expression profiling of liposarcoma identifies distinct biological types/subtypes and potential therapeutic targets in well-differentiated and dedifferentiated liposarcoma. Cancer Res 2007;67(14): 6626–36.
6. Singer SS. Histologic subtype and margin of resection predict pattern of recurrence and survival for retroperitoneal liposarcoma. Ann Surg 2003;238(3):52–65.
7. Heslin MJ, Lewis JJ, Nadler E, et al. Prognostic factors associated with long-term survival for retroperitoneal sarcoma: implications for management. J Clin Oncol 1997;15(8):2832–9.
8. Stoeckle E, Coindre JM, Bonvalot S, et al. Prognostic factors in retroperitoneal sarcoma: a multivariate analysis of a series of 165 patients of the French Cancer Center Federation Sarcoma Group. Cancer 2001;92(2):359–68.
9. Jaques DP, Coit DG, Hajdu SI, et al. Management of primary and recurrent soft-tissue sarcoma of the retroperitoneum. Ann Surg 1990;212(1):51–9.
10. Mendenhall WM, Zlotecki RA, Hochwald SN, et al. Retroperitoneal soft tissue sarcoma. Cancer 2005;104(4):669–75.
11. Bonvalot S, Rivoire M, Castaing M, et al. Primary retroperitoneal sarcomas: a multivariate analysis of surgical factors associated with local control. J Clin Oncol 2009;27(1):31–7.
12. Bremjit PJ, Jones RL, Chai X, et al. A contemporary large single-institution evaluation of resected retroperitoneal sarcoma. Ann Surg Oncol 2014;21(7):2150–8.
13. Erzen D, Sencar M, Novak J. Retroperitoneal sarcoma: 25 years of experience with aggressive surgical treatment at the Institute of Oncology, Ljubljana. J Surg Oncol 2005;91(1):1–9.
14. Gronchi A, Lo Vullo S, Fiore M, et al. Aggressive surgical policies in a retrospectively reviewed single-institution case series of retroperitoneal soft tissue sarcoma patients. J Clin Oncol 2009;27(1):24–30.
15. Miura JT, Charlson J, Gamblin TC, et al. Impact of chemotherapy on survival in surgically resected retroperitoneal sarcoma. Eur J Surg Oncol 2015;41(10): 1386–92.
16. Raut CP, Pisters PW. Retroperitoneal sarcomas: combined-modality treatment approaches. J Surg Oncol 2006;94(1):81–7.
17. Nussbaum DP, Speicher PJ, Gulack BC, et al. The effect of neoadjuvant radiation therapy on perioperative outcomes among patients undergoing resection of retroperitoneal sarcomas. Surg Oncol 2014;23(3):155–60.

18. Pawlik TM, Pisters PW, Mikula L, et al. Long-term results of two prospective trials of preoperative external beam radiotherapy for localized intermediate- or high-grade retroperitoneal soft tissue sarcoma. Ann Surg Oncol 2006;13(4):508–17.

19. Strauss DC. Available at: https://clinicaltrials.gov/ct2/show/NCT01344018?term=NCT01344018&rank=1.

20. Zlotecki RA, Katz TS, Morris CG, et al. Adjuvant radiation therapy for resectable retroperitoneal soft tissue sarcoma: the University of Florida experience. Am J Clin Oncol 2005;28(3):310–6.

21. Feng M, Murphy J, Griffith KA, et al. Long-term outcomes after radiotherapy for retroperitoneal and deep truncal sarcoma. Int J Radiat Oncol Biol Phys 2007; 69(1):103–10.

22. Le Pechoux C, Musat E, Baey C, et al. Should adjuvant radiotherapy be administered in addition to front-line aggressive surgery (FAS) in patients with primary retroperitoneal sarcoma? Ann Oncol 2013;24(3):832–7.

23. Choi AH, Barnholtz-Sloan JS, Kim JA. Effect of radiation therapy on survival in surgically resected retroperitoneal sarcoma: a propensity score-adjusted SEER analysis. Ann Oncol 2012;23(9):2449–57.

24. Tseng WH, Martinez SR, Do L, et al. Lack of survival benefit following adjuvant radiation in patients with retroperitoneal sarcoma: a SEER analysis. J Surg Res 2011;168(2):e173–80.

25. Bates JE, Dhakal S, Mazloom A, et al. The benefit of adjuvant radiotherapy in high-grade nonmetastatic retroperitoneal soft tissue sarcoma: a SEER analysis. Am J Clin Oncol 2015. [Epub ahead of print].

26. Zhou Z, McDade TP, Simons JP, et al. Surgery and radiotherapy for retroperitoneal and abdominal sarcoma: both necessary and sufficient. Arch Surg 2010; 145(5):426–31.

27. Nathan H, Raut CP, Thornton K, et al. Predictors of survival after resection of retroperitoneal sarcoma: a population-based analysis and critical appraisal of the AJCC staging system. Ann Surg 2009;250(6):970–6.

28. Sindelar WF, Kinsella TJ, Chen PW, et al. Intraoperative radiotherapy in retroperitoneal sarcomas. Final results of a prospective, randomized, clinical trial. Arch Surg 1993;128(4):402–10.

29. Alektiar KM, Hu K, Anderson L, et al. High-dose-rate intraoperative radiation therapy (HDR-IORT) for retroperitoneal sarcomas. Int J Radiat Oncol Biol Phys 2000; 47(1):157–63.

30. Petersen IA, Haddock MG, Donohue JH, et al. Use of intraoperative electron beam radiotherapy in the management of retroperitoneal soft tissue sarcomas. Int J Radiat Oncol Biol Phys 2002;52(2):469–75.

31. Pervaiz N, Colterjohn N, Farrokhyar F, et al. A systematic meta-analysis of randomized controlled trials of adjuvant chemotherapy for localized resectable soft-tissue sarcoma. Cancer 2008;113(3):573–81.

32. Bagaria SP, Wagie AE, Gray RJ, et al. Validation of a soft tissue sarcoma nomogram using a National Cancer Registry. Ann Surg Oncol 2015;22(Suppl 3): S398–403.

33. Tan MC, Brennan MF, Kuk D, et al. Histology-based classification predicts pattern of recurrence and improves risk stratification in primary retroperitoneal sarcoma. Ann Surg 2015;22(Suppl 3):S398–403.

34. Gronchi A, Miceli R, Allard MA, et al. Personalizing the approach to retroperitoneal soft tissue sarcoma: histology-specific patterns of failure and postrelapse outcome after primary extended resection. Ann Surg Oncol 2015;22(5):1447–54.

35. Pirayesh A, Chee Y, Helliwell TR, et al. The management of retroperitoneal soft tissue sarcoma: a single institution experience with a review of the literature. Eur J Surg Oncol 2001;27(5):491–7.
36. Karakousis CP, Velez AF, Emrich LJ. Management of retroperitoneal sarcomas and patient survival. Am J Surg 1985;150(3):376–80.

Management of Truncal Sarcoma

John E. Mullinax, MD, Ricardo J. Gonzalez, MD*

KEYWORDS

- Desmoid • Spermatic cord • Sentinel node biopsy • Liposarcoma

KEY POINTS

- Reconstruction following resection of truncal soft tissue sarcoma is complex due to the multiplanar forces exerted on this region.
- Desmoid tumors arise often in the trunk and have many options for management, including observation alone.
- Sarcoma of the inguinal region or spermatic cord offers unique surgical management decisions regarding the genitourinary system that can have significant psychosocial implications.

INTRODUCTION

Soft tissue sarcomas (STSs) were responsible for 11,930 new cases of cancer and 4870 deaths in 2015.[1] Sarcomas can occur throughout the body with most (40%) occurring in the extremity and approximately 20% in the retroperitoneum. The site of disease is important regarding prognosis. The 15-year survival rate is better for extremity STS (68.4%) than for primary retroperitoneal sarcoma (50%), and truncal sarcoma falls roughly in the middle (59.5%).[2] Sarcomas occurring within the layers of the abdominal or chest wall are considered truncal sarcomas. The anatomic boundaries that define the region include the entire circumference of the body bordered by the clavicles superiorly and the inguinal crease inferiorly. Approximately one-fifth of STSs originate within these boundaries.[3] The most common malignant histologies that occur in this region are, in descending order, undifferentiated pleomorphic sarcoma, liposarcoma, and myxofibrosarcoma.[4] Although there are certainly some similarities regarding the management of extremity and truncal STS, this article focuses on the unique histologies most associated with truncal sarcoma and the unique aspects of surgical management for patients with truncal sarcoma.

Disclosures: None.
Sarcoma Department, H. Lee Moffitt Cancer Center, 12902 Magnolia Drive, Tampa, FL 33606, USA
* Corresponding author.
E-mail address: ricardo.gonzalez@moffitt.org

General Principles

Initial evaluation of a patient with STS begins with a thorough history and physical examination. The history of the lesion itself is important, such as duration, temporal changes, and local symptoms, including weakness or neurovascular deficit. Family history can be especially important because the patient may be the proband for inherited conditions like Li Fraumeni (p53 mutation), Gardner syndrome (APC mutation), or Von Recklinghausen disease (NF1 mutation). Physical examination should be general enough to identify comorbid conditions to affect the perioperative morbidity and mortality but also focus on the lesion of interest. For truncal sarcoma, specific attention should be paid to prior surgical incisions around the lesion, prior surgical drain sites (such as tube thoracostomy), and the mobility of the lesion from the abdominal or chest wall. Palpation and movement of the truncal mass is a crucial finding for the operating surgeon because it helps to better define the invasive nature of the lesion related to bony structures, such as the pelvis or chest wall.

Before resection, it is essential to stage the patient adequately. Truncal lesions require imaging of the primary lesion in the form of computed tomography (CT) or MRI with contrast to plan the surgical resection (**Fig. 1**). Staging should include a CT scan of the chest for intermediate- or high-grade lesions or any lesion greater than 5 cm in size.[5] Intravenous contrast is important for both staging and diagnostic CT scans so as to better define the enhancement of any potential visceral lesions identified. The imaging characteristics are often suggestive of the histology (ie, lipomatous and myxoid tumors) and even the grade (ie, degree of necrosis/enhancement) of the tumor. These characteristics drive the decision regarding the need for preoperative biopsy of resectable tumors because those lesions under consideration for neoadjuvant chemotherapy or radiation require biopsy.

Preoperative biopsy of trunk lesions should be used when the diagnosis is unclear based on imaging, and in general, is recommended. Imaging findings that strongly suggest a high-grade lesion (increased contrast uptake or foci of necrosis) should prompt biopsy to better direct a multidisciplinary approach, which may require neoadjuvant chemotherapy or radiation. The method of biopsy should be image-guided core biopsy, and the operating surgeon should be involved in the biopsy planning. Image guidance is advocated so the radiologist can sample those areas of the tumor thought most likely to harbor the highest grade component of the lesion. Excisional biopsy can

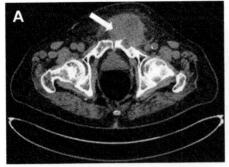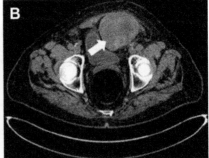

Fig. 1. CT scan of abdominal wall dedifferentiated liposarcoma in the left lower quadrant. (A) The solid, dedifferentiated component (*arrow*) involves the superior ramus of the pubis. (B) The solid component (*arrow*) demonstrated external compression of the bladder and remained entirely extraperitoneal.

also be considered for small (<3 cm) lesions. Incisional biopsies should be generally avoided because of the potential for local dissemination of malignant cells, which could impact the extent of resection required. One specific indication for incisional biopsy is when preoperative therapy is being considered but attempts at core biopsy are nondiagnostic. In this case, the surgeon responsible for the oncologic resection should perform the incisional biopsy to ensure that the incision is appropriately oriented for the definitive resection; meticulous hemostasis is achieved, and there is minimal dissection of tissue.

As stated previously, radical resection of the primary sarcoma is the standard therapy and that which offers the patient the greatest opportunity for long-term survival. Following adequate staging, the patient should be discussed in a multidisciplinary fashion and ideally referred to a center specializing in the treatment of sarcomas.

UNIQUE CONSIDERATIONS FOR TRUNCAL SARCOMA
Desmoid Tumors

Hyperproliferation of myofibroblasts can form lesions referred to as desmoid tumors, which are quite rare, representing only 0.03% of all neoplasms.[6] These lesions are generally indolent and have very little propensity for distant spread. They are often described as "aggressive fibromatosis" and can form at the site of prior trauma, including within the healed incision following an operation. These tumors arise in 3 general anatomic locations: intra-abdominal, extremity, and the trunk (within chest or abdominal wall). Some locations that present unique management decisions include the shoulder girdle, low pelvic incisions (following cesarean section), and the bowel mesentery. Symptoms present at the time of presentation are often either neurologic due to sensory nerve involvement within a given dermatome or mechanical due to compression of viscera in the case of intraperitoneal disease. Evaluation with axial imaging is standard, but biopsy is not generally necessary. Desmoid tumors have very characteristic findings on axial imaging, such as fibrous bundles, lack of defined border, hypointense to muscle on T1, and hyperintense to muscle on T2 phases of MRI.[7,8] Despite these findings, biopsy confirmation can be helpful to ensure the correct diagnosis before a plan for surveillance or systemic therapy is undertaken.

Patients with intraperitoneal desmoid tumors should be screened for familial adenomatous polyposis syndrome. Although only 2% to 5% of desmoid tumors are associated with this germline mutation, the diagnosis has important implications for other sites of disease and other family members of the index patient.[9,10] For this reason, a thorough family history is vital to the care of these patients, and any upper or lower gastrointestinal malignancy in relatives increases the likelihood of a germline APC mutation in these patients. There is a 20% incidence of desmoid tumors in those with the mutation.[9] Upper and lower endoscopy should be performed in patients with any gastrointestinal symptoms associated with an intra-abdominal desmoid in an effort to identify primary malignant disease in other organs at risk such as the colon and duodenum.

The treatment of desmoid tumors has evolved, and there is literature to support a wide array of approaches. Early work supported the aggressive resection of these lesions with wide margins, similar to the resection for any other soft tissue malignancy. Aggressive resection was based on the knowledge that these tumors were unlikely to generate distant disease, and therefore, radical resection could be curative.[10–12] More recent experience has shown that the indolent nature of desmoid tumors often appears to outweigh the morbidity of resection, and therefore, a "nonoperative approach" has been proposed.[6,13] A recent large experience of an observational approach to extra-abdominal desmoid tumors by Briand and colleagues[6] demonstrated failure of this approach in only 9% of patients with median follow-up of 73 months. The reason for dropout from observation was progressive disease that was completely resected in the majority (80%) of patients, and systemic therapy was given for progression in the remaining patients. In another report, the 5-year progression-free survival was 53.4% for patients who were observed with median follow-up of 33 months.[13] Finally, the spontaneous regression of desmoid tumors has been described, although the incidence in one large series was only 2%.[13]

The data regarding resection versus observation can be difficult to interpret based on the heterogeneity of datasets and retrospective nature of institutional experience. Many times, intra-abdominal and abdominal wall lesions are grouped together, and other times extremity patients are included in reports comparing these approaches. In an effort to describe context, one report of a large institutional series illustrated the conflicting nature of retrospective reports. The authors of this large series presented 6 studies whereby 4 showed increased recurrence following resection with positive margins and 2 showed no difference.[14] Review of the available literature leaves the final conclusion that observation of small abdominal or chest wall lesions with CT or MRI scan every 6 months is safe with two-thirds of patients not requiring any surgical intervention.[13] Resection of large, symptomatic superficial desmoid tumors is generally favored and especially those resectable lesions involving bowel mesentery or other viscera due to the risk that progression with observation will lead to significant morbidity.

Systemic therapy for patients with unresectable or symptomatic desmoid tumors has been advocated. The observation that desmoid tumors stain positive for estrogen receptor-β led to the use of tamoxifen as a hormonal therapy.[15,16] Other noncytotoxic therapy includes nonsteroidal anti-inflammatory drugs (NSAIDs), which have been used because they are known to inhibit the Wnt-APC-β-catenin pathway, of which there are mutations in the CTNNB1 gene (β-catenin) in up to 85% of desmoid tumors[17] (**Fig. 2**). The largest experience with antiestrogen therapy and NSAIDs described 25 patients treated with tamoxifen and sulindac. In these series, 46% of patients with primary desmoid tumor had stable disease and 31% had an objective response (either complete or partial response) that lasted more than 6 months. The results were not as promising for the patients with recurrent disease because 75% had progressive disease with the same drug treatment.[9] The Children's Oncology Group experience with tamoxifen and sulindac for patients less than 19 years old demonstrated only

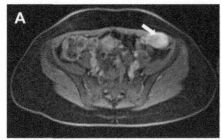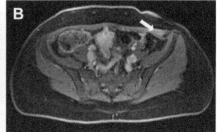

Fig. 2. Abdominal wall desmoid tumor treated with NSAID therapy. (*A*) Initial imaging with left lower quadrant abdominal wall desmoid tumor (*arrow*). (*B*) Near complete regression after 16 months of therapy with celexocib (*arrow*).

8% response rate and 36% 2-year progression-free survival.[18] One prospective report of 16 patients treated with neoadjuvant tamoxifen and sulindac demonstrated only a 12% response rate but obviated resection in 30% of patients.[19]

More recent reports of targeted therapy are encouraging. Sorafenib, a multityrosine kinase inhibitor, produced stable disease in 70% of patients and partial response in 25% with no complete responses.[20] Although not randomized, the percentage of patients with stable disease is higher than the reported series of patients observed for desmoid tumors. It should be noted that 57% of patients had a median of 2 prior systemic treatments, and 62% of the patients were treated for a recurrence, making this a group at high risk for progression.

Radiation therapy has also been described in the treatment of desmoid tumors. The largest report of desmoid tumor management has advocated against the use of radiation therapy on the basis of no improvement in recurrence-free survival. In this report, the management of 495 patients with desmoid tumors was evaluated from a retrospective database. The 5-year recurrence-free survival for patients with adjuvant radiation therapy was 68% compared with 72% for those patients without radiation therapy.[11] This report is limited by the retrospective approach and the combined experience of extremity intraperitoneal desmoid tumors. Furthermore, only a limited number of patients from the dataset received radiation therapy (12% for primary disease; 32% for recurrent disease). Despite these limitations, other large series report similar 5-year local control rates of 75%.[21]

Soft Tissue Sarcoma of the Inguinal Region

The inguinal region is the primary site of disease for 2.5% of patients with STS and is found incidentally on less than 0.01% of inguinal hernia pathology specimens. From analysis of the Surveillance, Epidemiology, and End Results database, the frequency of histology is liposarcoma (46%), followed by leiomyosarcoma (20%), undifferentiated pleomorphic sarcoma (13%), and rhabdomyosarcoma (9%).[22] The diagnosis of sarcoma is a very uncommon cause of an inguinal mass, and many times patients are diagnosed with an inguinal hernia initially. A large series of inguinal region sarcoma indicate that up to 16% were initially thought to have an inguinal hernia. Fortunately, the subsequent oncologic operation following an unexpected postoperative diagnosis did not change the prognosis. Patients operated on following an initial exploration for presumed inguinal hernia have the same disease-specific survival as those with an index operation for known STS of the inguinal region.[23]

There are unique considerations regarding the management of these lesions. First, the anatomy of this location encompasses the primary motor innervation along with the arterial and venous supply to the lower extremity. A study by Brooks and colleagues[23] of 88 patients with inguinal sarcoma described a large single-institution series of inguinal sarcomas whereby 20% of tumors involved the femoral neurovascular bundle. Although a limb-sparing approach was successful in 94% of the entire cohort, an amputation was required in 30% of those with neurovascular involvement. The spermatic cord may either be the site of primary tumor or intimately involved in an abdominal wall primary tumor. There are occasions when a primary or recurrent lesion involves the pelvic bones and concomitant resection is required (**Fig. 3**). Orchiectomy is required for all spermatic cord primary tumors and up to 10% of abdominal wall sarcomas of the inguinal region.[22–24] This aspect of the resection can bring about psychological stress in the patient, although it is of limited morbidity.

The reconstruction required after resection of inguinal region STS is another important consideration (**Fig. 4**). As mentioned, the neurovascular structures supplying the lower extremity are within the field of resection, and tissue coverage of these vital

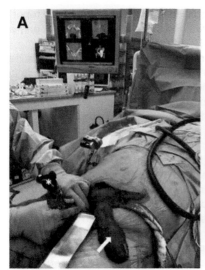
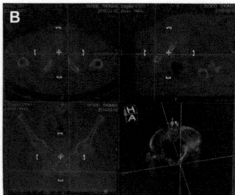

Fig. 3. Resection of the superior ramus of the pubis using navigational osteotome. (A) The navigational osteotome (*asterisk*) is aligned for the precise osteotomy. The primary tumor contained well-differentiated component that was contained within the retroperitoneum and extended along the spermatic cord, necessitating orchiectomy (*arrow*). (B) Osteotomies are guided by intraoperative CT scan performed before incision.

structures, if not resected, should be considered. Transposition of the sartorius muscle is the most commonly performed maneuver and is important because many of these patients will require adjuvant radiation for either large or high-grade tumors. Protection of the neurovascular structures mitigates the morbidity of wound

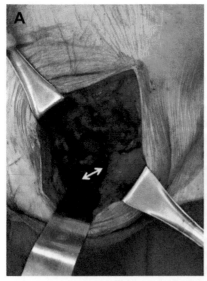
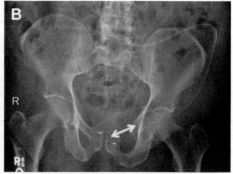

Fig. 4. Resection cavity following extirpation of the mass. (A) The tumor remained entirely extraperitoneal and required resection of the lower rectus abdominus muscle, external oblique, and radical orchiectomy. Arrow indicates resected superior ramus of the pubis. (B) Radiograph with arrow demonstrating resected portion of bone for comparison.

complications that may arise from radiation therapy. The inguinal canal itself should also be reconstructed so as to prevent herniation of the abdominal contents. Inguinal canal reconstruction is most often accomplished with synthetic mesh, and care should be taken to incorporate the mesh such that femoral and obturator hernias are prevented.

Finally, management of the pelvic and para-aortic lymph nodes is an important consideration for tumors involving the spermatic cord. Historical literature advocated for complete pelvic and retroperitoneal lymphadenectomy for any tumor involving the spermatic cord. This approach was based on a published report from 1970 that described the para-aortic location as the only site of recurrence in 17% of patients with spermatic cord tumors.[25] More recent publications indicate a recurrence rate of 38% with the resection site as the solitary site of recurrence in 60% of these patients.[24] Deep pelvic and para-aortic recurrence is the solitary site of recurrence in only 12.5% of patients with spermatic cord tumors, considering all histologies. Some specific histologies such as rhabdomyosarcoma have higher rates of lymph node dissemination but represent only 11% of tumors arising from the spermatic cord. These investigators advocate for radical resection to include orchiectomy followed by adjuvant radiation, with the radiation fields planned such that the pelvic and para-aortic nodes are treated.[24,26] Routine retroperitoneal lymphadenectomy is not advocated given the low incidence of solitary lymphatic recurrence (12.5%) and is reserved only for those histologies with known lymphatic dissemination.

Lymph Node Biopsy

Sentinel lymph node (SLN) biopsy or some form of nodal staging should be considered for those that are known to metastasize via lymphatic channels; these include clear cell sarcoma, angiosarcoma, rhabdomyosarcoma, and synovial sarcoma and epithelioid sarcoma.[27] Unlike cutaneous malignancies, the size of sarcoma can limit the feasibility of SLN biopsy. In addition, the lymphatic drainage is less predictable for truncal lesions when compared with extremity tumors of the same histology or cutaneous neoplasms. For this reason, lymphoscintigraphy or single-photon emission computed tomography scan can be performed before resection, which is helpful for 2 reasons. First, it identifies the number of SLNs with more specificity. Second, the draining basin at most risk for recurrence is identified, which can aid in surveillance. This imaging allows for precise localization of the SLN and target basins for biopsy. Imaging should be performed just before resection so that an intraoperative gamma-counter can be used to identify lymph nodes during the operation.

Chest Wall Sarcoma

STS that arises within the layers of the chest wall presents unique considerations regarding the reconstruction following complete resection. Preoperative planning, as with all complex resections, is essential, but there are 2 specific concerns related to chest wall sarcomas. First, involvement of a plastic surgeon early in the surgical planning is essential when it is anticipated that advanced tissue coverage will be required; this allows for precise planning and execution of the ablative portion of the operation, which can significantly affect the reconstructive options.[28] Second, the preoperative pulmonary function should be assessed thoroughly because it is very common to have some decrease in pulmonary function following these resections. Preoperative assessment allowing for appropriate counseling regarding the possibility of pulmonary complications, including prolonged mechanical ventilation, is essential.

The size of the planned defect is the primary determinant of reconstructive material for those tumors that involve the ribs or intercostal muscles. Typically, defects less than 5 cm or requiring less than 2 rib resections can be covered with soft tissue alone. For larger defects, a mesh construct will be required to achieve integrity of the reconstruction. Historical use of a methylmethacrylate and synthetic mesh "sandwich" has been used, but this approach is generally not used due to the rigidity of this approach and the postoperative discomfort often associated. Currently, synthetic or biologic mesh is used. Synthetic mesh is generally preferred for larger defects due to the increased rigidity but cannot be placed directly over the viscera. Biologic mesh can be placed in this position but has less structural integrity over time. A combined approach with a deep placement of biologic mesh and more superficial placement of synthetic mesh has been advocated. In one large series, the postoperative complication rate was found to be 11.1% with the most common complication being superficial infection at 8.6%.[29] Titanium plating can be used in cases where a significant length (>15 cm) of more than 3 ribs are resected. The overall complication rate is higher for this approach (37%) with a 7.4% major complication rate. Fracture of the rib plates occurred in 7.4% of patients with only one requiring reoperation.[30]

No matter the approach to structural reconstruction, there are various approaches to soft tissue coverage. For small defects, skin graft or rotational flaps can be used. For larger defects, a musculocutaneous rotational flap may be needed or even a free tissue transfer flap. Large defects are often covered with either pectoralis major advancement flaps or latissimus dorsi rotational flaps over which a fasciocutaneous advancement flap is used.[28]

Radiation-Associated Sarcoma

Radiation-associated angiosarcoma (RAAS) is a specific type of sarcoma that is often found in the trunk. The common presentation is in a woman following external beam radiation therapy for primary breast malignancy, and the median latency period is 7 years.[31,32] These patients present with small, violaceous, cutaneous nodules that can also be coalesced into larger plaques. The treatment is wide excision to include all subcutaneous tissue to the level of the pectoralis fascia. Mastectomy is generally required due to the large area of disease, but some have advocated for a more limited resection of only visible cutaneous disease rather than all skin within the radiation field. One large series compared a conservative (limited to only visible disease) approach to a more radical (all skin within prior radiation field) approach. A substantial difference in favor of a radical approach was noted in the local (23% vs 76%) and distant (18% vs 47%) recurrence rate. Five-year disease-specific survival was also improved with a more radical approach (86% vs 46%).[32]

Local recurrence is the primary concern with RAAS, and almost half of the patients will recur locally with a median time to recurrence up to 20 months.[31] One in 4 patients will occur with distant disease with a median time of 3 years. Multiple recurrences are common, and half of the patients with local recurrence will have multiple local recurrences despite optimal multimodal therapy.[31,32] The reconstruction principles are similar to those for chest wall sarcomas, but because these tumors do not generally involve the musculoskeletal portion of the chest wall, a rotation or advancement flap of tissue generally suffices for adequate tissue coverage.

Surveillance of Truncal Sarcoma

Following complete resection or after completion of adjuvant therapy, surveillance of the patient is essential to identify recurrence early, at a time when subsequent therapy will be most beneficial. Knowledge about recurrence patterns drives the recommendations for surveillance. The recurrence pattern of truncal sarcoma is more closely aligned with extremity lesions than retroperitoneal or visceral lesions. Local recurrence occurs in 25% of patients at 10 years from complete resection, but local recurrence after 10 years can occur in high-grade sarcomas. Grade is the most important determinant of distant recurrence risk with low-grade lesions having less than 10% 10-year distant recurrence rate and high-grade lesions of 40%.[4] To evaluate for local recurrence, patients are seen every 3 months with contrast-enhanced imaging of the primary tumor site. A contrast-enhanced CT of the chest is performed simultaneously every 3 months for those patients with a high-grade primary tumor to evaluate for distant disease. The visits are extended to 6 months after 2 years for a total of 5 years, and patients are seen annually in a survivorship clinic after 5 years free of disease.[5]

SUMMARY

The trunk, including the chest wall, back, and abdominal wall, represents the location for roughly one-fifth of the primary STS cases. Outcomes for truncal STS in terms of 5-year overall survival are better than retroperitoneal primary tumors but slightly worse than extremity tumors. Management of these tumors mirrors that of extremity STS with a few key differences. First, the larger surface area of the trunk offers more opportunity for wide resection, and reconstructive options are more abundant. Second, the inguinal region often demands resection of involved pelvis bone and radical orchiectomy to achieve negative margins. Fortunately, the neurovascular structures to the lower extremity can often be preserved, and amputation for inguinal region sarcomas is rare. Preoperative planning is essential and must include the reconstructive team to achieve optimal outcomes.

REFERENCES

1. American Cancer Society. Society AC. Cancer facts & figures 2015. Atlanta (GA): American Cancer Society; 2015.
2. Singer S, Corson JM, Demetri GD, et al. Prognostic factors predictive of survival for truncal and retroperitoneal soft-tissue sarcoma. Ann Surg 1995;1995(221):2.
3. Garonzik Wang JM, Leach SD. Truncal sarcomas and abdominal desmoids. Surg Clin North Am 2008;88(3):571–82, vi–vii.
4. Brennan MF, Antonescu CR, Moraco N, et al. Lessons learned from the study of 10,000 patients with soft tissue sarcoma. Ann Surg 2014;260(3):416–22.
5. von Mehren M, Randall RL, Benjamin RS, et al. Soft tissue sarcoma, version 2.2014. J Natl Compr Canc Netw 2014;12(4):473–83.
6. Briand S, Barbier O, Biau D, et al. Wait-and-see policy as a first-line management for extra-abdominal desmoid tumors. J Bone Joint Surg Am 2014;96(8):631–8.
7. Azizi L, Balu M, Belkacem A, et al. MRI features of mesenteric desmoid tumors in familial adenomatous polyposis. AJR Am J Roentgenol 2005;184:1128–35.
8. Lee JC, Thomas JM, Phillips S, et al. Aggressive fibromatosis: MRI features with pathologic correlation. AJR Am J Roentgenol 2006;186(1):247–54.
9. Hansmann A, Adolph C, Vogel T, et al. High-dose tamoxifen and sulindac as first-line treatment for desmoid tumors. Cancer 2004;100(3):612–20.
10. Sakorafas GH, Nissotakis C, Peros G. Abdominal desmoid tumors. Surg Oncol 2007;16(2):131–42.
11. Crago AM, Denton B, Salas S, et al. A prognostic nomogram for prediction of recurrence in desmoid fibromatosis. Ann Surg 2013;258(2):347–53.

12. Stojadinovic A, Hoos A, Karpoff H, et al. Soft tissue tumors of the abdominal wall analysis of disease patterns and treatment. Arch Surg 2001;136:70–9.

13. Fiore M, Rimareix F, Mariani L, et al. Desmoid-type fibromatosis: a front-line conservative approach to select patients for surgical treatment. Ann Surg Oncol 2009;16:2587–93.

14. Gronchi A. Quality of surgery and outcome in extra-abdominal aggressive fibromatosis: a series of patients surgically treated at a single institution. J Clin Oncol 2003;21(7):1390–7.

15. Leithner A, Gapp M, Radl R, et al. Immunohistochemical analysis of desmoid tumours. J Clin Pathol 2005;58(11):1152–6.

16. Deyrup AT, Tretiakova M, Montag AG. Estrogen receptor-beta expression in extraabdominal fibromatoses: an analysis of 40 cases. Cancer 2006;106(1):208–13.

17. Lazar AJ, Tuvin D, Hajibashi S, et al. Specific mutations in the beta-catenin gene (CTNNB1) correlate with local recurrence in sporadic desmoid tumors. Am J Pathol 2008;173(5):1518–27.

18. Skapek SX, Anderson JR, Hill DA, et al. Safety and efficacy of high-dose tamoxifen and sulindac for desmoid tumor in children: results of a Children's Oncology Group (COG) phase II study. Pediatr Blood Cancer 2013;60(7):1108–12.

19. Francis WP, Zippel D, Mack LA, et al. Desmoids: a revelation in biology and treatment. Ann Surg Oncol 2009;16(6):1650–4.

20. Gounder MM, Lefkowitz RA, Keohan ML, et al. Activity of Sorafenib against desmoid tumor/deep fibromatosis. Clin Cancer Res 2011;17(12):4082–90.

21. Guadagnolo BA, Zagars GK, Ballo MT. Long-term outcomes for desmoid tumors treated with radiation therapy. Int J Radiat Oncol Biol Phys 2008;71(2):441–7.

22. Rodriguez D, Barrisford GW, Sanchez A, et al. Primary spermatic cord tumors: disease characteristics, prognostic factors, and treatment outcomes. Urol Oncol 2014;32(1):52.e19-25.

23. Brooks A, Bowne W, Delgado R, et al. Soft tissue sarcomas of the groin: diagnosis, management, and prognosis. J Am Coll Surg 2001;193(2):130–6.

24. Ballo MT, Zagars GK, Pisters PW, et al. Spermatic cord sarcoma: outcome, patterns of failure and management. J Urol 2001;166:1306–10.

25. Banowsky LH, Shultz GN. Sarcoma of the spermatic cord and tunics: review of the literature, case report and discussion of the role of retroperitoneal lymph node dissection. J Urol 1970;103(5):628–31.

26. Kay MD, Desai A, Gourevitch D. Sarcomas of the spermatic cord and paratesticular tissues: our experience and review of current literature. Br J Med Surg Urol 2012;5(6):271–8.

27. Blazer DG, Sabel MS, Sondak VK. Is there a role for sentinel lymph node biopsy in the management of sarcoma? Surg Oncol 2003;12(3):201–6.

28. Momeni A, Kovach SJ. Important considerations in chest wall reconstruction. J Surg Oncol 2016;113(8):913–22.

29. Azoury SC, Grimm JC, Tuffaha SH, et al. Chest wall reconstruction: evolution over a decade and experience with a novel technique for complex defects. Ann Plast Surg 2016;76(2):231–7.

30. De Palma A, Sollitto F, Loizzi D, et al. Chest wall stabilization and reconstruction: short and long-term results 5 years after the introduction of a new titanium plates system. J Thorac Dis 2016;8(3):490–8.

31. Torres KE, Ravi V, Kin K, et al. Long-term outcomes in patients with radiation-associated angiosarcomas of the breast following surgery and radiotherapy for breast cancer. Ann Surg Oncol 2013;20(4):1267–74.
32. Li GZ, Fairweather M, Wang J, et al. Cutaneous radiation-associated breast angiosarcoma. Ann Surg 2016. [Epub ahead of print].

Management of Desmoids

Valerie P. Grignol, MD, Raphael Pollock, MD, PhD,
John Harrison Howard, MD*

KEYWORDS

- Desmoid fibromatosis • Beta-catenin • Management • Margins • Observation

KEY POINTS

- Desmoid fibromatosis is an infiltrative tumor that can be aggressive in nature because of its ability to locally invade adjacent structures.
- Mutations in β-catenin and APC genes are responsible for the development of most desmoid tumors.
- Wide local excision with negative margins is the standard surgical treatment of desmoid tumors.
- A variety of nonsurgical therapies are useful in the management of desmoid tumors, including radiation, chemotherapy, nonsteroidal antiinflammatory drugs, and hormonal therapy.
- Treatment algorithms are evolving with the observation that many tumors remain stable under a program of watchful waiting, and spontaneous regression has been observed.

INTRODUCTION

Desmoid tumors (also known as aggressive fibromatosis) are rare, with an incidence of 0.03% of all neoplasms and 3.0% of soft tissue tumors.[1] They are seen more commonly in women than men with a 2:1 predilection for women.[2–4] Young adults are the most commonly affected, and it is frequently in the 25- to 35-year-old demographic.[2,3] Most desmoid tumors occur sporadically, but they can be associated with familial adenomatous polyposis syndrome (FAP). In the FAP patient population there is not a sex predilection for these tumors.[5] Mutations in either the β-catenin or APC genes are usually the cause for the development of these tumors. Sporadic development of desmoid tumors has been associated with β-catenin mutations, whereas mutations in the APC gene pathway are associated with development of desmoids in the setting of FAP syndrome. It seems that these mutations are mutually exclusive.[6] Other factors that have been associated with development of desmoids include

Disclosures: none.
Division of Surgical Oncology, Department of Surgery, The Ohio State University, N924 Doan Hall, 410 West 10th Avenue, Columbus, OH 43210, USA
* Corresponding author.
E-mail address: John.Howard@osumc.edu

Surg Clin N Am 96 (2016) 1015–1030
http://dx.doi.org/10.1016/j.suc.2016.05.008
0039-6109/16/$ – see front matter © 2016 Elsevier Inc. All rights reserved.
surgical.theclinics.com

pregnancy, hormonal exposure, and physical factors, such as trauma and/or surgery.[3,4] Although desmoid tumors cannot be considered a true malignancy because of their inability to metastasize, they are aggressive in their ability to locally invade adjacent structures. Surgical resection has been the mainstay of treatment; however, recurrence rates range from 20% to 45%.[7–9] Because of the propensity for recurrence, multimodal therapies have been used, including hormonal therapy, nonsteroidal antiinflammatory drugs (NSAIDs), chemotherapy, and radiation. Recently the surgery-first approach has begun to evolve into a movement of watchful waiting, as observational studies have shown long-term stability of some tumors without treatment and even spontaneous regression in 5% to 10%[6,10] of cases.

Pathogenesis

Alterations in the Wnt signaling pathway seem to be the mechanism of tumorigenesis in the development of desmoid fibromatosis.[11] Genetic mutations that alter this pathway and are associated with the development of desmoid tumors have been identified in the β-catenin and APC genes. Both β-catenin and APC are part of the Wnt pathway suggesting that 2 separate mutations affecting the same end point are involved with the development of desmoid fibromatosis.[12] These mutations result in the development of intranuclear accumulation of β-catenin, which stimulates DNA transcription and cell proliferation.[11] Eighty-five percent of sporadic desmoid tumors have an activating mutation in the CTNNB1 gene coding for β-catenin, whereas the germline mutation of the APC gene leads to the development of desmoid tumors for patients with FAP.[11,13] More recently a genetic analysis looking at wild-type desmoids or those without the aforementioned known mutations found that with deep sequencing 95% of desmoids may have mutations that affect the Wnt/β-catenin pathway suggesting a near-universal relationship between desmoid tumors and the Wnt signaling.[14]

In sporadic desmoid tumors, mutations in the gene coding for β-catenin, CTNNB1, occur in 71% to 91% of tumors. The highest rate of mutation is found in intra-abdominal tumors.[13,15–19] The most common mutations are T41A and S45F. The discovery of genetic mutations in the development of desmoid tumors has been an important advancement as they have also been associated with prognosis, providing the opportunity to improve the ability to risk stratify patients. Several studies have shown a significantly higher chance of disease recurrence at 5 years despite complete resection for patients harboring a S45F mutation, which is likely exclusive to extra-abdominal desmoids.[13,17,19] The growing amount of data suggests that specific mutations within this gene do play a role in disease recurrence and provide the opportunity to influence clinical care in the future.

For those without a β-catenin gene mutation, APC gene mutations are suspected to be the source of development of desmoid tumors. APC mutations are most common among patients with FAP. Approximately 10% to 15% of patient with FAP develop desmoids, and intra-abdominal tumors have become the primary cause of death in patients with FAP who have previously had a prophylactic colectomy.[11,20] Despite a similar molecular end point for APC and β-catenin mutations, the phenotype between the two is different, as most tumors in FAP are intra-abdominal with involvement of the small bowel mesentery.[5]

Presentation

Desmoid tumors can occur anywhere in the body. They are divided into 3 general anatomic locations: extra-abdominal, intra-abdominal, and abdominal wall. There are important behavioral differences related to location that may affect specific treatment algorithms.

Extra-abdominal desmoid tumors are composed of tumors in the pelvic and shoulder girdles, head, neck, and extremities (**Fig. 1**A). They arise from deep fascia or within muscle, have an infiltrative growth pattern, and are often poorly circumscribed.[21] This location has been associated with a 2- to 3-fold increased rate of recurrence and 20% decrease in recurrence-free survival when compared with intra-abdominal or abdominal wall/trunk lesions.[6,7,22,23]

Intra-abdominal desmoids often arise in the mesentery of the small bowel or are located in the pelvis (see **Fig. 1**B). This location is more commonly associated with FAP but can also occur sporadically. In patients less than 40 years old found to have an intra-abdominal or abdominal wall desmoid, a colonoscopy should be performed to rule out polyposis.[6] Overall, FAP-associated desmoid tumors represent a small proportion (2%–15%) of all patients with desmoid tumors.[2,5,6,12] The management of intra-abdominal desmoids can be quite difficult because of size and location and frequently require resection of large amounts of small bowel for complete removal. In a study of patients with FAP and mesenteric desmoids that were treated surgically, small bowel resections were necessary in 87.5% of cases with an average of 45.6 cm of bowel removed.[24] In extreme cases this can lead to intestinal failure, chronic total parenteral nutrition, and possible need for small bowel transplantation. This location in particular may be optimal for nonsurgical approaches first in asymptomatic patients, as the consequences of extended resections can be devastating.

Lesions of the abdominal wall or trunk seem to have the most favorable prognosis of the 3 groups (see **Fig. 1**C). They have been associated with the lowest recurrence rates of 6% to 20%[7,25] and the highest likelihood of spontaneous regression.[10,26]

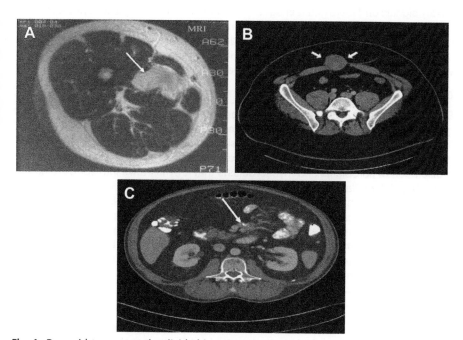

Fig. 1. Desmoid tumors can be divided into 3 anatomic locations: (A) extra-abdominal, (B) abdominal wall (C) intra-abdominal. Arrows depict tumor.

This location is also the most common for pregnancy-related desmoid tumors. There has been a reported association between pregnancy and the development or progression of desmoids. It is thought that this is related to the observation that these tumors stain strongly positive for estrogen-receptor β on immunohistochemistry.[27] In a recent study that evaluated desmoid fibromatosis and pregnancy, the investigators found that, although there was an increased risk of progression during pregnancy, patients could still be managed with standard therapies with minimal risk to the mother or child. The risk of progression was more prominent in patients who were diagnosed with desmoid fibromatosis before pregnancy (42%) versus the patients whose disease presented during pregnancy (13%). The rate of spontaneous regression in this population was 14%, which is higher than what is seen in other patient populations. They concluded that desmoid tumors during pregnancy have an indolent course, do not increase risk of obstetric complications, and should not be a contraindication for subsequent pregnancies.[28]

EVALUATION
Radiologic Evaluation

Imaging modalities useful in the diagnosis and surveillance of desmoid tumors include ultrasound, computed tomography (CT) scan, and MRI. For initial evaluation, cross-sectional imaging is most appropriate to evaluate tumor size and local invasion of adjacent anatomic structures. Contrast-enhanced CT scan is the preference for intra-abdominal tumors to evaluate proximity to adjacent intra-abdominal vasculature and organs. CT scan of intra-abdominal lesions reveals a soft-tissue density with radiating strands typically located in the mesenteric fat. MRI is the modality of choice for evaluating extremity and soft-tissue tumors often demonstrating a heterogeneous pattern due to the mixed fibrous and cellular components. Tumors appear as low intensity signals on T2-weighted images.[29] Linear extension along fascial planes known as the fascial tail sign is common. Ultrasound can be used to survey for recurrence or to follow lesions in the extremities and abdominal wall. Appearance on ultrasound is that of a hypoechoic lesion with posterior acoustic shadowing. They are often vascular, and a fascial tail sign may also be seen with this modality.

Diagnosis

Biopsy is mandatory to confirm the diagnosis before treatment is discussed. Image-guided core biopsies are the recommended approach with ultrasound being useful in performing biopsy of soft-tissue lesions and CT-guided biopsy for intra-abdominal disease. Pathologically desmoid fibromatosis appears as a low cellularity proliferation of fibroblasts and myofibroblasts that are infiltrative into surrounding tissues. The differential diagnosis of desmoid tumors includes scar tissue, low-grade fibromyxoid sarcoma, nodular fasciitis, and other benign fibroblast proliferations. Immunohistochemical stains aid in confirming the diagnosis. In particular intranuclear staining of β-catenin has been shown to be positive in 67% to 80% of cases.[30] As previously mentioned, these tumors also stain strongly positive for estrogen receptor β.[27] Cyclooxygenase-2 expression may also be present and can be useful to determine desmoid from healing scar.[31]

TREATMENT

The management of desmoid tumors has traditionally been a surgery-first approach. For patients whereby surgical removal would lead to significant morbidity or lesions that are unresectable on initial presentation, there are several nonoperative strategies.

A recent development in management includes watchful waiting as an initial approach, as studies have shown 50% progression-free survival (PFS) as well as spontaneous regression of tumors with no treatment.[32] Because of the complexity of management and the variety of treatment options as outlined later, treatment recommendations are best determined in a multidisciplinary setting.

Surgery

Wide local excision with negative margins has been the standard treatment of desmoid tumors. This treatment can prove to be challenging because of the infiltrative nature of these tumors. Retrospective studies have shown recurrence rates for margin negative (R0) resection ranging from 16% to 22% and 19% to 48% for microscopically positive margin (R1) resection.[22,23,33–35] The frequency of recurrences after surgical resection has led to multiple studies that have evaluated margin status as a prognostic indicator of recurrence. When examining the prognostic significance of microscopic margin status, the data are mixed; some have found it to be significantly associated with recurrence-free survival, whereas others have shown no prognostic significance when comparing R0 versus R1 resections in desmoid tumors (**Table 1**).[9,33,36–38] A study from the MD Anderson Cancer Center compared desmoid outcomes from 2

Table 1
Selected studies evaluating R0 versus R1 as prognostic factor for recurrence in desmoid tumor

Author	No. Patients	Tumor Types	Univariate Analysis	Multivariate Analysis
Mullen et al[33]	177	Intra-abdominal and Extra-abdominal	HR 0.42 (95% CI 0.22–0.79) P = .008	HR 0.39 (95% CI 0.19, 0.82) P = .012
Gronchi et al[23]	203	Extra-abdominal	—	Primary tumors HR 0.76 (95% CI 0.31, 1.88), recurrent tumors HR 1.92 (95% CI 0.80, 4.64) P = .14
Bertani et al[39]	62	Intra-abdominal and Extra-abdominal	—	HR 2.94 (95% CI 0.47, 18.20) P = .25
Huang et al[9]	198	Extra-abdominal and abdominal wall	—	HR 3.11 (95% CI 1.40, 6.93) P = .005
Peng et al,[7] 2012	211	Intra-abdominal and Extra-abdominal	HR 2.16 (95% CI 1.17, 4.01) P = .01	HR 1.51 (95% CI 0.85, 2.66) P = .16
Crago et al[37]	495	Intra-abdominal and Extra-abdominal	HR 1.18 (95% CI 0.78, 1.80) P = .42	HR 0.99 (95% CI 0.65, 1.52) P = .97
van Broekhoven et al[40]	132	Extra-abdominal	HR 1.22 (95% CI 0.38, 3.90) P = .736	—
Spear et al,[35] 1998	107	Extra-abdominal	NS	HR 3.00 P = .046

Abbreviations: CI, confidence interval; HR, hazard ratio.

distinct time frames: the first is 1965 to 1994 and a more modern cohort from 1995 to 2005. Interestingly, margin status was a significant predictor of disease recurrence in the older cohort but that significance was lost in the modern cohort despite similar rates of margin positive resections between the two groups (46% vs 47%).[22] Evaluating the current data, it is not clear that recurrence rates are significantly different with microscopically positive margins. The inability to clearly define margin status as a prognostic factor has led to the recommendation that effort should be made to perform an R0 resection but not at the expense of organ or limb function. Re-resection for recurrent disease has similar cure rates as those achieved for primary resection, even in multiply recurrent patients.[34] Thus, for recurrent disease that is technically resectable without unreasonable morbidity, surgery should still be offered as a viable option for cure.

Frozen-section analysis has been used to help improve margin clearance.[39,41] It is not clear whether this technique has led to improved R0 resection rates.[41] In cases of recurrence it is difficult to distinguish desmoid fibromatosis from scar on frozen section. Based on these findings, the use of intraoperative frozen-section analysis is not recommended for confirmation of margin negative resection, as it is unreliable.

The surgical challenges of desmoid tumors extend beyond their infiltrative nature and ability to adequately obtain clear margins. Removal of these tumors in the abdominal wall or extremity locations can leave large anatomic defects. The goal in these locations is to restore skin and musculofascial integrity. This restoration often requires myocutaneous flaps and/or mesh for the abdominal wall. The safety of mesh closure was demonstrated in a study of 50 patients with abdominal desmoid tumor. Although more than half had an R1 resection, the recurrence rate was low at 8% and repairs were durable.[25] For those tumors that extend into the intra-abdominal space, care must be taken to close the peritoneum to prevent fistulas; alternatively staged reconstruction with bioprosthetic mesh may be appropriate. For extremity tumors limb-salvage is the standard. In a review of 15 patients who would require amputation for resection of limb recurrence, patients were treated with a variety of adjuvant therapies as well as observation alone. No one developed significant disease progression requiring amputation supporting the recommendation that function-preserving management is safe.[42] Tumors of the extremity not amenable to R0 resection due to neurovascular involvement can often be resected in an R1 fashion using adjuvant systemic therapy or radiation to help achieve local control and avoid amputation. Multidisciplinary surgical approaches, including plastic and reconstructive surgery, are important in preoperative planning. Regional therapy with isolated limb infusion or perfusion has been used in a variety of skin and soft-tissue extremity tumors to control disease while avoiding amputation when other more conservative approaches have failed. The use of limb perfusion with tumor necrosis factor alpha and melphalan in desmoid tumors has been described and led to a response in 19 of 28 treatments in a cohort of 25 patients. Limb preservation was achieved in all but 3 patients.[43] This technique seems to be a viable approach for symptomatic, progressive tumors of the extremity. Given all of the aforementioned information, amputation is still appropriate in a select group of patients, including those with intractable pain, loss of function of the extremity, or complicated wounds.

Intra-abdominal tumors present a separate set of challenges, particularly those located in the mesentery of the bowel. Proximity to the superior mesenteric artery and vein may limit resectability. Efforts to obtain histologically negative margins can lead to significant loss of bowel length and does not improve recurrence rates or overall survival.[44] Surgical bypass may be preferable in symptomatic patients with extensive vascular involvement in an effort to limit morbidity and mortality.[45]

Historical data have suggested that recurrence rates for intra-abdominal tumors in patients with FAP were higher than those with sporadic disease; however, more recent data suggest that there is no difference.[24] The propensity for the FAP population to develop mesenteric tumors that are diffuse and difficult to resect may be the reason for previous findings. With more modern surgical and nonsurgical strategies, the algorithm for patients with FAP is the same as those with sporadic disease. Treatment decisions should be made in the context of a multidisciplinary review and use multimodality therapy with surgery reserved for those with impending loss of critical structures or symptoms.

Surgical resection with wide local excision can achieve cure or local control of disease for most desmoid tumors. The goal of surgical resection should be a margin negative resection with the preservation of function of surrounding involved organs and structures.

Systemic Therapy

Because of the propensity for recurrence and the morbidity of repeat resections, there has been a multitude of therapies used to treat desmoid tumors either in the adjuvant setting or as definitive treatment. Traditionally the use of systemic therapy has been in the unresectable, recurrent, or progressing desmoid tumors; but this is changing.

Hormonal and nonsteroidal antiinflammatory drugs

Antiestrogen agents and NSAIDs are considered first-line agents because of their effectiveness and relatively low side-effect profile.[2,38,46–48] Based on the observation that many desmoid tumors stain strongly positive for estrogen receptor, the use of antiestrogen therapy may have a biological basis. The most common antiestrogen agents are tamoxifen and raloxifene. Response rates to these agents are approximately 40% to 51%.[20,49] Sulindac is the most commonly used NSAID. The response rate to this NSAID is approximately 28%.[20]

To improve response rates, hormonal therapies and NSAIDs are typically used in combination. A report of 134 patients treated with both an antiestrogen agent and sulindac achieved an 85% response rate when used as either adjuvant or definitive therapy. In patients who had previously been resected, therapy could eventually be tapered with only one long-term recurrence.[50] This group contained patients with sporadic and FAP-related tumors. The high response rate and durability is encouraging for nonsurgical management of these tumors. However, an objective response may take several months to achieve stability of disease and decrease in associated symptoms.[46,47,50]

Chemotherapy

The response rate of chemotherapy in desmoid tumors has been reported to be as high as 79%.[20,47,51] Similar to hormonal and NSAID therapy, time to response can be variable. Because of the associated side effects, chemotherapy is generally considered second-line systemic therapy. For those with rapidly progressive disease, impending destruction of critical anatomic structures, or symptomatic, unresectable tumors, it should be considered as a first-line therapy.[20,47,51–53] Combinations using anthracyclines seem to be the most effective. Other commonly used agents include methotrexate, vinblastine, and cisplatin.

Anthracycline-based regimens have resulted in long PFS and even complete responses. In a retrospective study by the French Sarcoma Group evaluating the role of chemotherapy in desmoid tumors, response rates favored anthracycline-based regimens compared with other systemic therapies (54% vs 12% P = .0011). The anthracycline group contained only 13 patients; all experienced stable disease (46%) or a partial response (PR) (54%).[54] Others have confirmed these results with a PFS of 74 months in anthracycline-based therapy.[51] Toxicity is higher with this regimen resulting in grade 3 to 4 hematological toxicities in approximately 31% to 43% of patients.[51,54] Cardiotoxicity is a concern for this regimen particularly because of the young patient population. A pegylated liposomal formulation of doxorubicin, which improves drug delivery with decreased cardiotoxicity, has been reported. A small series has shown similar efficacy as all patients had either PR (36%) or stable disease (64%) with decreased toxicity.[55]

Another commonly used regimen for desmoids is termed low-dose chemotherapy, which consists of methotrexate and vinblastine. This regimen has consistently resulted in stable or responding disease in 67% to 100% of patients treated.[47,54,56] Low-dose chemotherapy has been associated with a durable response and 5-year PFS as high as 67%.[56] Similar to anthracycline-based regimens, toxicity results in patient intolerance and a 50% attrition rate. Neurotoxicity related to vinblastine is the most common side effect resulting in patient intolerance. Another Vinka alkaloid, vinorelbine, has been described as an effective alternative to vinblastine with less long-term neurotoxicity.[57,58] This alkaloid is also given with methotrexate and may be a useful regimen in patients who do not tolerate vinblastine.

Targeted therapy

The tyrosine kinase inhibitors (TKI) have been used for the treatment of desmoids resulting in stability of disease, limited toxicity, but low response rates. A phase II trial using imatinib reported a 1-year PFS of 66% but an objective response rate of only 6%.[59] In a heavily pretreated group of patients using higher doses of imatinib, Heinrich and colleagues[60] saw a 15.7% PR rate ($\geq$50% tumor shrinkage). The duration of response was greater than 1.5 years for all patients. In a third phase II trial using imatinib patients experienced progression free survival of 67% at 1 year.[61] Toxicity for all 3 of these trials was acceptable with very few grade 4 toxicities, which were treated effectively with dose reduction. In addition to these phase II trials, other small retrospective reviews have revealed stable or PR in 36% to 80% of patients treated with TKI and a median PFS of nearly 27 months by Response Evaluation Criteria in Solid Tumors (RECIST) criteria.[47]

Sunitinib, another TKI that also blocks vascular endothelial growth factor receptors, has also been investigated for use in the treatment of desmoid tumors. A phase II study showed an overall response rate of 26.3% and a 2-year PFS rate of 74.7%. Importantly, 3 of the 12 patients with mesenteric disease developed serious adverse events with the first dose of treatment, which presented as tumor bleeding, bowel perforation, and entero-tumoral fistula formation. The investigators postulate that all of these events could be explained by the drugs antiangiogenic affect with resultant tumor necrosis.[62] Although this report may signify sunitinib as a potent treatment of desmoids, the significance of adverse events with this therapy should be noted.

Other TKI and antiangiogenic drugs that have been evaluated and shown to have efficacy in treating desmoid tumors are sorafenib and pazopanib.[63,64] In a retrospective review of 26 patients treated with sorafenib, 70% of patient-reported improved symptoms and 95% of patients had either a PR or stable disease at 6 months.[63] Following the response seen from sorafenib, the antiangiogenic drug pazopanib has also shown promise as a potential option in treating desmoid tumors. Two case reports show that patients treated with pazopanib had improved symptoms, tumor shrinkage, and decreased tumor cellularity similar to results seen with sorafenib.[64]

Conclusions regarding these drugs' efficacy must be interpreted with caution until larger prospective clinical trials are performed to validate initial findings.

Novel therapies

Therapies are evolving as new information emerges on the pathophysiology of desmoid tumors. The NOTCH pathway drives several cancer-related processes in solid tumors and has recently been recognized as a potential therapeutic target in desmoid tumors. It can be blocked by γ-secretase inhibition. Desmoid tumor cell lines treated with a γ-secretase inhibitor showed decreased cell growth, migration, and invasion.[65] In an open-label phase I dose-escalation trial of a γ-secretase inhibitor, 5 of 7 patients with desmoid tumors that were treated showed an objective response rate of 71.4% with some patients achieving durable response.[66] These promising early data have led to an ongoing phase II trial.[67] Recently another target, hyaluronan (HA), a glycosaminoglycan in the stromal microenvironment involved with normal wound healing, has also been associated with desmoid tumorigenesis.[68] HA levels were shown to be overexpressed in desmoid tumor surgical specimens as well as in immortalized cell lines. By using an inhibitor of HA, tumor proliferation rates as well as HA levels were decreased, suggesting a novel therapeutic target in treating desmoid fibromatosis. As the pathways in desmoid tumorigenesis are elucidated, novel therapeutic targets will continue to emerge.

Radiation Therapy

The use of radiation therapy in desmoid tumors has been evaluated in several settings. It has been used as adjuvant therapy for margin positive resections and to decrease recurrence of completely resected tumors. Radiation has also been used successfully as a definitive treatment of unresectable tumors or for tumors whereby resection would be associated with unacceptable morbidity or functional deficit.

In a large meta-analysis of 22 studies evaluating patients treated with surgery, surgery plus radiation, or radiation alone revealed a superior local control rate with radiation or radiation plus surgery (78% and 75%, respectively) than patients treated with surgery alone (61%).[69] The investigators suggested that all patients with desmoid be treated with radiation. However, the radiation doses in this study were highly variable; this recommendation does not take into consideration the morbidity associated with radiation. Complication rates related to radiation for desmoid fibromatosis are 17% to 23%.[21,69,70] Radiation-induced malignancies are particularly relevant in a disease that often affects a younger cohort of patients.[70] In a more recent single-institution retrospective review of 95 patients, investigators found no difference in the rate of recurrence for surgery alone (14.8%), radiation alone (15.4%), and surgery plus radiation (32.1%) ($P = .300$). There was also no association between local control and radiation therapy in those patients with a positive margin.[71] They did find that the head and neck location was associated with increased recurrence in their patient population. The investigators concluded that a subset of patients with high risk for local failure can be identified that may benefit from adjuvant radiation, including those with head and neck location, recurrent disease after surgery, and possibly those with positive margins. Although there seems to be a real benefit of radiation for some patients, the true utility of radiation as an adjuvant therapy in desmoid fibromatosis has not been evaluated in a prospective, randomized trial. Most studies are small, retrospective, and do not have standardization of patient selection. Because of the lack of clearly defined indications for radiation, it is critical to make these decisions in large-volume multidisciplinary centers to properly select patients to optimize benefit and avoid unnecessary exposure and morbidity from this treatment.

Definitive radiation seems to be as effective as surgery for those that would otherwise need radical and disfiguring surgery. Radiation as the primary mode of therapy for unresectable disease offers a 70% to 80% chance of local control in retrospective studies.[21,72,73] The European Organization for Research and Treatment of Cancer conducted a phase II study that standardized treatment of 44 patients with unresectable disease to 56 Gy received in 28 fractions. At 3 years, local control was 81.5% with 13.6% of patients having a complete response. Notably, radiation response will continue beyond 3 years in some patients promoting the durability of this therapy for unresectable disease.[73] For patients treated unsuccessfully with definitive radiation, surgery or systemic therapy may be an option as salvage therapy.

The use of radiation for desmoid tumors in a neoadjuvant setting has not been investigated in a trial but has been reported. The proposed benefit would be for those patients who are initially deemed unresectable or when a response would allow preservation of critical structures decreasing the morbidity of surgical resection. Because of the small numbers of patients treated with neoadjuvant radiation followed by surgery, it is difficult to evaluate the true benefit of this approach, although it seems to be similar to either modality alone.[21] Radiation has also been used in combination with chemotherapy in the neoadjuvant setting in small series and was associated with a control rate of 85% to 90%.[74,75]

Watchful Waiting

The heterogeneous nature of desmoids has led to a variety of therapies used to treat and control the disease. In many large databases, there are patients who receive no treatment of their tumors but have shown no progression and sometimes even spontaneous regression. While evaluating the best initial therapy for primary desmoid tumors, Bonvalot and colleagues[26] compared a group of patients who were treated nonsurgically with those who underwent surgery as their initial therapy. Three-year event-free survival was similar between the groups (68% no surgery vs 65% surgery). The nonsurgical group included medically treated patients and patients who underwent observation only. To understand this observation further, a multi-institutional study to evaluate the wait-and-see approach was undertaken. Patients were stratified into an observation group or a medical therapy group from a prospective database. In the 83 patients treated with observation, the 5-year PFS was 49.9%, which was not different from the 58.6% PFS in the 59 medically treated patients.[32] Significant prognostic factors to identify progression were not identified. When progression occurred, it was in the first 2 years for most patients (89%). Based on these findings, the investigators have proposed close disease surveillance for 24 months. These data led to several notable European groups developing proposals to standardize desmoid tumor management such that a watchful-waiting strategy is the first step for all new tumors.[6,46] Patients will be followed closely by a multidisciplinary team, with escalation of care only if the tumor declares an aggressive phenotype and spare patients with indolent tumors the morbidity of aggressive therapy (**Fig. 2**).

This approach should not be confused with doing nothing and may not be appropriate for every tumor. It requires close follow-up and monitoring of the disease with appropriate imaging based on tumor location. The recommended imaging schedule is every month for 2 months, every 3 months for the first year, then every 6 months up to 5 years, and yearly thereafter.[46] It is most appropriate in patients with tumors that are asymptomatic and free of anatomically critical structures. For those with tumor adjacent to critically important anatomy, frequent imaging is critical so as to not lose an operative window.

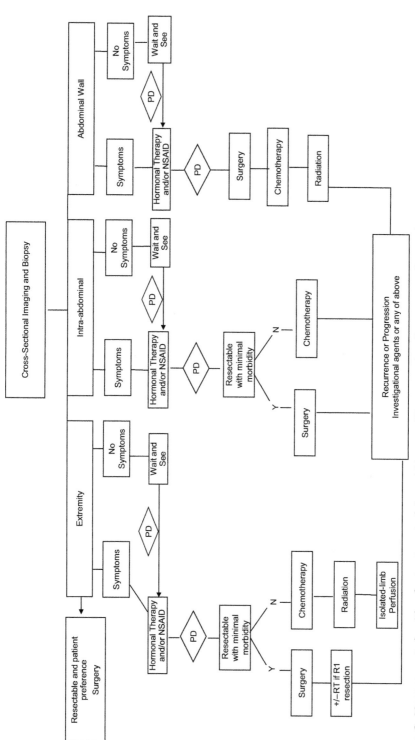

Fig. 2. Management algorithm for treatment of desmoid tumors. PD, progressive disease; RT, radiation therapy.

SURVEILLANCE

Recurrence for desmoid tumor typically occurs within the first 2 years.[22] After complete surgical resection or other definitive therapy, patients should be surveyed with appropriate imaging every 3 to 6 months for 2 to 3 years and then annually.[76]

SUMMARY

Because of the rarity of the disease and most data being retrospective, it is difficult to define a clear treatment algorithm. Many studies have had differing results in determining prognostic factors that lead to recurrence. Overall the treatment must be individualized and is best accomplished at large-volume centers with a multidisciplinary approach.

REFERENCES

1. Reitamo JJ, Hayry P, Nykyri E, et al. The desmoid tumor. I. incidence, sex-, age- and anatomical distribution in the Finnish population. Am J Clin Pathol 1982; 77(6):665–73.
2. Eastley NC, Hennig IM, Esler CP, et al. Nationwide trends in the current management of desmoid (aggressive) fibromatosis. Clin Oncol (R Coll Radiol) 2015;27(6): 362–8.
3. Eastley N, Aujla R, Silk R, et al. Extra-abdominal desmoid fibromatosis–a sarcoma unit review of practice, long term recurrence rates and survival. Eur J Surg Oncol 2014;40(9):1125–30.
4. Walczak BE, Rose PS. Desmoid: the role of local therapy in an era of systemic options. Curr Treat Options Oncol 2013;14(3):465–73.
5. Clark SK, Phillips RK. Desmoids in familial adenomatous polyposis. Br J Surg 1996;83(11):1494–504.
6. Kasper B, Baumgarten C, Bonvalot S, et al. Management of sporadic desmoid-type fibromatosis: a European consensus approach based on patients' and professionals' expertise - a sarcoma patients EuroNet and European organisation for research and treatment of cancer/soft tissue and bone sarcoma group initiative. Eur J Cancer 2015;51(2):127–36.
7. Peng PD, Hyder O, Mavros MN, et al. Management and recurrence patterns of desmoids tumors: a multi-institutional analysis of 211 patients. Ann Surg Oncol 2012;19(13):4036–42.
8. Ballo MT, Zagars GK, Pollack A, et al. Desmoid tumor: prognostic factors and outcome after surgery, radiation therapy, or combined surgery and radiation therapy. J Clin Oncol 1999;17(1):158–67.
9. Huang K, Fu H, Shi YQ, et al. Prognostic factors for extra-abdominal and abdominal wall desmoids: a 20-year experience at a single institution. J Surg Oncol 2009;100(7):563–9.
10. Bonvalot S, Ternes N, Fiore M, et al. Spontaneous regression of primary abdominal wall desmoid tumors: more common than previously thought. Ann Surg Oncol 2013;20(13):4096–102.
11. Lips DJ, Barker N, Clevers H, et al. The role of APC and beta-catenin in the aetiology of aggressive fibromatosis (desmoid tumors). Eur J Surg Oncol 2009;35(1): 3–10.
12. de Bree E, Keus R, Melissas J, et al. Desmoid tumors: need for an individualized approach. Expert Rev Anticancer Ther 2009;9(4):525–35.

13. Colombo C, Miceli R, Lazar AJ, et al. CTNNB1 45F mutation is a molecular prognosticator of increased postoperative primary desmoid tumor recurrence: an independent, multicenter validation study. Cancer 2013;119(20):3696–702.

14. Crago AM, Chmielecki J, Rosenberg M, et al. Near universal detection of alterations in CTNNB1 and wnt pathway regulators in desmoid-type fibromatosis by whole-exome sequencing and genomic analysis. Genes Chromosomes Cancer 2015;54(10):606–15.

15. Domont J, Salas S, Lacroix L, et al. High frequency of beta-catenin heterozygous mutations in extra-abdominal fibromatosis: a potential molecular tool for disease management. Br J Cancer 2010;102(6):1032–6.

16. Huss S, Nehles J, Binot E, et al. Beta-catenin (CTNNB1) mutations and clinicopathological features of mesenteric desmoid-type fibromatosis. Histopathology 2013;62(2):294–304.

17. Lazar AJ, Tuvin D, Hajibashi S, et al. Specific mutations in the beta-catenin gene (CTNNB1) correlate with local recurrence in sporadic desmoid tumors. Am J Pathol 2008;173(5):1518–27.

18. Mullen JT, DeLaney TF, Rosenberg AE, et al. Beta-catenin mutation status and outcomes in sporadic desmoid tumors. Oncologist 2013;18(9):1043–9.

19. van Broekhoven DL, Verhoef C, Grunhagen DJ, et al. Prognostic value of CTNNB1 gene mutation in primary sporadic aggressive fibromatosis. Ann Surg Oncol 2015;22(5):1464–70.

20. Desurmont T, Lefevre JH, Shields C, et al. Desmoid tumour in familial adenomatous polyposis patients: responses to treatments. Fam Cancer 2015;14(1):31–9.

21. Ballo MT, Zagars GK, Pollack A. Radiation therapy in the management of desmoid tumors. Int J Radiat Oncol Biol Phys 1998;42(5):1007–14.

22. Lev D, Kotilingam D, Wei C, et al. Optimizing treatment of desmoid tumors. J Clin Oncol 2007;25(13):1785–91.

23. Gronchi A, Casali PG, Mariani L, et al. Quality of surgery and outcome in extra-abdominal aggressive fibromatosis: a series of patients surgically treated at a single institution. J Clin Oncol 2003;21(7):1390–7.

24. Latchford AR, Sturt NJ, Neale K, et al. A 10-year review of surgery for desmoid disease associated with familial adenomatous polyposis. Br J Surg 2006; 93(10):1258–64.

25. Wilkinson MJ, Chan KE, Hayes AJ, et al. Surgical outcomes following resection for sporadic abdominal wall fibromatosis. Ann Surg Oncol 2014;21(7):2144–9.

26. Bonvalot S, Eldweny H, Haddad V, et al. Extra-abdominal primary fibromatosis: aggressive management could be avoided in a subgroup of patients. Eur J Surg Oncol 2008;34(4):462–8.

27. Deyrup AT, Tretiakova M, Montag AG. Estrogen receptor-beta expression in extra-abdominal fibromatoses: an analysis of 40 cases. Cancer 2006;106(1):208–13.

28. Fiore M, Coppola S, Cannell AJ, et al. Desmoid-type fibromatosis and pregnancy: a multi-institutional analysis of recurrence and obstetric risk. Ann Surg 2014; 259(5):973–8.

29. Walker EA, Petscavage JM, Brian PL, et al. Imaging features of superficial and deep fibromatoses in the adult population. Sarcoma 2012;2012:215810.

30. Carlson JW, Fletcher CD. Immunohistochemistry for beta-catenin in the differential diagnosis of spindle cell lesions: analysis of a series and review of the literature. Histopathology 2007;51(4):509–14.

31. Mignemi NA, Itani DM, Fasig JH, et al. Signal transduction pathway analysis in desmoid-type fibromatosis: transforming growth factor-beta, COX2 and sex steroid receptors. Cancer Sci 2012;103(12):2173–80.

32. Fiore M, Rimareix F, Mariani L, et al. Desmoid-type fibromatosis: a front-line conservative approach to select patients for surgical treatment. Ann Surg Oncol 2009;16(9):2587–93.
33. Mullen JT, Delaney TF, Kobayashi WK, et al. Desmoid tumor: analysis of prognostic factors and outcomes in a surgical series. Ann Surg Oncol 2012;19(13): 4028–35.
34. Merchant NB, Lewis JJ, Woodruff JM, et al. Extremity and trunk desmoid tumors: a multifactorial analysis of outcome. Cancer 1999;86(10):2045–52.
35. Spear MA, Jennings LC, Mankin HJ, et al. Individualizing management of aggressive fibromatoses. Int J Radiat Oncol Biol Phys 1998;40(3):637–45.
36. Salas S, Dufresne A, Bui B, et al. Prognostic factors influencing progression-free survival determined from a series of sporadic desmoid tumors: a wait-and-see policy according to tumor presentation. J Clin Oncol 2011;29(26):3553–8.
37. Crago AM, Denton B, Salas S, et al. A prognostic nomogram for prediction of recurrence in desmoid fibromatosis. Ann Surg 2013;258(2):347–53.
38. Huang K, Wang CM, Chen JG, et al. Prognostic factors influencing event-free survival and treatments in desmoid-type fibromatosis: analysis from a large institution. Am J Surg 2014;207(6):847–54.
39. Bertani E, Testori A, Chiappa A, et al. Recurrence and prognostic factors in patients with aggressive fibromatosis. The role of radical surgery and its limitations. World J Surg Oncol 2012;10:184.
40. van Broekhoven DL, Verhoef C, Elias SG, et al. Local recurrence after surgery for primary extra-abdominal desmoid-type fibromatosis. Br J Surg 2013;100(9): 1214–9.
41. Bertani E, Chiappa A, Testori A, et al. Desmoid tumors of the anterior abdominal wall: results from a monocentric surgical experience and review of the literature. Ann Surg Oncol 2009;16(6):1642–9.
42. Lewis JJ, Boland PJ, Leung DH, et al. The enigma of desmoid tumors. Ann Surg 1999;229(6):866–72 [discussion: 872–3].
43. van Broekhoven DL, Deroose JP, Bonvalot S, et al. Isolated limb perfusion using tumour necrosis factor alpha and melphalan in patients with advanced aggressive fibromatosis. Br J Surg 2014;101(13):1674–80.
44. Smith AJ, Lewis JJ, Merchant NB, et al. Surgical management of intra-abdominal desmoid tumours. Br J Surg 2000;87(5):608–13.
45. Berri RN, Baumann DP, Madewell JE, et al. Desmoid tumor: current multidisciplinary approaches. Ann Plast Surg 2011;67(5):551–64.
46. Gronchi A, Colombo C, Le Pechoux C, et al. Sporadic desmoid-type fibromatosis: a stepwise approach to a non-metastasising neoplasm–a position paper from the Italian and the French sarcoma group. Ann Oncol 2014;25(3):578–83.
47. de Camargo VP, Keohan ML, D'Adamo DR, et al. Clinical outcomes of systemic therapy for patients with deep fibromatosis (desmoid tumor). Cancer 2010; 116(9):2258–65.
48. Hansmann A, Adolph C, Vogel T, et al. High-dose tamoxifen and sulindac as first-line treatment for desmoid tumors. Cancer 2004;100(3):612–20.
49. Bocale D, Rotelli MT, Cavallini A, et al. Anti-oestrogen therapy in the treatment of desmoid tumours: a systematic review. Colorectal Dis 2011;13(12):e388–95.
50. Quast DR, Schneider R, Burdzik E, et al. Long-term outcome of sporadic and FAP-associated desmoid tumors treated with high-dose selective estrogen receptor modulators and sulindac: a single-center long-term observational study in 134 patients. Fam Cancer 2016;15(1):31–40.

51. Gega M, Yanagi H, Yoshikawa R, et al. Successful chemotherapeutic modality of doxorubicin plus dacarbazine for the treatment of desmoid tumors in association with familial adenomatous polyposis. J Clin Oncol 2006;24(1):102–5.

52. Okuno SH, Edmonson JH. Combination chemotherapy for desmoid tumors. Cancer 2003;97(4):1134–5.

53. Patel SR, Evans HL, Benjamin RS. Combination chemotherapy in adult desmoid tumors. Cancer 1993;72(11):3244–7.

54. Garbay D, Le Cesne A, Penel N, et al. Chemotherapy in patients with desmoid tumors: a study from the French sarcoma group (FSG). Ann Oncol 2012;23(1): 182–6.

55. Constantinidou A, Jones RL, Scurr M, et al. Pegylated liposomal doxorubicin, an effective, well-tolerated treatment for refractory aggressive fibromatosis. Eur J Cancer 2009;45(17):2930–4.

56. Azzarelli A, Gronchi A, Bertulli R, et al. Low-dose chemotherapy with methotrexate and vinblastine for patients with advanced aggressive fibromatosis. Cancer 2001;92(5):1259–64.

57. Bertagnolli MM, Morgan JA, Fletcher CD, et al. Multimodality treatment of mesenteric desmoid tumours. Eur J Cancer 2008;44(16):2404–10.

58. Weiss AJ, Horowitz S, Lackman RD. Therapy of desmoid tumors and fibromatosis using vinorelbine. Am J Clin Oncol 1999;22(2):193–5.

59. Chugh R, Wathen JK, Patel SR, et al. Efficacy of imatinib in aggressive fibromatosis: results of a phase II multicenter sarcoma alliance for research through collaboration (SARC) trial. Clin Cancer Res 2010;16(19):4884–91.

60. Heinrich MC, McArthur GA, Demetri GD, et al. Clinical and molecular studies of the effect of imatinib on advanced aggressive fibromatosis (desmoid tumor). J Clin Oncol 2006;24(7):1195–203.

61. Penel N, Le Cesne A, Bui BN, et al. Imatinib for progressive and recurrent aggressive fibromatosis (desmoid tumors): an FNCLCC/French sarcoma group phase II trial with a long-term follow-up. Ann Oncol 2011;22(2):452–7.

62. Jo JC, Hong YS, Kim KP, et al. A prospective multicenter phase II study of sunitinib in patients with advanced aggressive fibromatosis. Invest New Drugs 2014; 32(2):369–76.

63. Gounder MM, Lefkowitz RA, Keohan ML, et al. Activity of sorafenib against desmoid tumor/deep fibromatosis. Clin Cancer Res 2011;17(12):4082–90.

64. Martin-Liberal J, Benson C, McCarty H, et al. Pazopanib is an active treatment in desmoid tumour/aggressive fibromatosis. Clin Sarcoma Res 2013;3(1):13.

65. Shang H, Braggio D, Lee YJ, et al. Targeting the notch pathway: a potential therapeutic approach for desmoid tumors. Cancer 2015;121(22):4088–96.

66. Messersmith WA, Shapiro GI, Cleary JM, et al. A phase I, dose-finding study in patients with advanced solid malignancies of the oral gamma-secretase inhibitor PF-03084014. Clin Cancer Res 2015;21(1):60–7.

67. Hughes DP, Kummar S, Lazar AJ. New, tolerable gamma-secretase inhibitor takes desmoid down a notch. Clin Cancer Res 2015;21(1):7–9.

68. Briggs A, Rosenberg L, Buie JD, et al. Antitumor effects of hyaluronan inhibition in desmoid tumors. Carcinogenesis 2015;36(2):272–9.

69. Nuyttens JJ, Rust PF, Thomas CR Jr, et al. Surgery versus radiation therapy for patients with aggressive fibromatosis or desmoid tumors: a comparative review of 22 articles. Cancer 2000;88(7):1517–23.

70. Guadagnolo BA, Zagars GK, Ballo MT. Long-term outcomes for desmoid tumors treated with radiation therapy. Int J Radiat Oncol Biol Phys 2008;71(2):441–7.

71. Gluck I, Griffith KA, Biermann JS, et al. Role of radiotherapy in the management of desmoid tumors. Int J Radiat Oncol Biol Phys 2011;80(3):787–92.

72. Micke O, Seegenschmiedt MH. German Cooperative Group on radiotherapy for benign diseases. radiation therapy for aggressive fibromatosis (desmoid tumors): results of a national patterns of care study. Int J Radiat Oncol Biol Phys 2005;61(3):882–91.

73. Keus RB, Nout RA, Blay JY, et al. Results of a phase II pilot study of moderate dose radiotherapy for inoperable desmoid-type fibromatosis–an EORTC STBSG and ROG study (EORTC 62991-22998). Ann Oncol 2013;24(10):2672–6.

74. Francis WP, Zippel D, Mack LA, et al. Desmoids: a revelation in biology and treatment. Ann Surg Oncol 2009;16(6):1650–4.

75. Baliski CR, Temple WJ, Arthur K, et al. Desmoid tumors: a novel approach for local control. J Surg Oncol 2002;80(2):96–9.

76. NCCN guidelines. Soft tissue sarcoma. 2015. Available at: http://www.nccn.org/professionals/physician_gls/pdf/sarcoma.pdf. Accessed January 20, 2015.

Dermatofibrosarcoma Protuberans

Jeffrey Reha, MD[a], Steven C. Katz, MD[a,b],*

KEYWORDS

- Dermatofibrosarcoma • DFSP • Soft tissue sarcoma • Dermal sarcoma
- Tyrosine kinase inhibitor

KEY POINTS

- Dermatofibrosarcoma protuberans (DFSP) is a rare superficial soft tissue sarcoma with a propensity for local recurrence.
- DFSP management requires input from experts in oncology to guide multidisciplinary care.
- Wide surgical excision is the cornerstone of management for primary and recurrent DFSP.

INTRODUCTION

Dermatofibrosarcoma protuberans (DFSP) is a rare low-grade cutaneous malignancy first described in 1890 by Taylor.[1] Darier[2] was credited with establishing DFSP as a clinicopathologic entity in 1924 and Hoffman[3] established the term in 1925. The rarity of DFSP precludes large prospective studies, highlighting the importance of referral to highly specialized practitioners. The clinical diagnosis requires a high index of suspicion because the lesions often have a fairly innocuous gross appearance. After biopsy or excision, expert pathologic assessment with focused immunohistochemical testing is essential to differentiate DFSP from other superficial soft tissue neoplasms.

No definitive risk factors for the development of DFSP have been identified. Effective management requires a sound appreciation of tumor biology and the nature of infiltrative growth into surrounding tissues. Morphologic studies of DFSP have revealed highly irregular borders with fingerlike extensions into surrounding and deep tissues.[4] Although DFSP rarely metastasizes, there is a propensity for local recurrence that may be associated with substantial morbidity.[5] As such, aggressive surgical resection with widely negative margins is essential to proper management.

[a] Department of Surgery, Roger Williams Medical Center, 825 Chalkstone Avenue, Prior 4, Providence, RI 02908, USA; [b] Department of Surgery, Boston University School of Medicine, 72 East Concord Street, Boston, MA 02118, USA
* Corresponding author. Division of Surgical Oncology, Roger Williams Medical Center, 825 Chalkstone Avenue, Prior 4, Providence, RI 02908.
E-mail address: skatz@chartercare.org

Surg Clin N Am 96 (2016) 1031–1046
http://dx.doi.org/10.1016/j.suc.2016.05.006
0039-6109/16/$ – see front matter
surgical.theclinics.com

Radiotherapy may be indicated in special circumstances, including recurrent DFSP or when complete microscopic tumor clearance is not possible. An understanding of the molecular pathogenesis of DFSP has resulted in use of tyrosine kinase inhibitor therapy for patients with advanced disease. DFSP patients require long-term follow-up with expert oncology practitioners, and ideally, a multidisciplinary team.

EPIDEMIOLOGY AND SUBTYPES

DFSP has an annual incidence of 0.8 to 4.2 cases per million.[6] It represents 0.1% of all malignancies[7] and 18% of cutaneous soft tissue sarcomas.[8] There is a slight male preponderance to the disease[6] and African Americans have an incidence that is almost double that reported among Caucasians.[9] DFSP is most commonly seen in the third to fifth decades of life, but can also present in infancy or in the elderly. The anatomic distribution of these tumors varies by study, but DFSP most commonly arises in the trunk (42%), upper extremities (23%), lower extremities (18%), and head and neck (13%).[9] Infrequent sites of disease include the breast, vulva, and penis.[10] Owing to the wide range of potential primary sites, a dermal-based soft tissue tumor in any location should raise the possibility of DFSP.

There are multiple rare histologic variants of DFSP including myxoid, pigmented, atrophic, giant cell fibroblastoma (GCF), and DFSP with fibrosarcomatous change (DFSP-FS). The primary myxoid variant is described as containing more than 50% myxoid stroma.[11] Histologically, myxoid DFSP demonstrates the typical infiltrative growth pattern, honeycomb appearance, and CD34 positivity present in classic DFSP. Myxoid DFSP is distinguished by sheetlike, bland spindle cells with lobular proliferation and pale stroma. A report of 23 myxoid DFSP cases described presentations similar to classic DFSP, with a slight increase extremity and head and neck cases.[12] The clinical outcomes of patients with myxoid DFSP were similar to the classic DFSP.

The Bednar tumor or pigmented variant accounts for fewer than 1% of DFSPs.[9] This tumor is found most commonly in the pediatric population and African Americans.[13] As with classic DFSP, it presents most commonly on the trunk and extremities. The tumor was first described in 1957.[14] Histologically, Bednar tumors are similar to the classic DFSP, except for the presence of melanin.[15] The Bednar tumor is generally less aggressive with lower rates of local recurrence.[13] It is important to differentiate Bednar tumors from other pigmented lesions such as melanoma, because the management and clinical outcomes are quite different.

Although DFSP typically occurs in adults, GCF is a fibroblastic dermal tumor that arises in the pediatric population with distinctive perivascular extravasation of lymphocytes in an onionskin pattern.[16] GCF is considered benign owing to its low likelihood to metastasize, especially in its pure form, although there is a propensity for local recurrence. There have also been case reports of the DFSP and GCF occurring in the same lesion.[17] DFSP and GCF are both CD34 positive and share the same t(17;22) chromosomal abnormality, resulting in a COL1A1–PDGFB gene fusion.[18] Based on these findings, it is reasonable to consider GCF and DFSP as part of the same disease spectrum.

DFSP-FS has received attention owing to its purported capacity for hematogenous dissemination. DFSP-FS represents 7% to 16% of diagnosed DFSPs.[19] DFSP-FS and classic DFSP share the same chromosomal and molecular derangements, with similar susceptibility to targeted therapy with tyrosine kinase inhibitors. DFSP-FS is distinguished from classic DFSP by increased cellularity, cytologic atypia, mitotic activity, and rare expression of CD34.[20] Areas of classic DFSP are interspersed with a herringbone pattern with high mitotic activity, reminiscent of fibrosarcoma (**Fig. 1**).[21] Despite

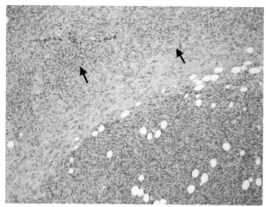

Fig. 1. Hematoxylin and eosin stain showing dermatofibrosarcoma protuberans (DFSP) with fibrosarcomatous change. Black arrows show fibrosarcomatous region; green arrow indicates classic DFSP infiltrating normal adipocytes.

the potential for DFSP-FS to behave in a more aggressive fashion, controversy exists as to the true outcome of this variant. When compared with classic DFSP, DFSP-FS has been reported to have a higher rate of local recurrence, distant metastases, and even death.[22] In a single report, the recurrence-free survival rate for DFSP-FS patients at 5 years was 42%.[23] Literature reviews have reported local recurrence rates of 36% and metastatic rates of 13%, which are notably higher than classic DFSP.[24] Bowne and associates[25] reported worse outcomes related to DFSP-FS, but Fields[26] found no association with disease-free survival and DFSP-FS using an updated database from the same institution. Although the propensity for distant dissemination is not universally accepted, we typically add chest imaging to the surveillance plans for DFPS-FS patients.

GENETICS

Genetic evaluation of DFSP tumors has led to significant advances in treatment of this disease. Cytogenetic analysis of DFSP specimens led to the identification of the t(17; 22) ring chromosome in a majority of these tumors.[27] The result of this translocation is a fusion of the collagen type I alpha 1 (*COL1A1*) and platelet-derived growth factor beta (*PDGFB*) genes, resulting in overexpression of *PDGFB*[28] and excessive PDGF receptor activity.[29] Identification of the supernumerary ring chromosome in DFSP occurred via cytogenic analysis[30] and fluorescence in situ hybridization.[31] Reverse transcriptase polymerase chain reaction has allowed for more accurate evaluation of the genetic rearrangements in DFSP. As noted, identification of the *COL1A1–PDGFB* fusion gene has enabled targeted molecular therapy with tyrosine kinase inhibitors.

RISK FACTORS

Although genetic studies have identified the t(17; 22) chromosomal abnormality associated with DFSP, clear clinical risk factors have yet been characterized. No familial association has been identified. Prior trauma has been hypothesized as a risk factor for the development of DFSP, but a mechanistic basis has been lacking. In a study of 12 African American patients, one-third of subjects reported a prior traumatic event at the site of disease.[32] Subsequent studies in similar populations showed no association with traumatic events.[33] There have also been studies showing association with surgical and burn scars, and even prior immunizations.[34] These studies cumulatively show roughly 10% of DFSP patients report prior trauma at the site of disease, but it is unclear if this association has any causative basis. The absence of clear risk factors emphasizes the critical importance of a high index of suspicion to drive appropriate tissue sampling and treatment in cases of DFSP.

DIAGNOSIS AND EVALUATION

DFSP usually presents as a slow growing dermal nodule, often with a violaceous coloring (**Fig. 2**). Clinical examination focuses on the visual and palpable extent of disease, in addition to fixation of the lesion to deeper structures. Although lymphatic dissemination is rare, clinical evaluation of the regional nodal basins is appropriate, particularly if the diagnosis of DFSP has not yet been established. If DFSP is suspected, early assessment of potential wound closure options will guide definitive planning. In addition to the need for complete tumor clearance, functional and cosmetic considerations factor into excision and reconstruction choices.

The differential diagnosis for lesions concerning for DFSP is extensive and includes neurofibroma, leiomyoma, malignant melanoma, morpheaform basal cell carcinoma, keloid, desmoid tumors, Kaposi sarcoma, fibrosarcoma, dermatofibroma (DF), nodular fasciitis, and sarcoidoisis.[35] Incisional or excisional biopsy of suspicious lesions is the cornerstone of a proper diagnostic evaluation. If smaller lesions are diagnosed by excisional biopsy, orientation of the scar should be made with subsequent wide excision in mind. In general, transverse incisions on extremities should be avoided. We strongly advocate early consultation with a surgical oncology team when DFSP is suspected on clinical grounds, to avoid compromising the definitive surgical excision and reconstruction.

DF is a common dermal-based cutaneous lesion and can be easily confused with DFSP, both grossly and on pathologic evaluation. DF is a benign lesion that presents typically as a small nodule on the lower extremities, whereas DFSP is typically larger than 5 cm, extends into the subcutaneous tissues, and is more commonly found on

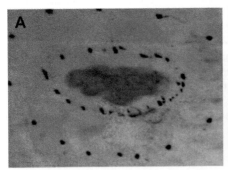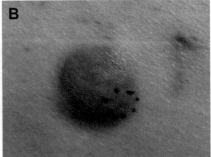

Fig. 2. Gross examples of 2 dermatofibrosarcoma protuberans lesions. (*A*) A large lower back lesion with the inner markings representing the lesion palpable beneath the skin and the outer markings representing the planned 3-cm surgical margins. MRI revealed that this lesion extended into the underlying paraspinal muscle fascia. (*B*) Smaller lesion from another patient, on the lower back, that was found to be confined to the superficial adipose tissue.

the trunk.[36] What makes DF difficult to differentiate from DFSP is that DF may extend into the subcutaneous fat.[37] In these cases, pathologic evaluation is the only means of differentiating the 2 lesions.

Whereas small lesions may be treated without formal imaging, imaging studies may provide better definition of the local extent of disease and enable more precise surgical planning. Computed tomography and MRI show a soft tissue mass that may enhance with contrast.[38] As with most extremity and trunk soft tissue sarcomas, we prefer MRI to define the extent of tissue infiltration and depth of involvement. MRI with short T1 inversion recovery and gadolinium contrast has been useful in evaluating location and extent owing to high signal enhancement of lesions.[39] Thornton and colleagues[40] showed that preoperative imaging with MRI altered the surgical management of patients in 20% of cases. MRI is the study of choice for evaluation of DFSP both in the preoperative setting as well as in postoperative surveillance. In larger or fixed tumors, MRI can show the extent the tumor extends beyond what is visible and the depth in relation to the underlying fascia and musculature (**Fig. 3**). This knowledge can aid in surgical planning and in choosing the most appropriate reconstruction strategy. Preoperative MRI can also provide baseline images to allow for differentiation between scar or postoperative change and recurrence.

PATHOLOGIC EVALUATION

Pathologic evaluation of DFSP is challenging given histologic similarities to other superficial fibroblastic soft tissue tumors. Histologically, the classic description by Taylor

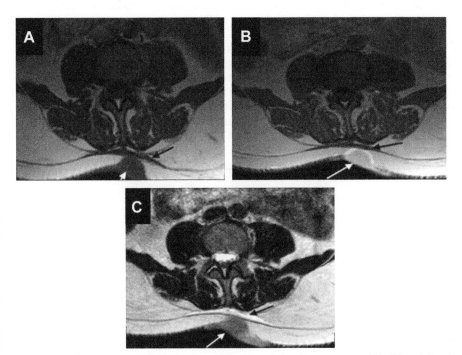

Fig. 3. MRI showing representative lesion on T1-weighted precontrast (*A*), T1-weighted postcontrast (*B*), and T2-weighted (*C*) images. On each image the tumor is marked by the white arrow and the fascia by the black arrow.

and Helwig[41] of DFSP is spindle cells in the deep dermis arranged in a cartwheel or storiform pattern, with infiltration of fingerlike projections into the adjacent tissue. This pattern can be seen using routine hematoxylin and eosin staining (**Fig. 4**). Despite this classic pattern, DFSP can be difficult to distinguish from other entities on hematoxylin and eosin staining, and may require immunohistochemical staining. A typical staining profile for DFSP includes expression of CD34 (**Fig. 5**) and vimentin, and the absence of factor XIIIa, which would be positive in DF.[42] Additional IHC stains that can aid with diagnosis include apolipoprotein, nestin, and cathepsin (**Table 1**).[43] The absence of S100 and CD56 immunoreactivity is useful for distinguishing from melanoma and neurogenic tumors, respectively.[44,45]

Margins are difficult to assess in DFSP specimens and are critically important in determining adequacy of resection and risk of recurrence.[26] DFSP has been described as the "iceberg tumor" owing to the extensive degree of microscopic tumor extension not appreciated visually or by palpation from the surface. Grossly, DFSP may seem to be well-circumscribed, but often extends beyond gross borders into the subcutaneous tissue or deeper structures.[46] These tentaclelike extensions are what make pathologic assessment difficult, because sampling error is a potential pitfall.[47] Standard evaluation of pathologic specimens involves bread loafing the specimen followed by evaluation of a representative sample of the margin. This results in about 10% of the margin being assessed, making this method for margin evaluation susceptible to false-negative results. En face evaluation is more time consuming, particularly for large tumors, but allows for a more thorough assessment of the surgical margins. Using en face assessments, along with immunohistochemical staining for CD34, Farma and colleagues[48] reported a local recurrence rate of 1% and positive margin rate of only 3%. Based on its infiltrative growth, en face pathologic assessment of the specimen is a rational strategy for maximizing DFSP margin assessment accuracy and thereby minimizing local recurrence.

Unfortunately, intraoperative frozen section assessments are not reliable. Stojadinovic and coworkers[49] reported that frozen section was inaccurate for determining margin status with a 57% false-negative rate. Massey and associates[50] also showed that it can be difficult to assess margins for the presence of tumor on frozen section, because benign dermal spindle cells are challenging to distinguish from DFSP by this process. Due to concerns regarding inaccuracy, decisions regarding margin status

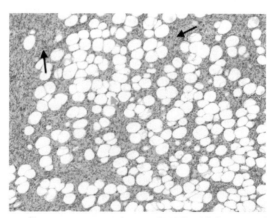

Fig. 4. Classic dermatofibrosarcoma protuberans (DFSP) with hematoxylin and eosin stain. The black arrows represent infiltrating DFSP; the green arrow represents normal adipocytes.

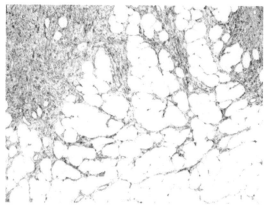

Fig. 5. Immunohistochemical analysis of dermatofibrosarcoma protuberans demonstrating diffuse CD34 expression.

should not be based on frozen sections. As noted, wide excision and open wound management is a viable option in cases where margins are in doubt.

TREATMENT
Surgery for Primary Tumors

The preferred management for primary DFSP is wide surgical excision. The primary concern in DFSP is local recurrence, because the tumor is locally aggressive and widely infiltrative. The principal goal of surgical therapy is resection to negative margins. Surgical excision can be achieved with standard wide local excision or Mohs micrographic surgery (MMS). Individual tumor, patient, anatomic, functional, and cosmetic considerations will dictate the most appropriate surgical approach in each instance. When planning surgical excision, reconstructive issues should be weighed early in the process. When DFSP is suspected, we strongly advocate referral to a surgical team with specific expertise in the management and biologic assessment of soft tissue sarcoma.

Early experiences with DFSP were associated with very high local recurrence rates, in excess of 25%.[51] Taylor and Helwig,[41] in a 1963 case series, reported recurrence rates of 49%. In 1967, McPeak and colleagues[34] reported 63 recurrences in 82 patients. In these earlier studies, there were no standards for clinical margins and it is likely that patients rarely underwent adequately wide R0 resection. Fields showed that the depth, anatomic location, and margin status (R0 resection) were predictors of local recurrence.[26] Lindner and colleagues[52] reported high rates of local recurrence after an inadequate primary resection at almost 57%. In this study, 7 patients had inadequate margins after re-resection and 4 received radiation with no recurrences.

Table 1	
Immunohistochemical assessment of dermatofibrosarcoma protuberans	
Present	**Absent**
CD34	Factor XIIIa
Nestin	Stromelysin 3
Apolipoprotein D	Cathepsin K

In contrast, the local recurrence rates with R0 resection are between 0.5% and 19% (**Table 2**).[25] Bogucki and colleagues[35] reviewed pooled data from several studies and showed a local recurrence rate of 0% to 11% for wide local excision with margins between 1 and 5 cm. Using a standard surgical approach and en face evaluation of the pathologic margins, Farma and associates[48] reported a local recurrence rate of less than 1% with the use of 2-cm margins. Definitive closure of the defect was postponed until final margins were negative, a practice we routinely use to avoid reoperation after a difficult or complex reconstruction. Currently, there is no standard margin for resection, but generally a 2- to 3-cm margin is recommended for DFSP, except when tissue is limited, as it is in head and neck lesions.[49]

MMS is a rational approach when preservation of tissue and cosmesis is a priority, as for head and neck lesions near critical structures. Serial sectioning during MMS allows creation of 3-dimensional maps of the lesion and its margins. Hobbs and colleagues[53] evaluated MMS in the excision of 10 DFSP patients, and there were no local recurrences at a median follow-up of 38 months. Loghdey and coworkers[54] reported similar findings from 76 patients, with 91% cleared and a 1.5% local recurrence rate, with a median follow-up of 50 months. A recent series evaluating MMS evaluated 74 patients with an average tumor size of 12 cm^2 and an average surgical defect after the procedure of 28 cm^2.[55] The local recurrence rate was 3% with a median follow-up of 59 months. A review of 23 papers evaluating MMS showed an overall local recurrence rate between 0% and 8%, in keeping with modern reports of standard wide excision.[56] Gloster and colleagues[57] reviewed 11 MMS studies and compared the recurrence rates with those reported in 15 wide excision studies. The local recurrence rates were lower on average in the MMS studies, but limitations of this analysis warrant caution. Older wide excision series may not have rigorously applied current surgical techniques, including wide margins, delayed closure, and en face pathologic assessments. With respect to MMS reports, limited oncologic follow-up and referral or selection bias may have impacted the local recurrence rates.

Unfortunately, most studies evaluating MMS for DFSP excisions are limited by short follow-up.[53] The importance of long-term follow-up after MMS for DFSP is underscored by a report indicating 25% of local recurrences are detected beyond 5 years.[58] In addition, the studies of MMS for DFSP tend to have smaller lesions and have greater percentages of head and neck tumors.[59] Proponents of MMS discuss smaller defect sizes compared with wide local excision, but a study by Kimmel and colleagues[60] showed similar defects sizes after excisions were completed. Additional concerns arise regarding the reliability of frozen section margin assessments for DFSP.[61] Regardless of the technique used for surgical treatment of DFSP, the involvement

Table 2
Local recurrence rates with wide local excision

Author, Year	Journal	Patients	Recurrent at Referral	R0 (%)	Recurrence Rate (%)
Stojadinovic et al,[49] 2000	Annals of Surgical Oncology	33	12	67	9
Bowne et al,[25] 2000	Cancer	159	48	68	21
Chang et al,[82] 2004	European Journal of Surgical Oncology	60	UNK	95	16
Farma et al,[48] 2010	Annals of Surgical Oncology	204	32	99	1

Data from Refs.[25,48,49,82]

of practitioners with formal oncologic training is of paramount importance. Proper care for DFSP patients requires a detailed understanding of tumor biology and disease natural history, in addition to technical expertise.

Reconstruction of Dermatofibrosarcoma Protuberans Surgical Defects

As noted, wide surgical excision of these tumors often results in large defects. Owing to the locally aggressive nature and difficulty in assessing margins, management of these defects can be complicated. Delayed wound management has become an effective strategy in these instances.[48,62] Pending assessment of final wound margins by pathology, the open wound can be managed using a negative pressure device or temporary placement of an allogeneic dermal graft. Negative pressure devices afford the additional advantage of decreasing defect size and facilitating granulation to minimize the depression if skin grafting will be used. Once the final pathologic margins are confirmed to be negative on permanent section, final closure can be performed. It is our practice to close wounds primarily if possible and to use delayed closure if grafts or complex flaps will be required.

In general, the need for complex closures can be anticipated at the time of initial evaluation based on the lesion size, location, and preoperative imaging. Preoperative planning should include consultation with a reconstructive surgeon if complex closure is anticipated, thus allowing for preservation of pedicles that may be required for flaps. Additionally, extensive undermining of uninvolved tissues should be avoided because it can result in seeding of the tumor beneath the flaps or closures.[59] This preoperative planning before the intervention has been shown improve both oncologic and cosmetic outcomes.[63] Skin grafts are also an option in large defects when there is still a concern regarding margin status, because surveillance for recurrence is not impeded. As noted, delayed wound closure when tissue transfer will be required and preoperative planning with a reconstructive surgeon are highly recommended for complicated cases.

Surgery for Recurrent Tumors

Proper surgical treatment and pathologic assessment of primary of DFSP typically results in high R0 resection rates and low local recurrence risk. Despite these advances, locally recurrent DFSP will affect a subset of patients and present formidable management challenges. Multiple options exist to manage recurrent DFSP including re-resection, radiotherapy, and targeted molecular therapy. The latter 2 options are discussed in sections below. In most cases, resection of the local recurrence remains the best treatment option. Lindner and colleagues[52] showed that surgical treatment of recurrences can be highly successful, with an 80% R0 resection rate and a local recurrence rate of 8%. Several other studies have also shown the ability to successfully perform resection of local recurrences in patients with negative margins.[25] There have also been rare cases where resection of recurrent disease has failed and clearance of the tumor would require amputation.[64]

Radiotherapy

DFSP, as with many sarcomas, has been shown to be radiosensitive. Radiotherapy can be a useful adjunct in the treatment of DFSP. Radiotherapy can be used as a primary treatment for unresectable disease or as an adjuvant therapy after resection. Yang and associates[65] evaluated 91 patients treated with adjuvant radiotherapy for a variety of soft tissue sarcomas and showed a significant reduction in the rate of local recurrence. Although this study did show a significant benefit for patients with soft tissue sarcomas, there were only 4 DFSP patients in the study. Adjuvant treatment with radiation has been recommended in patients with recurrent DFSP or in cases of positive margins when R0 re-excision cannot be achieved.[66] Typical radiation doses delivered for the treatment of DFSP are between 50 and 65 Gy, but vary depending on the platform used for treatment. Standard external beam radiation therapy uses parallel opposed beams to the affected area with large margins and a variable amount of normal tissue included.[67] Intensity-modulated radiation therapy has the ability to conform photon beams to the shape of target area and reduces the dose to normal tissue.[68] Currently there is no evidence to specifically support the use of intensity-modulated radiation therapy in DFSP, but data support its role in soft tissue sarcoma in general, in terms of efficacy and sparing of surrounding structures.[67,69] On occasion, electron beam therapy is recommended for DFSP given its finite range and high dose concentration in superficial structures.

Several studies have evaluated the clinical outcomes of DFSP patients treated with radiation therapy. Early small studies demonstrated that radiation therapy was beneficial in DFSP patients who were unresectable or in those with positive margins.[70] Haas and colleagues[71] reviewed 38 patients with DFSP and reported that adjuvant radiation therapy decreased the local recurrence rate from 33% to 18%, although the results were not statistically significant. Castle and coworkers[66] reviewed the records of 53 patients with DFSP, many of whom had recurrent disease, who underwent resection and either neoadjuvant or adjuvant radiation and showed a 10-year local control rate of 93%. However, these recurrence rates are similar to those demonstrated in modern series of wide surgical excision. A recent meta-analysis by Chen and colleagues[72] evaluated the use of radiotherapy in DFSP and there was no local recurrence benefit with adjuvant treatment. Even so, they recommend adjuvant radiation in patients with large or recurrent tumors, especially in the setting where R0 resection would result in functional or cosmetic deficit. In the absence of clear evidence-based support for adjuvant radiation after resection of DFSP, an individualized approach is necessary.

The most common complications associated with radiotherapy are wound related. Complications reported in DFSP patients include fibrosis and skin graft failures with necrosis requiring reoperation.[73] Chronic complications can include fibrosis, edema, joint stiffness, and even fracture. Sequencing of radiation therapy can also alter the complication pattern, with neoadjuvant use increasing the risk of wound complications that require operative intervention.[74] Use of radiation therapy for DFSP should be limited to highly selected cases, including patients with unresectable disease and in those where negative margins are unattainable.

Systemic Therapy

Systemic cytotoxic therapy for locally advanced or metastatic DFSP plays a limited role in treatment. Historically, soft tissue sarcoma treatment regimens have been used in cases of metastatic DFSP. The most common regimens used in the cases included doxorubicin and ifosfamide. Case reports using methotrexate and vinblastine or vincristine, actinomycin, and cyclophosphamide have shown little to no effect in treating DFSP.[42] Overall, there is minimal role for conventional chemotherapy in the treatment of DFSP; response rates and clinical outcomes have been poor.[47]

Although systemic therapy has been shown to be ineffective in treating DFSP, molecular targeted therapy has proven to be more promising. Identification of the t(17;22) translocation and resulting PDGFB hyperactivity opened the possibility of tyrosine kinase inhibitor treatment similar to gastrointestinal stromal tumor. Based on the clinical experience of treating gastrointestinal stromal tumors with imatinib, Rubin and colleagues[75] evaluated the response of a 25-year-old patient with metastatic DFSP. The patient was treated for 4 months, resulting in a significant reduction in tumor volume. Subsequent resection showed no residual viable tumor. McArthur and colleagues[76] evaluated the use of imatinib in the treatment of 8 patients with locally advanced DFSP, with 4 of the 8 patients showing complete responses.

Multiple phase II trials have followed, further evaluating the efficacy of imatinib in DFSP patients. Rutkowski and associates[77] reviewed the results of the European Organization for Research and Treatment of Cancer (EORTC) and Southwest Oncology Group (SWOG) phase II trials evaluating imatinib in locally advanced and metastatic DFSP. Twenty-four patients were enrolled and the objective response rate approached 50%. The Dermatologic Cooperative Oncology Group (DeCOG) trial evaluated the neoadjuvant use of imatinib in advanced primary and locally recurrent DFSP, with 57% showing complete or partial responses.[78] Wicherts and colleagues[79] also showed the ability to use imatinib in neoadjuvant fashion, allowing for complete resection of a recurrent, locally advanced periclavicular DFSP. Sunitinib was recently evaluated in 30 patients with imatinib-resistant DFSP, and 40% of patients showed a partial or complete response after failing treatment with imatinib.[80] Sorafenib, a B-raf and vascular endothelial growth factor receptor inhibitor, has shown activity in DFSP as well.[81] Tyrosine kinase inhibitor therapy is useful addition to the armamentarium for DFSP patients with recurrent or metastatic disease.

METASTATIC DISEASE

Metastatic disease is uncommon in DFSP. Regional metastases to lymph nodes are rare, occurring in approximately 1% of cases.[7] The low rate of metastasis to the regional lymph nodes negates the need for standard surgical evaluation of these areas, with no role for sentinel node mapping. Distant metastases are also rare, occurring in fewer than 5% of cases.[7] Like other sarcomas, when DFSP is associated with distant disease, it usually involves the lung. The low rate of distant metastases renders routine chest imaging unnecessary, except in the case of aggressive variants. As noted previously, there is controversy regarding the metastatic potential of DFSP-FS.[25] We favor imaging to detect pulmonary metastases in DFSP-FS patients given the uncertainty and availability of effective molecular therapy.

FOLLOW-UP AND SURVEILLANCE

Patients diagnosed with DFSP require long-term follow-up. Local recurrences are problematic and can occur more than 5 years out from initial treatment. Patients should be seen initially every 3 to 6 months for a clinical examination to evaluate for local recurrence, depending on individual tumor and patient features. For those individuals with large, deep, or with aggressive variants, surveillance imaging may be appropriate. Because MRI has been shown to be effective in the preoperative evaluation of these patients, it may be appropriate for surveillance in patients at high risk for local recurrence at locations not easily assessed on physical examination.[39] If MRI will be used for surveillance of those patients with large or deep tumors, we recommend obtaining a baseline study in the early postoperative period to allow for better differentiation of postoperative changes from local recurrence. Any abnormalities should be biopsied for confirmation. As noted, metastatic disease is rare, but surveillance with chest imaging is reasonable in patients with particularly aggressive histologic features.

SUMMARY

DFSP is a rare dermal neoplasm with an aggressive and unpredictable tendency for wide and deep tissue infiltration. Despite its locally aggressive nature, regional and distant metastases are unusual. Multiple variants exist, with DFSP-FS being the most aggressive, and all share the t(17; 22) translocation resulting in hyperactivation of PDGFB. No definitive clinical risk factors for its development have been identified. Diagnosis requires a high index of suspicion, with a low threshold for tissue sampling. Despite classic or typical histologic features of DFSP, immunohistochemistry is an important component of the pathologic diagnosis.

Wide surgical excision remains the mainstay of management and the best chance for cure. MMS is useful in special situations, including head and neck tumors. Open wound management is an important strategy for cases in which margins are in doubt or complex reconstruction is required. Detailed assessment of resection margins is important for defining adequacy of excision and minimizing the risk of local recurrence. Radiation is offered in the adjuvant setting when margins are positive and re-excision is not feasible, or in cases of unresectable disease. Conventional chemotherapy has no role in treatment, but molecular targeted therapy has contributed to the management of metastatic or locally advanced disease. Above all else, involvement of specialty trained oncologic experts is essential for proper management of this rare entity.

REFERENCES

1. Taylor R. Sarcomatous tumor resembling in some respects keloid. Arch Dermatol 1890;8:384–7.
2. Darier J. Dermatofibromes progressifs et recidivants ou fibrosarcomes de la peu. Ann Dermatol Syphiligr 1924;5:545–62.
3. Hoffman E. Uber das knollentreibende fibrosarkom der haut (Dermatofibrsarkoma protuberans). Dermat Ztschr 1925;43:1–28.
4. McGregor JK. Role of surgery in the management of dermatofibrosarcoma protuberans. Ann Surg 1961;154:255–8.
5. Ratner D, Thomas CO, Johnson TM, et al. Mohs micrographic surgery for the treatment of dermatofibrosarcoma protuberans. Results of a multiinstitutional series with an analysis of the extent of microscopic spread. J Am Acad Dermatol 1997;37(4):600–13.
6. Monnier D, Vidal C, Martin L, et al. Dermatofibrosarcoma protuberans: a population-based cancer registry descriptive study of 66 consecutive cases diagnosed between 1982 and 2002. J Eur Acad Dermatol Venereol 2006; 20(10):1237–42.
7. Rutgers EJ, Kroon BB, Albus-Lutter CE, et al. Dermatofibrosarcoma protuberans: treatment and prognosis. Eur J Surg Oncol 1992;18(3):241–8.
8. Rouhani P, Fletcher CD, Devesa SS, et al. Cutaneous soft tissue sarcoma incidence patterns in the U.S. : an analysis of 12,114 cases. Cancer 2008;113(3): 616–27.
9. Criscione VD, Weinstock MA. Descriptive epidemiology of dermatofibrosarcoma protuberans in the United States, 1973 to 2002. J Am Acad Dermatol 2007;56(6): 968–73.
10. Zlatnik MG, Dinh TV, Lucci JA 3rd, et al. Dermatofibrosarcoma protuberans of the vulva: report of two new cases and review of the literature. J Low Genit Tract Dis 1999;3(2):135–8.
11. Frierson HF, Cooper PH. Myxoid variant of dermatofibrosarcoma protuberans. Am J Surg Pathol 1983;7(5):445–50.
12. Reimann JD, Fletcher CD. Myxoid dermatofibrosarcoma protuberans: a rare variant analyzed in a series of 23 cases. Am J Surg Pathol 2007;31(9):1371–7.

13. Marcus JR, Few JW, Senger C, et al. Dermatofibrosarcoma protuberans and the Bednar tumor: treatment in the pediatric population. J Pediatr Surg 1998;33(12): 1811–4.
14. Bednar B. Storiform neurofibromas of the skin, pigmented and nonpigmented. Cancer 1957;10(2):368–76.
15. Enzinger FM, Weiss SW, editors. Soft tissue tumors. 1st edition. St Louis (MO): Mosby; 1988. p. 252–300.
16. Shmookler BM, Enzinger FM. Giant cell fibroblastoma: a peculiar childhood tumor. Lab Invest 1982;46.
17. Maeda T, Hirose T, Furuya K, et al. Giant cell fibroblastoma associated with dermatofibrosarcoma protuberans: a case report. Mod Pathol 1998;11(5):491–5.
18. Terrier-Lacombe MJ, Guillou L, Maire G, et al. Dermatofibrosarcoma protuberans, giant cell fibroblastoma, and hybrid lesions in children: clinicopathologic comparative analysis of 28 cases with molecular data–a study from the French Federation of Cancer Centers Sarcoma Group. Am J Surg Pathol 2003;27(1):27–39.
19. Goldblum JR. CD34 positivity in fibrosarcomas which arise in dermatofibrosarcoma protuberans. Arch Pathol Lab Med 1995;119(3):238–41.
20. Kuzel P, Mahmood MN, Metelitsa AI, et al. A clinicopathologic review of a case series of dermatofibrosarcoma protuberans with fibrosarcomatous differentiation. J Cutan Med Surg 2015;19(1):28–34.
21. Palmerini E, Gambarotti M, Staals EL, et al. Fibrosarcomatous changes and expression of CD34+ and apolipoprotein-D in dermatofibrosarcoma protuberans. Clin Sarcoma Res 2012;2(1):4.
22. Liang CA, Jambusaria-Pahlajani A, Karia PS, et al. A systematic review of outcome data for dermatofibrosarcoma protuberans with and without fibrosarcomatous change. J Am Acad Dermatol 2014;71(4):781–6.
23. Hoesly PM, Lowe GC, Lohse CM, et al. Prognostic impact of fibrosarcomatous transformation in dermatofibrosarcoma protuberans: a cohort study. J Am Acad Dermatol 2015;72(3):419–25.
24. Voth H, Landsberg J, Hinz T, et al. Management of dermatofibrosarcoma protuberans with fibrosarcomatous transformation: an evidence-based review of the literature. J Eur Acad Dermatol Venereol 2011;25(12):1385–91.
25. Bowne WB, Antonescu CR, Leung DH, et al. Dermatofibrosarcoma protuberans: a clinicopathologic analysis of patients treated and followed at a single institution. Cancer 2000;88(12):2711–20.
26. Fields RC, Hameed M, Qin LX, et al. Dermatofibrosarcoma protuberans (DFSP): predictors of recurrence and the use of systemic therapy. Ann Surg Oncol 2011; 18(2):328–36.
27. Naeem R, Lux ML, Huang SF, et al. Ring chromosomes in dermatofibrosarcoma protuberans are composed of interspersed sequences from chromosomes 17 and 22. Am J Pathol 1995;147(6):1553–8.
28. Patel KU, Szabo SS, Hernandez VS, et al. Dermatofibrosarcoma protuberans COL1A1-PDGFB fusion is identified in virtually all dermatofibrosarcoma protuberans cases when investigated by newly developed multiplex reverse transcription polymerase chain reaction and fluorescence in situ hybridization assays. Hum Pathol 2008;39(2):184–93.
29. Sirvent N, Maire G, Pedeutour F. Genetics of dermatofibrosarcoma protuberans family of tumors: from ring chromosomes to tyrosine kinase inhibitor treatment. Genes Chromosomes Cancer 2003;37(1):1–19.
30. Bridge JA, Neff JR, Sandberg AA. Cytogenetic analysis of dermatofibrosarcoma protuberans. Cancer Genet Cytogenet 1990;49(2):199–202.

31. Pedeutour F, Coindre JM, Nicolo G, et al. Ring chromosomes in dermatofibrosarcoma protuberans contain chromosome 17 sequences: fluorescence in situ hybridization. Cancer Genet Cytogenet 1993;67(2):149.

32. Kneebone RL, Melissas J, Mannell A. Dermatofibrosarcoma protuberans in black patients. S Afr Med J 1984;66(24):919–21.

33. Ani AN, Attah EB, Ajayi OO. Dermatofibrosarcoma protruberans: analysis of eight cases in an African population. Am Surg 1976;42(12):934–40.

34. McPeak CJ, Cruz T, Nicastri AD. Dermatofibrosarcoma protuberans: an analysis of 86 cases–five with metastasis. Ann Surg 1967;166(5):803–16.

35. Bogucki B, Neuhaus I, Hurst EA. Dermatofibrosarcoma protuberans: a review of the literature. Dermatol Surg 2012;38(4):537–51.

36. Zelger B, Sidoroff A, Stanzl U, et al. Deep penetrating dermatofibroma versus dermatofibrosarcoma protuberans. A clinicopathologic comparison. Am J Surg Pathol 1994;18(7):677–86.

37. Li N, McNiff J, Hui P, et al. Differential expression of HMGA1 and HMGA2 in dermatofibroma and dermatofibrosarcoma protuberans: potential diagnostic applications, and comparison with histologic findings, CD34, and factor XIIIa immunoreactivity. Am J Dermatopathol 2004;26(4):267–72.

38. Zhang L, Liu QY, Cao Y, et al. Dermatofibrosarcoma protuberans: computed tomography and magnetic resonance imaging findings. Medicine (Baltimore) 2015;94(24):e1001.

39. Torreggiani WC, Al-Ismail K, Munk PL, et al. Dermatofibrosarcoma protuberans: MR imaging features. AJR Am J Roentgenol 2002;178(4):989–93.

40. Thornton SL, Reid J, Papay FA, et al. Childhood dermatofibrosarcoma protuberans: role of preoperative imaging. J Am Acad Dermatol 2005;53(1):76–83.

41. Taylor HB, Helwig EB. Dermatofibrosarcoma protuberans. A study of 115 cases. Cancer 1962;15:717–25.

42. Lemm D, Mügge LO, Mentzel T, et al. Current treatment options in dermatofibrosarcoma protuberans. J Cancer Res Clin Oncol 2009;135(5):653–65.

43. Lisovsky M, Hoang MP, Dresser KA, et al. Apolipoprotein D in CD34-positive and CD34-negative cutaneous neoplasms: a useful marker in differentiating superficial acral fibromyxoma from dermatofibrosarcoma protuberans. Mod Pathol 2008;21(1):31–8.

44. Haycox CL, Odland PB, Olbricht SM, et al. Immunohistochemical characterization of dermatofibrosarcoma protuberans with practical applications for diagnosis and treatment. J Am Acad Dermatol 1997;37(3 Pt 1):438–44.

45. Rekhi B. Perineurial malignant peripheral nerve sheath tumor in the setting of multiple soft tissue perineuriomas: a rare presentation of an uncommon tumor. J Cancer Res Ther 2013;9(1):131–4.

46. Pack GT, Tabah EJ. Dermato-fibrosarcoma protuberans. A report of 39 cases. AMA Arch Surg 1951;62(3):391–411.

47. Gloster HM Jr. Dermatofibrosarcoma protuberans. J Am Acad Dermatol 1996; 35(3 Pt 1):355–74 [quiz: 375–6].

48. Farma JM, Ammori JB, Zager JS, et al. Dermatofibrosarcoma protuberans: how wide should we resect? Ann Surg Oncol 2010;17(8):2112–8.

49. Stojadinovic A, Karpoff HM, Antonescu CR, et al. Dermatofibrosarcoma protuberans of the head and neck. Ann Surg Oncol 2000;7(9):696–704.

50. Massey RA, Tok J, Strippoli BA, et al. A comparison of frozen and paraffin sections in dermatofibrosarcoma protuberans. Dermatol Surg 1998;24(9):995–8.

51. Rowsell AR, Poole MD, Godfrey AM. Dermatofibrosarcoma protuberans: the problems of surgical management. Br J Plast Surg 1986;39(2):262–4.

52. Lindner NJ, Scarborough MT, Powell GJ, et al. Revision surgery in dermatofibrosarcoma protuberans of the trunk and extremities. Eur J Surg Oncol 1999;25(4): 392–7.

53. Hobbs ER, Wheeland RG, Bailin PL, et al. Treatment of dermatofibrosarcoma protuberans with Mohs micrographic surgery. Ann Surg 1988;207(1):102–7.

54. Loghdey MS, Varma S, Rajpara SM, et al. Mohs micrographic surgery for dermatofibrosarcoma protuberans (DFSP): a single-centre series of 76 patients treated by frozen-section Mohs micrographic surgery with a review of the literature. J Plast Reconstr Aesthet Surg 2014;67(10):1315–21.

55. Serra-Guillen C, Llombart B, Nagore E, et al. Mohs micrographic surgery in dermatofibrosarcoma protuberans allows tumour clearance with smaller margins and greater preservation of healthy tissue compared with conventional surgery: a study of 74 primary cases. Br J Dermatol 2015;172(5):1303–7.

56. Foroozan M, Sei JF, Amini M, et al. Efficacy of Mohs micrographic surgery for the treatment of dermatofibrosarcoma protuberans: systematic review. Arch Dermatol 2012;148(9):1055–63.

57. Gloster HM Jr, Harris KR, Roenigk RK. A comparison between Mohs micrographic surgery and wide surgical excision for the treatment of dermatofibrosarcoma protuberans. J Am Acad Dermatol 1996;35(1):82–7.

58. Snow SN, Gordon EM, Larson PO, et al. Dermatofibrosarcoma protuberans: a report on 29 patients treated by Mohs micrographic surgery with long-term follow-up and review of the literature. Cancer 2004;101(1):28–38.

59. DuBay D, Cimmino V, Lowe L, et al. Low recurrence rate after surgery for dermatofibrosarcoma protuberans: a multidisciplinary approach from a single institution. Cancer 2004;100(5):1008–16.

60. Kimmel Z, Ratner D, Kim JY, et al. Peripheral excision margins for dermatofibrosarcoma protuberans: a meta-analysis of spatial data. Ann Surg Oncol 2007; 14(7):2113–20.

61. Garcia C, Viehman G, Hitchcock M, et al. Dermatofibrosarcoma protuberans treated with Mohs surgery. A case with CD34 immunostaining variability. Dermatol Surg 1996;22(2):177–9.

62. Bertolli E, Campagnari M, Molina AS, et al. Artificial dermis (Matriderm(R)) followed by skin graft as an option in dermatofibrosarcoma protuberans with complete circumferential and peripheral deep margin assessment. Int Wound J 2015; 12(5):545–7.

63. Buck DW 2nd, Kim JY, Alam M, et al. Multidisciplinary approach to the management of dermatofibrosarcoma protuberans. J Am Acad Dermatol 2012;67(5): 861–6.

64. Kraemer BA, Fremling M. Dermatofibrosarcoma protuberans of the toe. Ann Plast Surg 1990;25(4):295–8.

65. Yang JC, Chang AE, Baker AR, et al. Randomized prospective study of the benefit of adjuvant radiation therapy in the treatment of soft tissue sarcomas of the extremity. J Clin Oncol 1998;16(1):197–203.

66. Castle KO, Guadagnolo BA, Tsai CJ, et al. Dermatofibrosarcoma protuberans: long-term outcomes of 53 patients treated with conservative surgery and radiation therapy. Int J Radiat Oncol Biol Phys 2013;86(3):585–90.

67. Stewart AJ, Lee YK, Saran FH. Comparison of conventional radiotherapy and intensity-modulated radiotherapy for post-operative radiotherapy for primary extremity soft tissue sarcoma. Radiother Oncol 2009;93(1):125–30.

68. Alektiar KM, Brennan MF, Healey JH, et al. Impact of intensity-modulated radiation therapy on local control in primary soft-tissue sarcoma of the extremity. J Clin Oncol 2008;26(20):3440–4.

69. Wang J, Wang S, Song Y, et al. Postoperative intensity-modulated radiation therapy provides favorable local control and low toxicities in patients with soft tissue sarcomas in the extremities and trunk wall. Onco Targets Ther 2015;8:2843–7.

70. Marks LB, Suit HD, Rosenberg AE, et al. Dermatofibrosarcoma protuberans treated with radiation therapy. Int J Radiat Oncol Biol Phys 1989;17(2):379–84.

71. Haas RL, Keus RB, Loftus BM, et al. The role of radiotherapy in the local management of dermatofibrosarcoma protuberans. Soft Tissue Tumours Working Group. Eur J Cancer 1997;33(7):1055–60.

72. Chen YT, Tu WT, Lee WR, et al. The efficacy of adjuvant radiotherapy in dermatofibrosarcoma protuberans: a systemic review and meta-analysis. J Eur Acad Dermatol Venereol 2016;30(7):1107–14.

73. Sun LM, Wang CJ, Huang CC, et al. Dermatofibrosarcoma protuberans: treatment results of 35 cases. Radiother Oncol 2000;57(2):175–81.

74. El-Bared N, Wong P, Wang D. Soft tissue sarcoma and radiation therapy advances, impact on toxicity. Curr Treat Options Oncol 2015;16(5):19.

75. Rubin BP, Schuetze SM, Eary JF, et al. Molecular targeting of platelet-derived growth factor B by imatinib mesylate in a patient with metastatic dermatofibrosarcoma protuberans. J Clin Oncol 2002;20(17):3586–91.

76. McArthur GA, Demetri GD, van Oosterom A, et al. Molecular and clinical analysis of locally advanced dermatofibrosarcoma protuberans treated with imatinib: Imatinib Target Exploration Consortium Study B2225. J Clin Oncol 2005;23(4): 866–73.

77. Rutkowski P, Van Glabbeke M, Rankin CJ, et al. Imatinib mesylate in advanced dermatofibrosarcoma protuberans: pooled analysis of two phase II clinical trials. J Clin Oncol 2010;28(10):1772–9.

78. Ugurel S, Mentzel T, Utikal J, et al. Neoadjuvant imatinib in advanced primary or locally recurrent dermatofibrosarcoma protuberans: a multicenter phase II DeCOG trial with long-term follow-up. Clin Cancer Res 2014;20(2):499–510.

79. Wicherts DA, van Coevorden F, Klomp HM, et al. Complete resection of recurrent and initially unresectable dermatofibrosarcoma protuberans downsized by Imatinib. World J Surg Oncol 2013;11:59.

80. Fu Y, Kang H, Zhao H, et al. Sunitinib for patients with locally advanced or distantly metastatic dermatofibrosarcoma protuberans but resistant to imatinib. Int J Clin Exp Med 2015;8(5):8288–94.

81. Kamar FG, Kairouz VF, Sabri AN. Dermatofibrosarcoma protuberans (DFSP) successfully treated with sorafenib: case report. Clin Sarcoma Res 2013;3(1):5.

82. Chang CK, Jacobs IA, Salti GI. Outcomes of surgery for dermatofibrosarcoma protuberans. Eur J Surg Oncol 2004;30(3):341–5.

Management of Breast Sarcoma

Cary Hsu, MD[a],*, Susan A. McCloskey, MD[b], Parvin F. Peddi, MD[c]

KEYWORDS

• Breast • Sarcoma • Multidisciplinary • Surgery • Radiation • Chemotherapy

KEY POINTS

• The natural history and biologic behavior of breast sarcomas is similar to sarcomas at other sites.
• Total mastectomy is frequently necessary because of tumor size and anatomic considerations, but partial mastectomy does not compromise outcomes if adequate margins can be attained.
• Lymph node metastases occur rarely; thus, routine axillary surgery provides no benefit and is not indicated.
• Adjuvant chemotherapy and radiation are considered for high-risk patients, particularly those with large and/or high grade sarcomas.

Breast sarcoma is a rare clinical entity that represents less than 1% of all breast malignancies and less than 5% of all sarcomas.[1,2] The published literature on breast sarcomas is predominantly composed of single institution retrospective analyses and case reports. These studies include patients with a wide variety of histologies, treated over many decades with great variability in surgical approaches, and inconsistencies in the use of adjuvant therapies. Owing to the rarity and heterogeneity of breast sarcomas, there are no published randomized trials that validate any particular treatment strategy. However, the literature in aggregate does provide valuable information about the biology and natural history of the disease. The anatomic site is an important variable and certainly influences the clinical decisions for this disease process. This paper discusses the management of breast sarcoma in the context of the studies that have defined current practices.

Disclosure Statement: The authors have nothing to disclose.
[a] Department of Surgery, Baylor College of Medicine, One Baylor Plaza, MS 390, Houston, TX 77030, USA; [b] Department of Radiation Oncology, University of California, Los Angeles, Los Angeles, CA 90095, USA; [c] Division of Hematology & Oncology, Department of Medicine, University of California, Los Angeles, Los Angeles, CA 90095, USA
* Corresponding author.
E-mail address: Cary.Hsu@bcm.edu

Surg Clin N Am 96 (2016) 1047–1058
http://dx.doi.org/10.1016/j.suc.2016.05.004
0039-6109/16/$ – see front matter © 2016 Elsevier Inc. All rights reserved.
surgical.theclinics.com

CLINICAL PRESENTATION AND INITIAL EVALUATION

Primary breast sarcomas occur almost exclusively in female patients and are typically diagnosed in the fifth or sixth decades of life. Most patients present with a solitary, firm, well-circumscribed, painless breast mass. In contrast with patients with benign soft tissue masses of the breast, patients often report a history of rapid growth over several months.[1,3] Historically, breast sarcomas are relatively large at the time of presentation with a median size of 5 cm, although it seems likely that smaller lesions will be detected increasingly as the use of routine screening mammography continues to increase.

Secondary breast sarcomas infrequently develop after prior treatment with external beam radiation for conditions such as non-Hodgkin lymphoma or breast carcinoma with a reported incidence rate of 0.2% for breast cancer patients. The peak incidence is approximately 5 to 10 years after radiotherapy, but the range is substantial. A wide array of histologic subtypes has been reported and these sarcomas are morphologically identical to primary sarcomas by histopathologic analysis. It has been noted that patients with radiation-induced sarcomas tend to present with more advanced disease than patients with primary sarcomas; this may be related to delay in diagnosis because physical examination is often difficult because of changes after radiotherapy. Angiosarcoma is the most common postradiation secondary breast sarcoma and has a median latency period of 6 to 7 years.[4–6] Radiation-associated angiosarcoma typically develops in cutaneous tissues and presents as skin discoloration and thickening, which may be subtle in the earliest stages of the disease.[7]

The initial evaluation for primary breast sarcoma includes standard diagnostic imaging used for women presenting with a breast mass. This evaluation includes mammography, ultrasonography, and occasionally breast MRI. Most often, mammograms reveal masses with a round, oval, or lobular shape. Approximately 30% of the mammograms demonstrate architectural distortion without a discrete mass. Calcifications or spiculated lesions are uncommon, but occasionally seen. On ultrasound imaging, most breast sarcomas are hypoechoic and without posterior attenuation. On MRI, breast sarcomas are heterogeneously hypointense on T1-weighted images and hyperintense on T2-weighted images. Intense enhancement is seen after contrast administration. Imaging findings associated with breast sarcoma have considerable overlap with findings that may be seen in breast carcinoma; thus, imaging alone is not diagnostic.[8]

Definitive diagnosis is critical because the management of epithelial malignancy is profoundly different and because the histologic subtype of the sarcoma may influence clinical decisions. Fine-needle aspiration cytology is of little usefulness and is inadequate for determining the subtype or grade of the lesion. Determination of histologic subtype and grade can almost always be achieved with image-guided core needle biopsy.[9,10] In the rare instance that a core biopsy is not able to provide a histologic diagnosis, incisional biopsy can be considered. Surgical biopsy incisions must be oriented in a manner such that the biopsy scar can be removed completely during the definitive surgical resection. Meticulous attention to hemostasis is paramount because postoperative hematomas may disseminate malignant cells throughout the biopsy cavity. Occasionally, small and presumably benign lesions are excised and return with the unexpected diagnosis of sarcoma; in this situation, the excision must be regarded as inadequate even if the operative report and pathology report suggest that the lesion has been completely removed.

Historically, there have been inconsistencies and some controversy in the reporting and classification of breast sarcomas. Many of the published series include patients with histologies such as dermatofibrosarcoma protuberans, carcinosarcoma, and malignant phyllodes tumors, which fall outside of the strict clinicopathologic definition of sarcoma.[11] The most common histologic subtypes reported in the literature are angiosarcomas followed by pleomorphic sarcomas (previously called malignant fibrous histiocytoma); these 2 subtypes account for approximately 50% of the cases in most series.[11–14] Fibrosarcoma, stromal sarcoma, osteogenic sarcoma, liposarcoma, and leiomyosarcoma are also represented in many of the series, but at a lower frequency.

Once the diagnosis of sarcoma has been established, appropriate cross-sectional imaging is indicated for operative planning and to rule out distant metastatic disease. Either computed tomography or MRI with an appropriate contrast agent provides anatomic information necessary to guide surgical resection. Cross-sectional imaging should also include the chest because the lungs are the most common site of metastasis for the majority of breast sarcomas. In a Radiology Diagnostic Oncology Group study, computed tomography and MRI were equally accurate in the local staging of soft tissue neoplasms with no difference in the ability to detect involvement of bone, joint, and neurovascular structures.[15] ^{18}F-fluorodeoxyglucose PET is considered investigational in the treatment of sarcomas, but its role is rapidly expanding. PET scans can provide useful information in staging and restaging, distinguishing between benign and malignant disease, assessing for both local and distant recurrence, and monitoring responses to systemic and regional therapy.[16]

MULTIDISCIPLINARY MANAGEMENT

Data are limited regarding management in general and particularly limited with regard to optimal adjuvant therapies. Effective treatment requires thorough pretreatment planning and coordinated care by an experienced, multidisciplinary team of physicians. This team should include surgical oncologists, reconstructive surgeons, medical oncologists, radiation oncologists, pathologists, and radiologists. A number of studies have documented patient benefit from the improved treatment of rare tumors, including soft tissue sarcomas, at specialty centers.[17,18] An additional benefit of a multidisciplinary approach is that it gives patients with large, high-grade sarcomas the opportunity to be enrolled in protocol-driven therapy, which may answer important clinical questions and drive the field forward. Many of these protocols involve the administration of neoadjuvant therapy (chemotherapy, targeted therapies, radiation therapy) to high-risk sarcomas.

SURGICAL MANAGEMENT

Complete surgical excision is of foremost importance in achieving local control and the only potentially curative therapy for breast sarcomas. The objectives of surgical resection are straightforward: complete removal of the tumor with microscopically negative margins, preservation of function, and secure wound closure. Skin incisions are typically made along the longest axis of the tumor. The skin surrounding the prior biopsy sites should be removed en bloc with the specimen because seeding of malignant cells along the biopsy tract has been reported.[16] With angiosarcoma as an exception, direct extension of the tumor into the skin is uncommon, but when it occurs, the involved skin is taken en bloc with the rest of the specimen. If the mass is large, a generous incision should be used to facilitate a wide resection. When surgical drains are used, they should exit the skin near the resection bed because the drain tract will need to be included in the radiation portals if adjuvant radiation is used.

Soft tissue sarcomas typically expand spherically along tissue planes and compress surrounding tissues creating a pseudocapsule of surrounding tissue; malignant cells can penetrate this pseudocapsule.[19,20] As such, there continues to be controversy in defining what constitutes an adequate margin of resection. Historically, sarcoma operations were described in which the entire anatomic compartment housing the tumor was resected. This has been abandoned and the current practice is to obtain a negative margin by dissecting through adjacent, uninvolved tissues away from the tumor. In general, a microscopically negative margin, or R0 resection, is considered adequate. For trunk and extremity sarcomas, there are conflicting data on whether margins wider than microscopically negative offer superior local control.[21–24] Currently, a margin of greater than 1 cm has been encouraged when feasible for all soft tissue sarcomas.[25] This question has not been addressed specifically for breast sarcomas, but a margin of greater than 1 cm is also recommended.[3] In contrast with most other breast sarcomas, angiosarcomas are often multicentric and infiltrative; these tumors frequently extend well beyond radiographically or grossly discernable boundaries. A widely negative margin is notoriously difficult to achieve for angiosarcomas; thus, it has been suggested that a 3-cm clinical margin (the gross distance from visible or palpable abnormality) may be more appropriate for this histologic subtype.[3]

The breast is a relatively favorable site for surgical management of sarcoma. For the majority of patients, there are no critical bony or neurovascular structures limiting the planned resection. Extensive soft tissue resections can often be undertaken with no disability and without the need for complex closure. There is considerable flexibility in the ability to tailor a mastectomy incision to center and orient it directly over the long axis of the tumor. In most reported series, the vast majority of patients presenting with primary breast sarcomas presented with resectable disease and had microscopically negative margins after surgery.[14,26–28]

Total mastectomy had long been regarded as the gold standard in surgical therapy for breast sarcomas.[29] Subsequently, numerous institutions have published retrospective analyses indicating that a wide excision to negative margins provides comparable local control in selected patients.[12–14,27,30–32] From a practical standpoint, the operative options will be dictated by the size and location of the tumor, the patient's breast size, and patient preference. Because the median presenting size of breast sarcomas is greater than 5 cm, mastectomy is often the most straightforward way to achieve the goal of a wide margin; however, selected patients can be managed safely with partial mastectomy. Surgical clips should be placed to mark the boundaries of the resection bed and any margins of concern; this may facilitate the planning of radiation portals if it is determined that adjuvant radiation therapy is indicated.

Frozen section analysis tends to be unreliable for mesenchymal malignancies, particularly when they are low to intermediate grade, and is not routinely used to assess margin status. Occasionally, we find frozen section useful when looking at a focal margin of interest in the setting of a high-grade lesion. If close or positive margins result after resection, reexcision or a completion mastectomy (if partial mastectomy was performed) should be undertaken if it can be accomplished without prohibitive morbidity. Likewise, breast sarcoma patients previously treated with nononcologic resections for presumed benign disease or resection with undocumented margins should be considered for reexcision or mastectomy, because such patients are likely to harbor residual disease from the initial operation.[33,34]

Soft tissue sarcomas are known to spread via the hematogenous route; thus, lymph node involvement is exceedingly rare.[35] As alluded to previously, reported series of breast sarcoma patients often span many decades and include an era in which axillary lymphadenectomy was performed routinely for all malignant lesions of the breast. It is well-documented that breast sarcoma patients who underwent axillary lymphadenectomy rarely had positive lymph nodes and most frequently this was seen in the context of disseminated disease.[11–14,27] Axillary lymphadenectomy confers no survival benefit.[12,36] Furthermore, for patients undergoing axillary dissection, the size of the radiation portal must be extended to include the axillary lymph node basin and this increases the risk of treatment-associated morbidity, particularly lymphedema.[37] There are histologic subtypes of sarcoma with potential for spread to the regional lymph nodes, particularly angiosarcoma, rhabdomyosarcoma, clear cell sarcoma, synovial sarcoma, and epithelioid sarcoma.[35,38] The axilla should be evaluated with axial imaging preoperatively. If nodal metastases are suspected, a biopsy should be obtained because reactive lymphadenopathy may be seen in up to 25% of breast sarcoma patients.[39] If axillary lymph node metastases are confirmed or if the primary tumor extends into the axilla, axillary lymphadenectomy should be part of the comprehensive treatment strategy. Otherwise, there are no indications for routine sentinel lymph node biopsy or axillary lymphadenectomy.

Reconstructive surgeons play a critical role in the surgical management of breast sarcomas and should be engaged early in the process of formulating the plan of care. Sarcoma surgery frequently results in complex wounds. When large or recurrent tumors are resected, there may not be adequate redundancy in the native tissues to close the incision primarily. In addition, sarcoma patients frequently receive radiation therapy, which compromises wound healing. The reconstructive surgeon brings expertise and a sophisticated array of techniques, from primary closure to free tissue transfer, to reliably restore integrity and form after extensive resection procedures.[40] Increasingly, breast reconstruction is being undertaken for breast sarcoma patients. The full range of reconstructive procedures used for epithelial breast cancers have been used, including oncoplastic techniques, breast implants, and local and free tissue flaps.[41] Importantly, breast reconstruction for sarcoma patients can be accomplished with low complication rates and without compromising the oncologic outcomes.[28] For patients with epithelial breast cancers, reconstruction has been shown to improve body image, sense of physical well-being, and quality of life; it is suspected that the same is true for sarcoma patients. Crosby and colleagues[41] have reported an extensive experience with reconstruction for breast sarcoma and have proposed an algorithm for clinical decisions regarding reconstructive options; the authors suggest that delayed, autologous tissue reconstruction minimizes complication rates and results in the best outcomes. Subtleties exist in patient selection, timing, and choice of reconstructive procedure; having a plastic surgeon involved in the multidisciplinary planning will help to identify patients who are appropriate candidates for breast reconstruction.

RADIATION THERAPY

Several single institutions have reviewed their experience with the treatment of primary breast sarcoma and, owing to exceedingly small numbers and heterogeneity in treatment selection, no definitive conclusions have been reached regarding the role of adjuvant radiation therapy. However, general conclusions regarding outcomes and specific risk factors for local recurrence have been informative.

Investigators at MD Anderson Cancer Center examined outcomes among 59 patients over 43 years with primary breast sarcoma, 16 of whom underwent segmental resection and 38 of whom underwent mastectomy. Four of 16 received radiation after segmental mastectomy and 13 of 38 received radiation after mastectomy. Owing to small numbers, no differences were detected by treatment modality; however, the authors did report that 14% failed locally after segmental resection alone versus 0% after segmental resection followed by radiation and 34% and 13% failed after mastectomy alone versus after mastectomy followed by radiation, respectively. Based on these findings, along with the findings that tumor size and surgical margins were significantly predictive of local failure, the investigators concluded that radiation is likely indicated for larger tumor size and positive margins.[26] Investigators at the National Institutes of Health observed no local failures among 10 patients with high-grade sarcoma who were treated with mastectomy and postoperative radiation with a median follow-up of 99 months, thus concluding that radiation therapy should be used for high-grade breast sarcomas.[42] Investigators at Princess Margaret Hospital in Toronto examined disease-specific and overall survival outcomes among 78 patients with breast sarcoma over 32 years. Twenty-six patients received radiation and 52 did not. In examining factors affecting prognosis, extent of surgery was not predictive of survival or local recurrence, but margin status was a significant predictor of local recurrence and radiation dose (>48 vs <48 Gy/no radiation therapy) significantly impacted cause-specific survival. The authors concluded that optimal outcomes were achieved with margin-negative surgical resection and that either lumpectomy or mastectomy achieved excellent local control if negative margins were achieved. This series stressed the importance of radiation given to appropriate dose.[31] The Institute Gustav-Roussey experience reviewing outcomes among 83 patients with breast sarcoma treated over 37 years similarly concluded that radiation may improve outcomes and should be considered for large and/or high-grade breast sarcomas or after conservative surgery.[14] Washington University investigators examined outcomes among 13 patients treated over 20 years with primary breast sarcoma and concluded that radiation should be considered in all cases owing to high rates of local recurrence, 54% in their series.[27] Most recently, Dutch investigators published a 35-year retrospective review examining outcomes among 42 patients with primary breast sarcoma in which they concluded size and grade to be prognostic and suggested high rates of observed local recurrence warrant aggressive surgery and consideration of postoperative radiation.[43] Finally, a Rare Cancer Network series exploring outcomes and prognostic factors in breast sarcomas suggested management should mirror that of extremity sarcoma.[12]

Thus, published series are suggestive of a role for radiation therapy in the setting of documented prognostic factors for local failure, which include close/positive surgical margins, high grade, and larger tumor size (most commonly >5 cm). Radiation has been used after both segmental resection and mastectomy in the presence of these risk factors and, unlike in the setting of epithelial breast malignancies, radiation therapy is typically not indicated for sterilization of microscopic nodal disease owing to the infrequency of nodal metastases. These considerations are in line with those used to guide decision making for extremity sarcoma and, indeed, radiation therapy recommendations for breast sarcoma are often extrapolated from general principles of radiation therapy for extremity sarcomas. Prospective randomized data have demonstrated that radiation therapy significantly improves local control for extremity soft tissue sarcoma.[44,45]

Regarding preoperative radiation therapy, there are no specific data to guide its use in the treatment of primary breast sarcoma, but it may be used for large or inoperable tumors at presentation and may also be of value in terms of optimizing target localization for radiation planning and potentially decreasing late effects of radiation. Preoperative versus postoperative radiation has been studied in the setting of extremity sarcoma and equivalent efficacy has been documented; however, there are toxicity tradeoffs with preoperative radiation associated with increased short-term wound complications but fewer long-term complications, including fibrosis, edema, and joint stiffness.[46,47] These tradeoffs can certainly be weighed in the multidisciplinary management of primary breast sarcoma.

Regarding radiation therapy delivery specifics, treatment fields have generally encompassed the anatomic breast borrowing from field design principles for epithelial breast malignancies. In terms of nodal coverage, it has been traditionally advisable that sarcoma fields encompass the surgical bed given the possibility of seeding surgical scars. Thus, although axillary dissection is not recommended owing to infrequency of nodal spread, if an axillary dissection was performed, consideration for extending the radiation fields to encompass the axillary surgical bed is advisable.[26] Regarding dose, Princess Margaret investigators among others advise microscopic tumoricidal dose of 50 Gy to the whole breast and at least 60 Gy to the tumor bed.[31] Extrapolating again from management principles for extremity sarcoma, the dose should be escalated according to margin status with doses of greater than 60 Gy recommended for microscopically or macroscopically positive margins. In the preoperative setting, 50 Gy has been used conventionally.

Angiosarcoma of the breast is a subtype that is most often radiation induced and thus special consideration is given. Cumulative radiation dose and associated toxicity is a consideration but not prohibitive of reirradiation. A systematic review published by Dutch investigators in 2014 examined treatment and prognostic factors of radiation-associated angiosarcoma. Data for 222 patients across 74 publications were included in the review. Seventeen percent (n = 37) of patients in the series received reirradiation, 30% of whom received hyperthermia with radiation. The 5-year local recurrence rate was improved in those patients receiving radiation, 34% versus 57%.[6] This and other single institution series indicated local recurrence approximating 60% for surgery alone for treatment of radiation associated angiosarcoma, thus justifying consideration of reirradiation.[48,49] In addition to examining reirradiation for the treatment of radiation-associated sarcoma, more novel reirradiation approaches including hyperthermia and hyperfractionation have also been explored and have shown promise.[50,51]

CHEMOTHERAPY

There are no prospective trials specifically assessing the benefit of adjuvant chemotherapy in breast sarcomas. Therefore, treatment recommendations for breast sarcomas are generally derived from trials on all soft tissue sarcomas or from retrospective studies. In a retrospective study of 60 patients with primary breast sarcoma treated at MD Anderson, adjuvant chemotherapy and/or radiotherapy was associated with prolonged disease-free survival ($P = .015$).[13] Other retrospective studies have not shown a similar benefit, although they included phyllodes tumors that are thought to be even less responsive to chemotherapy than breast sarcomas.[12,52] Adjuvant chemotherapy is therefore considered on an individual basis depending on patient age, comorbidities, tumor grade, and size. Given the unclear response rate to chemotherapy, we recommend neoadjuvant therapy only for large, high-grade sarcomas for which obtaining a negative margin may be challenging. However, limited data indicate that patients presenting with unresectable breast sarcomas are not likely to become surgical candidates after neoadjuvant chemotherapy.[14] Similar to other sarcomas, the recommended regimen is generally anthracycline and ifosfamide based. We recommend treatment on a case-by-case basis for high-grade sarcomas larger than 5 cm.

Radiation-induced sarcomas represent a particularly challenging subset of breast sarcomas because reradiation can be controversial given cumulative risk of toxicity, thereby leaving chemotherapy as the only option in addition to surgery. In one retrospective study of 95 patients with radiation-induced angiosarcoma at MD Anderson, adjuvant chemotherapy reduced risk of local recurrence significantly ($P = .0003$).[4]

Chemotherapy regimens varied and included ifosfamide, anthracyclines, taxanes, and gemcitabine. In another retrospective study in France of 80 patients with radiation-induced sarcoma, 42% of which were in the breast, no benefit was seen with the addition of chemotherapy to surgery.[53]

Angiosarcomas also deserve special mention, given their unique susceptibility to taxane chemotherapy. They represent less than 0.05% of all breast cancers and are not related to radiation therapy.[54] Taxanes are generally ineffective in sarcomas. However, in a phase II trial of 50 patients with inoperable angiosarcomas, 49% of whom had breast angiosarcomas, weekly paclitaxel resulted in a median overall survival of 19 months.[55] Similar results were seen in several other prospective and retrospective studies.[56–58] Weekly taxol is more active than therapy given every 3 weeks in 1 report, similar to studies in breast and gynecologic cancers.[56] Doxorubicin is also active, similar to other sarcomas.[59] It is unclear which chemotherapy is more efficacious for treatment of angiosarcomas and either is a reasonable option. Neoadjuvant chemotherapy is considered frequently for angiosarcomas because of the potential for chemosensitivity and the difficulty associated with achieving a negative margin with up-front surgery.[60,61]

CLINICAL OUTCOMES AND PROGNOSTIC FACTORS

There is considerable variability in reported clinical outcomes. The range for 5-year overall survival is 55% to 73% and the range for 5-year disease-free survival is 29.2% and 68%.[1] Many of the series have small numbers of patients and each series has considerable variability in the histologic subtypes that are represented. Furthermore, there is substantial variability in the treatment administered. Studies have most consistently identified size,[11–14,26,27] tumor grade,[12,14] and margin status[12,14,26,62] as important prognostic factors for disease-free and overall survival. Angiosarcoma has frequently been reported as a histologic subtype with a particularly poor prognosis; however, in 2 series from MD Anderson, patients with angiosarcoma actually had a relatively favorable prognosis.[12–14,26] The 5-year survival rate for radiation induced sarcomas is in the range of 27% to 48% and the poor prognosis has largely been attributed to a higher proportion of patients presenting with advanced clinical stage disease.[7] It seems likely that there is more to the biology of radiation-induced sarcomas than delayed diagnosis; indeed, genetic alterations unique to radiation-induced angiosarcomas have been characterized.[63]

Two of the largest series provide many insights on the natural history of the disease and it is worth highlighting some of the specific findings. In 2003, Zelek and colleagues[14] reported on 90 primary breast sarcoma patients treated at the Institut Gustave-Roussy. This series spanned approximately 40 years. Nearly 70% of patients had malignant fibrous histiocytomas and 10% had angiosarcomas. Approximately two-thirds of the patients were treated with surgery alone. The 10-year overall survival was 62% and 10-year disease-free survival was 50%. Tumor size and grade were the identified as prognostic factors for survival. The survival curves, stratified by grade and size, paralleled survival curves reported for extremity sarcomas. Most recurrences manifested within 5 years. Most recurrences seen in patients with low-grade sarcomas (7/8) were local (breast or chest wall). In contrast, approximately one-half of the recurrences associated with high-grade sarcomas were to distant sites. All of the patients with distant metastases had lung metastases (and some additional sites as well). Every patient with local recurrence related to grade 1 tumors achieved long-term survival after salvage surgery. In multivariate analysis, poorer survival was observed for patients with angiosarcoma. In 2007, Bousquet and colleagues[12] reported a retrospective study of 103 patients from the Rare Cancer Network, representing the largest series in the literature. Angiosarcoma was the most common histology in this cohort and represented 41% of the patients in the series. The 5-year overall survival was 55% and 5-year disease-free survival was 44%. Surgical margins of at least 1 cm was a favorable prognostic factor for local control and disease free survival. One-third of the patients underwent breast-conserving surgery and it was noted that the extent of surgery did not affect local failure rates. Angiosarcoma patients in this series had a 10-year disease-free survival of 12% versus 52% for the other histologies combined ($P = .0014$).

SUMMARY

Many issues specific to breast sarcomas have been addressed through observational studies. Most patients in reported series were able to undergo upfront surgery without neoadjuvant therapies and, for many patients, surgery was the only treatment modality. Mastectomy was the most frequently used operation, but partial mastectomy was found to be a safe alternative for patients with smaller tumors. Lymph node metastases are uncommon and thus routine lymphadenectomy is contraindicated. Adjuvant radiation and/or chemotherapy is considered for high-risk patients with the goals of enhancing local control and treating subclinical metastatic disease. The benefits of adjuvant therapies have been difficult to quantify owing to the heterogeneity of the disease and variability in treatments. Angiosarcoma stands out from the other histologic subtypes for the diffuse pattern of growth, multicentricity, cutaneous invasion, chemosensitivity, and prognosis. In general, breast sarcomas demonstrate biological behavior that is similar to sarcomas at other anatomic sites. The rarity and heterogeneity of breast sarcomas will likely preclude study in the context of prospective clinical trials. The current thinking is that sarcomas are better defined by histologic subtype and molecular profile, as opposed to the anatomic site of origin. Development of novel therapies will depend on the discovery of histology-specific strategies that exploit biologic behavior, molecular pathways, and drug sensitivities unique to the sarcoma subtype.

REFERENCES

1. Lim SZ, Ong KW, Tan BK, et al. Sarcoma of the breast: an update on a rare entity. J Clin Pathol 2016;69(5):373–81.
2. Pollard SG, Marks PV, Temple LN, et al. Breast sarcoma. A clinicopathologic review of 25 cases. Cancer 1990;66:941–4.
3. Al-Benna S, Poggemann K, Steinau HU, et al. Diagnosis and management of primary breast sarcoma. Breast Cancer Res Treat 2010;122:619–26.
4. Torres KE, Ravi V, Kin K, et al. Long-term outcomes in patients with radiation-associated angiosarcomas of the breast following surgery and radiotherapy for breast cancer. Ann Surg Oncol 2013;20:1267–74.
5. Yap J, Chuba PJ, Thomas R, et al. Sarcoma as a second malignancy after treatment for breast cancer. Int J Radiat Oncol Biol Phys 2002;52:1231–7.
6. Depla AL, Scharloo-Karels CH, de Jong MA, et al. Treatment and prognostic factors of radiation-associated angiosarcoma (RAAS) after primary breast cancer: a systematic review. Eur J Cancer 2014;50:1779–88.
7. Sheth GR, Cranmer LD, Smith BD, et al. Radiation-induced sarcoma of the breast: a systematic review. Oncologist 2012;17:405–18.
8. Surov A, Holzhausen HJ, Ruschke K, et al. Primary breast sarcoma: prevalence, clinical signs, and radiological features. Acta Radiol 2011;52:597–601.

9. Hoeber I, Spillane AJ, Fisher C, et al. Accuracy of biopsy techniques for limb and limb girdle soft tissue tumors. Ann Surg Oncol 2001;8:80–7.

10. Heslin MJ, Lewis JJ, Woodruff JM, et al. Core needle biopsy for diagnosis of extremity soft tissue sarcoma. Ann Surg Oncol 1997;4:425–31.

11. Adem C, Reynolds C, Ingle JN, et al. Primary breast sarcoma: clinicopathologic series from the Mayo Clinic and review of the literature. Br J Cancer 2004;91: 237–41.

12. Bousquet G, Confavreux C, Magne N, et al. Outcome and prognostic factors in breast sarcoma: a multicenter study from the rare cancer network. Radiother Oncol 2007;85:355–61.

13. Gutman H, Pollock RE, Ross MI, et al. Sarcoma of the breast: implications for extent of therapy. The M. D. Anderson experience. Surgery 1994;116:505–9.

14. Zelek L, Llombart-Cussac A, Terrier P, et al. Prognostic factors in primary breast sarcomas: a series of patients with long-term follow-up. J Clin Oncol 2003;21: 2583–8.

15. Panicek DM, Gatsonis C, Rosenthal DI, et al. CT and MR imaging in the local staging of primary malignant musculoskeletal neoplasms: report of the Radiology Diagnostic Oncology Group. Radiology 1997;202:237–46.

16. Schwartz HS, Spengler DM. Needle tract recurrences after closed biopsy for sarcoma: three cases and review of the literature. Ann Surg Oncol 1997;4:228–36.

17. Rydholm A. Improving the management of soft tissue sarcoma. Diagnosis and treatment should be given in specialist centres. BMJ 1998;317:93–4.

18. Ray-Coquard I, Thiesse P, Ranchere-Vince D, et al. Conformity to clinical practice guidelines, multidisciplinary management and outcome of treatment for soft tissue sarcomas. Ann Oncol 2004;15:307–15.

19. Bowden L, Booher RJ. The principles and technique of resection of soft parts for sarcoma. Surgery 1958;44:963–77.

20. Kawaguchi N, Ahmed AR, Matsumoto S, et al. The concept of curative margin in surgery for bone and soft tissue sarcoma. Clin Orthop Relat Res 2004;(419): 165–72.

21. Baldini EH, Goldberg J, Jenner C, et al. Long-term outcomes after function-sparing surgery without radiotherapy for soft tissue sarcoma of the extremities and trunk. J Clin Oncol 1999;17:3252–9.

22. Dickinson IC, Whitwell DJ, Battistuta D, et al. Surgical margin and its influence on survival in soft tissue sarcoma. ANZ J Surg 2006;76:104–9.

23. McKee MD, Liu DF, Brooks JJ, et al. The prognostic significance of margin width for extremity and trunk sarcoma. J Surg Oncol 2004;85:68–76.

24. Sampo M, Tarkkanen M, Huuhtanen R, et al. Impact of the smallest surgical margin on local control in soft tissue sarcoma. Br J Surg 2008;95:237–43.

25. Byerly S, Chopra S, Nassif NA, et al. The role of margins in extremity soft tissue sarcoma. J Surg Oncol 2016;113(3):333–8.

26. Barrow BJ, Janjan NA, Gutman H, et al. Role of radiotherapy in sarcoma of the breast–a retrospective review of the M.D. Anderson experience. Radiother Oncol 1999;52:173–8.

27. Fields RC, Aft RL, Gillanders WE, et al. Treatment and outcomes of patients with primary breast sarcoma. Am J Surg 2008;196:559–61.

28. Toesca A, Spitaleri G, De Pas T, et al. Sarcoma of the breast: outcome and reconstructive options. Clin Breast Cancer 2012;12:438–44.

29. Berg JW, Decrosse JJ, Fracchia AA, et al. Stromal sarcomas of the breast. A unified approach to connective tissue sarcomas other than cystosarcoma phyllodes. Cancer 1962;15:418–24.

30. North JH Jr, McPhee M, Arredondo M, et al. Sarcoma of the breast: implications of the extent of local therapy. Am Surg 1998;64:1059–61.
31. McGowan TS, Cummings BJ, O'Sullivan B, et al. An analysis of 78 breast sarcoma patients without distant metastases at presentation. Int J Radiat Oncol Biol Phys 2000;46:383–90.
32. Blanchard DK, Reynolds CA, Grant CS, et al. Primary nonphylloides breast sarcomas. Am J Surg 2003;186:359–61.
33. Giuliano AE, Eilber FR. The rationale for planned reoperation after unplanned total excision of soft-tissue sarcomas. J Clin Oncol 1985;3:1344–8.
34. Zagars GK, Ballo MT, Pisters PW, et al. Surgical margins and reresection in the management of patients with soft tissue sarcoma using conservative surgery and radiation therapy. Cancer 2003;97:2544–53.
35. Fong Y, Coit DG, Woodruff JM, et al. Lymph node metastasis from soft tissue sarcoma in adults. Analysis of data from a prospective database of 1772 sarcoma patients. Ann Surg 1993;217:72–7.
36. Gullett NP, Delman K, Folpe AL, et al. National surgical patterns of care: regional lymphadenectomy of breast sarcomas. Am J Clin Oncol 2007;30:461–5.
37. Warren LE, Miller CL, Horick N, et al. The impact of radiation therapy on the risk of lymphedema after treatment for breast cancer: a prospective cohort study. Int J Radiat Oncol Biol Phys 2014;88:565–71.
38. Sherman KL, Kinnier CV, Farina DA, et al. Examination of national lymph node evaluation practices for adult extremity soft tissue sarcoma. J Surg Oncol 2014;110:682–8.
39. Christensen L, Schiodt T, Blichert-Toft M, et al. Sarcomas of the breast: a clinico-pathological study of 67 patients with long term follow-up. Eur J Surg Oncol 1988; 14:241–7.
40. Langstein HN, Robb GL. Reconstructive approaches in soft tissue sarcoma. Semin Surg Oncol 1999;17:52–65.
41. Crosby MA, Chike-Obi CJ, Baumann DP, et al. Reconstructive outcomes in patients with sarcoma of the breast. Plast Reconstr Surg 2010;126:1805–14.
42. Johnstone PA, Pierce LJ, Merino MJ, et al. Primary soft tissue sarcomas of the breast: local-regional control with post-operative radiotherapy. Int J Radiat Oncol Biol Phys 1993;27:671–5.
43. Holm M, Aggerholm-Pedersen N, Mele M, et al. Primary breast sarcoma: a retrospective study over 35 years from a single institution. Acta Oncol 2016;55(5): 584–90.
44. Pisters PW, Harrison LB, Leung DH, et al. Long-term results of a prospective randomized trial of adjuvant brachytherapy in soft tissue sarcoma. J Clin Oncol 1996;14:859–68.
45. Yang JC, Chang AE, Baker AR, et al. Randomized prospective study of the benefit of adjuvant radiation therapy in the treatment of soft tissue sarcomas of the extremity. J Clin Oncol 1998;16:197–203.
46. Davis AM, O'Sullivan B, Turcotte R, et al. Late radiation morbidity following randomization to preoperative versus postoperative radiotherapy in extremity soft tissue sarcoma. Radiother Oncol 2005;75:48–53.
47. O'Sullivan B, Davis AM, Turcotte R, et al. Preoperative versus postoperative radiotherapy in soft-tissue sarcoma of the limbs: a randomised trial. Lancet 2002;359:2235–41.
48. Billings SD, McKenney JK, Folpe AL, et al. Cutaneous angiosarcoma following breast-conserving surgery and radiation: an analysis of 27 cases. Am J Surg Pathol 2004;28:781–8.

49. Seinen JM, Styring E, Verstappen V, et al. Radiation-associated angiosarcoma after breast cancer: high recurrence rate and poor survival despite surgical treatment with R0 resection. Ann Surg Oncol 2012;19:2700–6.

50. de Jong MA, Oldenborg S, Bing Oei S, et al. Reirradiation and hyperthermia for radiation-associated sarcoma. Cancer 2012;118:180–7.

51. Palta M, Morris CG, Grobmyer SR, et al. Angiosarcoma after breast-conserving therapy: long-term outcomes with hyperfractionated radiotherapy. Cancer 2010;116:1872–8.

52. Confavreux C, Lurkin A, Mitton N, et al. Sarcomas and malignant phyllodes tumours of the breast–a retrospective study. Eur J Cancer 2006;42:2715–21.

53. Lagrange JL, Ramaioli A, Chateau MC, et al. Sarcoma after radiation therapy: retrospective multiinstitutional study of 80 histologically confirmed cases. Radiation Therapist and Pathologist Groups of the Federation Nationale des Centres de Lutte Contre le Cancer. Radiology 2000;216:197–205.

54. Bordoni D, Bolletta E, Falco G, et al. Primary angiosarcoma of the breast. Int J Surg Case Rep 2016;20S:12–5.

55. Ray-Coquard IL, Domont J, Tresch-Bruneel E, et al. Paclitaxel given once per week with or without bevacizumab in patients with advanced angiosarcoma: a randomized phase II trial. J Clin Oncol 2015;33:2797–802.

56. Fury MG, Antonescu CR, Van Zee KJ, et al. A 14-year retrospective review of angiosarcoma: clinical characteristics, prognostic factors, and treatment outcomes with surgery and chemotherapy. Cancer J 2005;11:241–7.

57. Penel N, Bui BN, Bay JO, et al. Phase II trial of weekly paclitaxel for unresectable angiosarcoma: the ANGIOTAX Study. J Clin Oncol 2008;26:5269–74.

58. Schlemmer M, Reichardt P, Verweij J, et al. Paclitaxel in patients with advanced angiosarcomas of soft tissue: a retrospective study of the EORTC soft tissue and bone sarcoma group. Eur J Cancer 2008;44:2433–6.

59. Skubitz KM, Haddad PA. Paclitaxel and pegylated-liposomal doxorubicin are both active in angiosarcoma. Cancer 2005;104:361–6.

60. Vorburger SA, Xing Y, Hunt KK, et al. Angiosarcoma of the breast. Cancer 2005;104:2682–8.

61. Oxenberg J, Khushalani NI, Salerno KE, et al. Neoadjuvant chemotherapy for primary cutaneous/soft tissue angiosarcoma: determining tumor behavior prior to surgical resection. J Surg Oncol 2015;111:829–33.

62. Pandey M, Mathew A, Abraham EK, et al. Primary sarcoma of the breast. J Surg Oncol 2004;87:121–5.

63. Guo T, Zhang L, Chang NE, et al. Consistent MYC and FLT4 gene amplification in radiation-induced angiosarcoma but not in other radiation-associated atypical vascular lesions. Genes Chromosomes Cancer 2011;50:25–33.

Management of Gastrointestinal Stromal Tumors

Margaret von Mehren, MD

KEYWORDS

- GIST • KIT • PDGFRA • SDH-deficient GIST • Tyrosine kinase inhibitors
- Adjuvant therapy • Neoadjuvant therapy • Metastasectomy

KEY POINTS

- Gastrointestinal stromal tumors are malignant mesenchymal tumors of the intestinal tract that have varied behavior based on the molecular underpinnings of an individual tumor.
- Resection is the primary therapy for primary disease, with decisions on the type of surgery and need for neoadjuvant therapy influenced by tumor size, location, and molecular profile.
- Adjuvant therapy with imatinib therapy is indicated for tumors of high risk for recurrence.
- The role of resection in advanced disease is evolving but has been shown to be safe and seems to provide some benefit in progression-free survival in selected patients.

INTRODUCTION

Gastrointestinal stromal tumors (GISTs), once known as gastrointestinal (GI) leiomyosarcomas, represent 1% of GI malignancies with an incidence of 0.32 per 100,000 in the United States.[1] They had the reputation for poor outcomes because of their lack of response to interventions other than surgery. The discovery of gain-of-function mutations involving the receptor tyrosine kinases (RTKs) *KIT* or platelet-derived growth factor alpha (*PDGFRA*)[2,3] significantly altered the biological understanding and management of this disease. Beginning in 2000, advances in the management of these tumors occurred with the availability of tyrosine kinase inhibitors (TKIs), including imatinib, sunitinib, and regorafenib. With the availability of systemic therapy has come increased understanding about the disease and those cases that require therapy and those that do not. This article reviews the role of surgery and systemic therapy based on a broad definition of risk, including risk of recurrence but also risk of lack of response. Decisions on how to treat an individual patient is based on the

Disclosure Statement: The author has served as a paid consultant in the past to Norvatis and Pfizer; The author do not currently have any relationships to disclose.
Department of Hematology/Oncology, Fox Chase Cancer Center, C-218, 333 Cottman Avenue, Philadelphia, PA 19111, USA
E-mail address: Margaret.vonmehren@fccc.edu

stage of disease and pathologic characteristics, including the mutation status of the tumor, which has implications on prognosis.

MOLECULAR PATHOLOGIC CHARACTERISTICS OF GASTROINTESTINAL STROMAL TUMOR

GISTs, when viewed from the perspective of genetic changes, are relatively simple tumors. They have karyotypes with few genetic changes, particularly a subset of tumors that arise in the stomach.[4] Hirota and colleagues[5] were the first to identify that these tumors are driven by activating mutations in *KIT*. Since their discovery, it has become clear that most tumors contain mutations in *KIT* (85%) with an additional 5% to 10% having mutations in *PDGFRA*.[6] Mutations in *KIT* are found most commonly found in exon 11, followed by exons 9, 13, and 17, with rare reports of tumors in exon 14. *PDGFRA* mutations are found in exons 12 and 18, which are homologous with *KIT* exons 11 and 17. Rare cases of GIST, typically arising in the small bowel, have been associated with mutations in B-RAF or N-RAS.[6] GIST can be associated with neurofibromatosis in which, in addition to their *NF-1* mutation, the tumors can but do not always have typical *KIT* or *PDGFRA* mutations.[6,7]

More recently, gastric GIST without *KIT* or *PDGFRA* mutations, often arising in the stomach, have been recognized to contain defects in the Krebs cycle family of enzymes known as succinate dehydrogenase (SDH), either as a result of mutation or altered gene methylation. These tumors, formerly known as wild-type GIST, are now termed SDH-deficient GIST.[7,8]

PATHOLOGIC CHARACTERISTICS OF GASTROINTESTINAL STROMAL TUMOR

GISTs can develop anywhere along the GI tract. Although they can arise in any portion of the gut wall, most often they are found in the submucosa or muscularis propria. Typically, GISTs are well circumscribed with overlying mucosa intact but can be multinodular or ulcerated. Microscopically, tumors appear to have spindle cells, epithelioid cells, or a combination, with the epithelioid phenotype common in the stomach but not elsewhere.[9] Assessment of the number of mitoses per 50 high-power fields (HPF) is a critical component of pathologic assessment because it has implications for tumor prognosis.[10,11]

Immunohistochemistry

The most useful immunohistochemistry tests for GIST are CD117, DOG-1, and CD34. Ninety percent to 95% of GIST from all sites show strong cytoplasmic CD117 staining,[10,12] whereas CD34 stains up to 70% of spindle cell and epithelioid GISTs, especially colorectal and esophageal primaries. The DOG1 marker is particularly useful in tumors that histologically appear to be GIST but are negative for CD117.[13–15] A tumor that stains positive for desmin should be assessed closely because the most GISTs do not express this marker and the tumor likely represents another entity.

More recently, staining for succinate dehydrogenase B (SDHB) has been identified as useful in the assessment of gastric tumors.[7] Loss of SDHB staining is correlated with tumors that lack the common activating mutations in *KIT* or *PDGFRA*. These tumors contain mutations in the genes for the SDH family of proteins or alterations in methylation that result in deficiencies in SDHB production.[8,16] With loss of SDH, there is an accumulation of succinate that inhibits alpha-ketoglutarate-dependent dioxygenase enzymes and ultimately leads to a reduction of 5-hydroxymehtyl cytosine, which is required for DNA-demethylation.[17]

Molecular Pathologic Features

GISTs were first recognized to be driven by a mutation in *KIT* but it is now clear that tumors can contain mutations in other genes, including *PDGFRA, B-RAF, NF-1* and the *SDH* family of enzymes. There is some correlation with mutation and the primary location of a GIST. In addition, knowing the mutation of a tumor has implications for prognosis, response to TKIs, and the potential need for genetic testing. Studies have suggested that for those SDHB-deficient tumors that do not contain mutations in SDH family genes, the oncologic driver of malignancy is altered methylation affecting the transcription of genes. **Table 1** summarizes pathologic features and associations with GIST diagnosis, prognosis, and response to therapy.

Micro–Gastrointestinal Stromal Tumor

Increasingly, with the use of endoscopic ultrasound, small asymptomatic GISTs are being identified in the wall of the stomach. Importantly, it seems that as humans age, GIST may become the most common neoplasm found in the stomach but most are less than 1 cm in size. Micro-GISTS described by Scherubl and colleagues[18] are often identified on endoscopic ultrasound examination as submucosal protrusions. They differ from GISTs in that become clinically relevant because their rate of proliferation is very low and they have a different spectrum of KIT mutations than seen in larger tumors. For example, the rate of exon 11 mutations is lower than seen in series of larger tumors, as well as unique KIT and PDGFRA mutations not reported in clinically relevant GIST.[19] There is no report to date of progression of these small tumors.[20]

Table 1		
Associations with molecular pathologic features		
Pathologic Marker		**Associations**
IHC	KIT	Positive in most tumors, exception may be *PDGFRA*-mutated GIST
	DOG-1	Positive in almost all tumors
	Loss of SDHB staining	Loss seen in tumors with mutations in SDH family of enzyme genes or with altered methylation; associated with gastric primaries and more indolent behavior
		GIST may be part of the Carney triad or Carney-Stratakis dyad
		Limited response to imatinib but better disease control with VEGFR targeting TKIs
Mutations	*KIT*	Exon 11: best and longest duration of response with imatinib in advanced disease
		Exon 9: shorter duration of response with imatinib and overall poorer survival in advanced disease; most commonly in small bowel GIST
	PDGFRA	Similar response and outcomes as *KIT* mutations with the exception of *PDGFRA* D842V that has very limited response to standard kinase therapy; most commonly in gastric GIST
	SDH family of enzymes	Referral for genetic counseling to assess for Carney-Stratakis dyad
	NF-1	GIST can also contain a *KIT* or *PDGFRA* mutation
		May present with multifocal small volume disease, often indolent in nature
		Referral to genetic counseling if not previously known to be NF-1 carrier
	B-RAF, N-RAS	Very rare, usually of small bowel location

MANAGEMENT OF PRIMARY GASTROINTESTINAL STROMAL TUMOR
Clinical Presentation

Patients may present with symptoms, including abdominal pain, early satiety, anemia, or other signs of GI bleeding, leading to an evaluation. Other times, patients are identified with a mass in the stomach or elsewhere along the intestinal tract incidentally during an endoscopic examination or abdominal pelvic imaging. Biopsy of the mass is not required before resection unless preoperative therapy is indicated. Because tumors may be friable and bleed, endoscopic approaches are encouraged. Infrequently, patients may present with an acute abdomen following perforation of the GIST and should be managed as other intra-abdominal emergencies. Imaging of the abdomen and pelvis with computer-assisted tomography with contrast or MRI with and without contrast is appropriate. If the diagnosis of GIST is known, chest and bone imaging should be performed based on patient symptoms. Untreated GISTs are typically well visualized on 18F-fluorodeoxyglucose (FDG)-PET imaging. Typically, limited additional information is provided and should not be used routinely.

There are some presentations that are unique and associated with specific subtypes of GIST. The Carney triad, first reported in 1983, contains GIST most commonly arising in the stomach, functioning extra-adrenal paraganglioma, and pulmonary chondromas.[21] More recently, esophageal leiomyomas and adrenal cortical adenomas have been added as components of the syndrome.[22,23] Patients with this presentation are commonly diagnosed before the age of 30 years and are predominantly female. These tumors are SDHB-negative and represent tumors associated with altered methylation, previously described. The Carney-Stratakis dyad includes GIST and paragangliomas, again arising in younger patients with stomach primaries predominating. These tumors also are SDHB-deficient but have been found to contain mutations in SDH family members that are inherited and thus are a group of patients that require referral for genetic counseling and possible testing because of the risk of malignant multifocal paragangliomas, which can be screened for by MRI.[24]

Surgery

Surgery remains the gold standard for the management of primary disease. GIST can be friable and surgery should be performed, avoiding violating the tumor pseudocapsule or causing tumor rupture. A primary gastric GIST should be resected by wedge resection or larger resection obtaining a 1 to 2 cm margin, whereas small bowel tumor resections require segmental resections. Tumors of the rectum require different approaches based on the location. Those in the upper rectum will require a low anterior resection, whereas those in the lower third can be addressed by a full-thickness transanal resection, understanding that there is a greater risk for a resected margin (R) that is not R0 and for higher recurrence rates,[24–26] which, with the use of adjuvant and/or neoadjuvant therapy, have been shown to provide effective disease control (see later discussion).

Surgical resection maybe performed using laparoscopic approaches. Retrospective reports in the literature summarize not only on the safety of this approach but also report low recurrence rates, short inpatient hospital stays, and low morbidity.[27–32] Most reports describe this approach for gastric primaries that are 8 cm or less, although there are also limited data on small bowel tumors (**Table 2**). Long-term outcomes seem to be comparable to open surgical procedures, with shorter postoperative recovery. As with other laparoscopic resections for cancer, the use of a protective plastic bag to remove tumors and minimize the risk of port site recurrence is required.

Author	Subjects (Number)	Size	Location	Outcome
Novitsky et al,[29] 2006	50	1.0–8.5	Gastric	100% negative margins (2 cm-45 mm) at 36 mo follow-up, 92% NED
Otani et al, [30] 2006	35	2–5 cm	Gastric	No recurrences in tumors 4 cm or less
Nishimura et al,[31] 2007	39	—	Gastric	No difference in outcomes to open resections (n = 28)
Nakamori et al,[32] 2008	56	2–5 cm	Gastric	Retrospective review: open (66%) vs laparoscopic surgery (44%)
Nguyen et al,[33] 2006	43	Mean size: 4.6 (gastric) 3.5 cm (small bowel)	Gastric and small bowel	Retrospective review noting feasibility and safety

Table 2
Laparoscopic surgery

For larger tumors, open procedures may be more appropriate with consideration of neoadjuvant therapy.

Unlike other GI carcinomas, the role of lymphadenectomy is very limited. The risk of lymph node involvement by GIST is very low at presentation. Exceptions to this are the SDH-deficient tumors that often may present with a gastric mass and lymphadenopathy. This clinical scenario is associated with limited response to standard agents and frequent recurrences but often an indolent natural history with long-term survivors. Therefore, the surgical approach with this group of patients, often female presenting in the pediatric age group, with gastric primaries should be measured with the goal of controlling lesions that are causing bleeding or other difficulties, yet avoiding drastic approaches such as total gastrectomy. The likelihood of recurrence may be as high as 70% following initial resection but, despite this, these patients have prolonged survivals. For those tumors lacking KIT and PDGFRA mutations found in the small bowel or esophagus, complete resection of disease should be performed.[34]

Although the goal of surgery should always be to aim for an R0 resection, a recent analysis assessed the impact of positive margins from the adjuvant therapy trials.[35] This retrospective study included a review of pathologic findings and operative reports from 819 subjects who underwent surgical resection before enrollment on to the American College of Surgical Oncology Group (ACOSOG) adjuvant studies (Z9000 and Z9001). R1 resections were associated with larger tumor size (>10 cm), rectal primaries, and tumor rupture. In this analysis, 9% of subjects enrolled in these studies had an R1 resection and there was no significant difference in recurrence-free survival (RFS) irrespective of adjuvant therapy. This finding may suggest that outcome is depends more on inherent biological differences rather tumor resection status. Z9001, in particular, included subjects whose risk of recurrence would not currently lead to the use of adjuvant therapy. Alternatively, given that these trials gave imatinib for 1 year, the lack of difference in outcome may be a reflection of the length of adjuvant therapy. This seems less likely because the greatest impact of adjuvant therapy in Z9001 was noted for tumors with the highest risk of recurrence based on size and mitotic count.

Neoadjuvant Therapy

Given the efficacy of TKIs and minimal side effects, consideration of preoperative therapy is reasonable. The Radiation Therapy Oncology Group (RTOG) 0512 with the American College of Radiology Imaging Network (ACRIN) 6665 prospectively demonstrated the safety of this approach with minimal increase in surgical morbidity.[36] In a retrospective analysis of rectal GIST treated with neoadjuvant therapy, median tumor size decreased by 54%, with approximately 80% of those undergoing resection achieving sphincter preservation.[37] Patients should be selected for neoadjuvant approach carefully. Preoperative biopsies are often small and provide only limited diagnostic pathologic material. The assessment of mitoses per 50 HPF, an important prognostic criterion, is limited in a small sample and may not reflect the entirety of the tumor. In addition, in the setting of a good treatment response, the final tumor specimen will be altered and no longer provide prognostic information. Thus the risk of morbidity from a large resection should be balanced against the likelihood of giving prolonged adjuvant therapy to a patient with limited information on the tumor biology and risk of recurrence. Neoadjuvant therapy is, therefore, recommended for those situations in which resection of the primary tumor would result in a morbid procedure, such as a Whipple procedure, or for primary tumors of the rectum.

Adjuvant Therapy

Before the age of targeted therapy, it was evident that not all primary GIST resections were curative. A series from Memorial Sloan Kettering documented a 40% recurrence rate in 80 subjects who underwent resection, with a median follow-up of 2 years.[38] Adjuvant therapy has been studied and demonstrated to have benefit in several studies (**Table 3**).[38–44] To date, all studies have used imatinib at 400 mg daily irrespective of mutation status of the tumor. Studies have assessed treatment lasting for 12, 24, and 36 months and primarily have assessed RFS as their endpoint. The trial that did not was the European Organisation for Research and Treatment of Cancer (EORTC) trial that initially had overall survival as the primary endpoint. With ongoing experience, it became clear that many years of follow-up would be required to determine this endpoint. Therefore this study changed its primary endpoint to the time at which a subject became refractory to imatinib therapy.

These adjuvant trials have been analyzed for factors associated with benefit from therapy, as well as factors associated with recurrence. As demonstrated by Z9001,[45] which enrolled any resected GIST larger than 3 cm in size, the larger the tumors the greater the benefit of therapy. Other risk features also associated with an increased benefit from adjuvant treatment were small bowel primaries and tumors with mitoses greater than 5 per 50 HPF. Similar factors were identified in the analysis of the Scandinavian Sarcoma Group (SSG) XVIII trial, which included tumor rupture as an additional factor associated with recurrence in subjects receiving adjuvant imatinib.[46]

Assessment of Risk for Recurrence

Systematic analyses have been performed by various groups, which have all recognized the following as predictive of recurrence or metastatic: tumor location, size, and mitotic rate.[10,11,47,48] The initial National Institutes of Health (NIH) consensus classification system focused on the size of tumors and the mitotic rate, and was relatively simple to use.[10] Miettinen[11] further refined this classification system, noting the importance of tumor location for risk of recurrence.[11] Features that impart an improved

Table 3
Adjuvant therapy trials

Study	Criteria	Design	Primary Endpoint	Outcome	Reference
Z9000	Any of the following: 1. Tumor ≥10 cm 2. Rupture/hemorrhage 3. Multiple tumors (<5) Complete resection	Phase II open-label treatment with imatinib 400 mg daily for 12 mo	RFS	RFS at 1, 3, and 5 y is 96, 60% and 40%	DeMatteo et al,[39] 2013
Z9001	Tumor ≥3 cm complete resection	Phase III placebo-controlled double-blind study of 12 mo of adjuvant therapy	RFS	Improved RFS of 98% vs 83% with median follow-up of 19.7 mo	DeMatteo et al,[40] 2009
China Gastrointestinal Cooperative Group	Any of the following: 1. Tumor >5 cm 2. Mitotic rate >5/50 HPF	Phase II, adjuvant imatinib for 12 mo	RFS	Limited follow-up; 2 patients relapsed at 350 and 680 d postresection	Zhan et al,[41] 2007
SSGXVIII	>10.0 cm, >10 mitoses/50 HPF, >5 cm and >5 mitoses/50 HPF, or tumor rupture	Open-label randomized trial of 3 y vs 1 y adjuvant imatinib	RFS	5 y RFS: 65.5% vs 47.9%, HR 0.46 in favor of 3 y of therapy	Joensuu et al,[42] 2012
EORTC 62024	Any of the following: 1. Tumor >5 cm 2. Mitotic rate >10 3. Tumor <5 cm + mitotic count 6–10/50 HPF Complete resection	Phase III randomized trial of imatinib for 24 mo vs observation	Time to second-line therapy	Confirmed benefit of imatinib in RFS; Trend towards improved time to second line therapy in high risk patients	Casali et al,[43] 2015
Korea	Any of the following: 1. Tumor >5 cm + mitotic count >5/50 HPF 2. Tumor >10 cm 3. Mitotic count >10/50 HPF complete resection	Phase II open-label study of adjuvant imatinib for 24 mo	RFS	RFS 58.9 mo	Kang et al,[44] 2013
CSIT571BUS282	Any of the following: 1. Tumor ≥2 cm + mitotic count ≥5/50 HPF 2. Any nongastric tumor ≥5 cm Complete resection	Phase II open-label study of adjuvant imatinib for 60 mo	RFS	Study completed, not reported	

prognosis include gastric origin, size smaller than 5 cm, and a mitotic count of less than 5 per 50 HPF. More recently, tumor rupture at the time of initial resection has also been noted as a very important feature.[48] **Table 4** provides references and resources for predicting risk of recurrence. Two predictive tools developed more recently are the GIST nomogram that provides information on the likelihood of being free of recurrence at 2 and 5 years. This Web-based program is very easy to use; however, as with the NIH consensus and Miettinen classification systems, size of tumors and mitotic counts are primarily dichotomous variables; that is, size is either smaller or larger than 2 cm or 5 cm and mitotic count is less than 5 or 5 or more mitoses per 50 HPF. The prognostic contour maps, developed by Joensuu and colleagues,[47] provide information for individual patients using all known prognostic factors with greater granularity.[47] It allows for incorporation of discreet information about tumor size and mitotic rate, in addition to information on tumor rupture. To date, tumor mutations have not been incorporated into these modes. There are data to suggest that mitotic rate may be less predictive of aggressive biology in SDH-deficient tumors,[33] and some *KIT* exon 11 mutations have a greater risk of recurrence compared with other exon 11 alterations (Spanish Group for Sarcoma Research [GEIS]).[50]

Recommendations for adjuvant therapy should be based on the available data and only recommended to patients with high-risk GIST. Typically, this represents a patient with a large gastric tumor with high mitotic rate, or a patient whose tumor areas in other parts of the GI tract that have a high mitotic rate and/or is large. Using predictive tools, the risk should be greater than 20%. In the United States, a minimum of 3 years of therapy is considered standard. Results from the nonrandomized, phase II, trial of imatinib for 5 years will determine if prolonged therapy provides additional benefit in terms of progression-free survival and overall survival.

MANAGEMENT OF RECURRENT OR METASTATIC GASTROINTESTINAL STROMAL TUMOR
Systemic Therapy

Imatinib remains the gold standard for management of most patients that present with advanced GIST. Clinical trials have assessed response rates in advanced unresectable disease using a broad range of doses (**Table 5**).[51–56] Phase I and II trials demonstrated the safety and efficacy of doses up to 400 mg twice a day, with doses

Table 4
References and for predicting prognosis at presentation of primary gastrointestinal stromal tumor

Resource	Information provided	Reference
MSKCC Nomogram	Likelihood of being recurrence-free at 2 and 5 y postresection based on size, location and mitotic rate <5 or >5 mitoses/50HPF	49 https://www.mskcc.org/ nomograms/gastrointestinal
Joensuu Contour maps	10 y risk of recurrence based on size, location, number of mitoses and evidence of perforation	47
Miettinen criteria	Risk of metastatic potential following resection based on size, location and mitoses	11

Data from Refs.[11,47,49]

Table 5
Response rates to imatinib therapy at different doses

Dose	Complete Response (%)	Partial Response (%)	Stable Disease (%)	Progressive Disease (%)	Not Evaluable or Unknown (%)
400 mg daily	0–5	40–68.5	13.7–32	12–15.1	2.7–10
300 mg twice a day	2.7	64.9	17.6	8.1	6.8
400 mg twice a day	3–6	42–48	22–32	10–9	5–15
500 mg twice a day	0	57	29	14	0

higher than that associated with excess toxicity, particularly nausea, vomiting, and edema. The 2 large randomized phase III trials of imatinib were conducted testing imatinib at 400 mg daily compared with 400 mg twice daily. Meta-analysis of these 2 trials documented that lower dose therapy is as an effective therapy for patients with GIST as the higher dose treatment, with the exception of tumors with exon 9 mutations in which progression-free survival was longer in those receiving higher dose therapy.[57] Overall survival for both groups was similar because the study allowed for crossover to the higher dose arm at the time of disease progression. These studies demonstrated a 5-year overall survival, which was a significant improvement in subject outcomes compared with the 12 months noted in subjects treated with surgery when no other effective therapy was available. Factors associated with long-term disease control have been reported and include female gender, tumors with KIT exon 11 mutations, and normal neutrophil counts and albumin levels at baseline.[58] Long-term follow-up has demonstrated that 18% of subjects enrolled in the initial phase II trial of imatinib remain without disease progression on therapy at 9.4 years median follow-up.[59]

Pathologic variables can be determinants of outcome. Although histologic and immunophenotypic factors have not been correlated with outcome, there is a correlation with the tumor mutations status. Progression-free survival and overall survival are prolonged in tumors carrying an KIT exon 11 mutation, whereas those with KIT exon 9 mutations have shorter progression-free survival. An initial report had suggested that tumors without KIT or PDGFRA mutations had the poorest outcomes on imatinib but subsequent larger phase III studies no longer found this correlation.[60,61] It should be noted that in these studies tumors have not been reassessed for absence of SDHB expression, mutations in SDH enzymes or mutations in alternative kinases. The randomized phase III studies did suggest that the only populations of patients that require higher dose therapy are those with KIT exon 9 mutations, patients treated at 400 mg experienced a shorter progression-free survival. Retrospective data on response and disease control in patients whose tumors have mutations in PDGFRA D842V suggest that response is minimal and progression-free survival is short; there is currently no clear role for treatment with imatinib in this subgroup of GIST.[62]

Therapy Beyond Imatinib

Sunitinib and regorafenib are both approved for the management of GIST following progression on prior TKIs. Both sunitinib and regorafenib are multitargeted TKIs with activity against KIT, PDGFR, vascular endothelial growth factor (VEGFR) 1 to 3, and Fms-related tyrosine kinase (FLT)-3. The initial development of sunitinib was based on phase 1 studies that tested several doses and schedules to identify a maximum tolerated dose of 50 mg orally for 28 days followed by 14 days of rest, which was instituted to manage toxicities.[63] Response data in the early trials and the placebo-controlled, phase III trial demonstrated limited response rates with only partial response seen in 7% to 13% of subjects.[63–65] In addition, the phase I and II trials of sunitinib used PET scans that demonstrated rapid metabolic response during the 4 weeks of treatment but recurrence of metabolic activity during the 2-week washout. In addition, some subjects experienced symptoms of disease during the 2-week treatment break. A phase II trial tested the feasibility and efficacy of continuous daily dosing starting at 37.5 mg daily.[64] The study demonstrated the safety and tolerability of this approach, as well as similar response rates to prior studies, and has become the preferred regimen for many practitioners.

Responses and clinical benefit were observed more frequently in subjects with mutations that are less sensitive to imatinib such as *KIT* exon 9, wild-type *KIT*, compared with those with exon 11 mutations.[65,66] Time to progression was longest for subjects whose tumors contained a *KIT* exon 9 mutation, followed by wild-type, exon 11, and worst for a tumor with both an exon 11 mutation and a new mutation. Subjects with *KIT* exon 9 and wild-type mutations had the best overall survival. This does not suggest that sunitinib is inactive in exon 11 tumors; rather, it represents that subjects with exon 11 mutations who have progressed on imatinib have developed resistance and, typically, have clones with additional mutations. Further study has shown that secondary mutations involving *KIT* exons 13 or 14 are sensitive to sunitinib, whereas those with exon 17 and 18 secondary mutations tend to be resistant to sunitinib. Regorafenib, the most recently approved agent, is also a multikinase inhibitor that has meaningful activity KIT, PDGFRA, RET, RAF1, BRAF, VEGFR 1 to 3, TEK, and FGFR.[67] An initial phase II trial in advanced GIST that had progressed on at least imatinib and sunitinib demonstrated partial response in 12% and stable disease for longer than 16 weeks in 65% of subjects.[68] Most subjects had tumors with primary exon 11 mutations (56%), with the next most common subgroup being those without identifiable mutations in KIT or PDGFRA (24%). This study suggested that subjects with primary exon 11 mutations benefited more from regorafenib than those with primary exon 9 mutations, although the sample size for the latter group was very small. In the phase III international GRID trial, progression-free survival in subjects receiving regorafenib was compared with those receiving placebo.[67] Subjects on regorafenib received therapy for a median duration of 20.2 weeks compared with those on placebo who were on treatment for a median of 7 weeks. There was a statistically significant improvement in median progression-free survival of 4.8 months compared with 0.9 months on regorafenib compared with placebo. The partial response rate was 4.5%, with no complete responses observed. Disease control at 12 weeks was 52.6% with regorafenib compared with 9.1% with placebo. Overall survival did not differ in the arms because crossover was allowed from placebo to regorafenib at the time of disease progression. When comparing baseline characteristics, the only factor that was associated with a shorter progression-free survival on regorafenib compared with other groups was subjects who progressed on imatinib in less than 6 months. In this larger study there was no difference between tumors whose primary mutations were in *KIT* exon 11 or exon 9.

Evaluation of benefit of these agents in specific GIST mutation subtypes has been less studied. Because most patients receiving sunitinib, and certainly regorafenib, have been previously treated, these tumors are found to contain additional genetic alterations. The primary changes noted have been secondary mutations in the *KIT* or *PDGFRA* gene. Studies from subjects undergoing surgical resection have demonstrated that there can be multiple different secondary mutations, thus the role of repeat biopsy to assess genetic changes is limited.[69,70] Some studies have begun to incorporate assessment of circulating DNA as a research tool.[71]

Surgical Metastasectomy

Before the availability of tyrosine kinase therapy, treatment of progressive disease was primarily surgical. Patients in whom complete resection was not feasible had very poor outcomes with a median survival of less than 12 months.[38] The initial benefits seen with imatinib in advanced disease lead some clinicians to minimize the role of surgery for the management of advanced disease. However, as patients' disease began to progress on therapy, and other therapies for advanced disease demonstrated more modest benefits, the role of surgery has again become part of management of advanced disease.

The current standard of care for frontline management of advanced disease is treatment with imatinib. There are, however, various clinical scenarios that suggest surgery as an alternative option or an adjunct to therapy. The first scenario involves patients with GIST resistant to imatinib, such as tumors with *PDGFRA* D842V mutations. Interestingly, although a large proportion of patients at diagnosis have primary GIST with *PDGFRA* mutations, few progress with metastatic disease.[61,72] Those with advanced disease and D842V mutations have limited benefit from imatinib.[62] Therefore, consideration of surgical resection of metastatic disease is appropriate. For those with less responsive disease, surgery versus expectant observation should be well considered, as previously discussed.

Another consideration is the role of surgery following stabilization or response to imatinib. The rationale for considering resection at this time are data from the initial phase II trial of imatinib in advanced disease, which identified that tumor bulk was correlated with progression-free survival.[59] The greater the bulk of disease present, the shorter the time to progression. This is hypothesized to be due to a decreased likelihood of imatinib-resistant clones emerging when there is a smaller tumor volume and resection of disease might lead to prolonged time to progression on imatinib and improved overall survival. Retrospective data has demonstrated prolonged overall survival in patients that achieve R0 or R1 resections with imatinib therapy compared with those only able to have R2 resections.[73] This question was asked in 2 prospective clinical trials, both of which closed due to poor accrual.

As therapy with TKIs evolved, resistance began to be observed. One form of resistance seen is localized progression; in particular, an increase in an enhancing nodule within a responding hypodense lesion is evidence of local progression.[74] Most patients develop TKI resistance within 2 years[55,56] with evidence of either focal or limited disease growth or generalized progression.[75,76] For patients who progress on imatinib, retrospective series have demonstrated that the benefit of surgical resection for the management of progressive disease is observed when surgery is done when they are continuing to have disease control with imatinib (partial response or stable disease) or have limited progression rather than generalized progression. This benefit was measured in greater numbers of subjects able to undergo R0 or R1 resections, as well as prolonged disease-free survival in subjects with responding or limited progression compared with those with generalized disease growth. At 1 year following surgery, progression-free survival rates for subjects whose disease was controlled by imatinib was 70% to 96%, whereas only 0% to 14% of subjects who had generalized progression had lack of disease progression.[75–77] Importantly, at 1 year, overall survival was almost 100% in subjects with partial response or stable disease, or limited progression before resection compared with only 0% to 60% for those who had generalized progression.

Surgery for patients who have progressed beyond imatinib is more challenging given disease progression, as well as agents that are associated with inhibition of the VEGFR pathway, and may lead to complications in the perioperative period. Data from retrospective series of surgery for subjects on sunitinib are mixed regarding correlations between outcomes, including overall survival, and the status of the disease at the time of surgery.[78,79] The lack of correlation is most likely related to subject selection rather than to inherent differences in subjects undergoing surgery when having progression, be it focal or generalized, on sunitinib.

Focal Modalities for Management of Metastatic Disease

For disease in the liver, surgery, embolization with or without chemotherapy, cryotherapy, and radiofrequency ablation (RFA) were commonly used before the era of TKIs.[80–82] Radiation has also been reported to provide a symptomatic benefit for patients with pain or bleeding.[83] These modalities provide palliation in the areas treated in this manner. There were attempts at liver transplantation that were unsuccessful and this modality should not be considered.[84]

SUMMARY

GIST has been a paradigm for the use of targeted therapy for the management for a solid tumor. Resection still remains the mainstay of primary tumor management, with minimally invasive techniques used for smaller tumors. Risk-based adjuvant therapy for a minimum of 3 years is the standard of care in the United States. The initial impressive results with imatinib in the advanced setting raised the question regarding the ultimate role of surgery in this disease. Over the past 15 years, it has become appreciated that, although very effective, there continue to be recurrences after primary resection and a growing body of data to support that surgery plays an adjunctive role in advanced disease.

REFERENCES

1. Rubin JL, Sanon M, Taylor DC, et al. Epidemiology, survival, and costs of localized gastrointestinal stromal tumors. Int J Gen Med 2011;4:121–30.
2. Rubin BP, Singer S, Tsao C, et al. KIT activation is a ubiquitous feature of gastrointestinal stromal tumors. Cancer Res 2001;61(22):8118–21.
3. Heinrich MC, Corless CL, Duensing A, et al. PDGFRA activating mutations in gastrointestinal stromal tumors. Science 2003;299(5607):708–10.
4. Corless CL. PDGFRA mutations in gastrointestinal stromal tumors: frequency, spectrum and in vitro sensitivity to imatinib. J Clin Oncol 2005;23(23):5357–64.
5. Hirota S, Isozaki K, Moriyama Y, et al. Gain-of-function mutations of c-kit in human gastrointestinal stromal tumors. Science 1998;279(5350):577–80.
6. Miranda C, Nucifora M, Molinari F, et al. KRAS and BRAF mutations predict primary resistance to imatinib in gastrointestinal stromal tumors. Clin Cancer Res 2012;18(6):1769–76.
7. Janeway KA, Kim SY, Lodish M, et al. Defects in succinate dehydrogenase in gastrointestinal stromal tumors lacking KIT and PDGFRA mutations. Proc Natl Acad Sci U S A 2011;108(1):314–8.
8. Killian JK, Kim SY, Miettinen M, et al. Succinate dehydrogenase mutation underlies global epigenomic divergence in gastrointestinal stromal tumor. Cancer Discov 2013;3(6):648–57.
9. Yantiss RK, Rosenberg AE, Selig MK, et al. Gastrointestinal stromal tumors: an ultrastructural study. Int J Surg Pathol 2002;10(2):101–13.

10. Fletcher CD, Berman JJ, Corless C, et al. Diagnosis of gastrointestinal stromal tumors: a consensus approach. Hum Pathol 2002;33(5):459–65.

11. Miettinen M, Lasota J. Gastrointestinal stromal tumors: pathology and prognosis at different sites. Semin Diagn Pathol 2006;23(2):70–83.

12. Miettinen M, Sobin LH, Sarlomo-Rikala M. Immunohistochemical spectrum of GISTs at different sites and their differential diagnosis with a reference to CD117 (KIT). Mod Pathol 2000;13(10):1134–42.

13. Espinosa I, Lee CH, Kim MK, et al. A novel monoclonal antibody against DOG1 is a sensitive and specific marker for gastrointestinal stromal tumors. Am J Surg Pathol 2008;32:210–8.

14. Lopes LF, West RB, Bacchi LM, et al. DOG1 for the diagnosis of gastrointestinal stromal tumor (GIST): comparison between 2 different antibodies. Appl Immunohistochem Mol Morphol 2010;18:333–7.

15. Liegl B, Hornick JL, Corless CL, et al. Monoclonal antibody DOG1.1 shows higher sensitivity than KIT in the diagnosis of gastrointestinal stromal tumors, including unusual subtypes. Am J Surg Pathol 2009;33:437–46.

16. Belinsky MG, Skorobogatko YV, Rink L, et al. High density DNA array analysis reveals distinct genomic profiles in a subset of gastrointestinal stromal tumors. Genes Chromosomes Cancer 2013;52(2):214–24.

17. Mason EF, Hornick JL. Succinate dehydrogenase deficiency is associated with decreased 5-hydroxymethylcytosine production in gastrointestinal stromal tumors: implications for mechanisms of tumorigenesis. Mol Pathol 2013;26(11):1492–7.

18. Scherubl H, Faiss S, Knoefel WT, et al. Management of early asymptomatic gastrointestinal stromal tumors of the stomach. World J Gastrointest Endosc 2014;6(7):266–71.

19. Rossi S, Gasparotto D, Toffolatti L, et al. Molecular and clinicopathologic characterization of gastrointestinal stromal tumors (GISTs) of small size. Am J Surg Pathol 2010;34:1480–91.

20. Bennett JJ, Rubino MS. Gastrointestinal Stromal Tumors of the Stomach. Surg Oncol Clin N Am 2012;21:21–33.

21. Carney JA. The triad of gastric epithelioid leiomyosarcoma, pulmonary chondroma, and functioning extra-adrenal paraganglioma: a five-year review. Medicine (Baltimore) 1983;62(3):159–69.

22. Carney JA. Gastric stromal sarcoma, pulmonary chondroma, and extra-adrenal paraganglioma (Carney Triad): natural history, adrenocortical component, and possible familial occurrence. Mayo Clin Proc 1999;74(6):543–52.

23. Knop S, Schupp M, Wardelmann E, et al. A new case of Carney triad: gastrointestinal stromal tumours and leiomyoma of the oesophagus do not show activating mutations of KIT and platelet-derived growth factor receptor alpha. J Clin Pathol 2006;59(10):1097–9.

24. Jasperson KW, Kohlmann W, Gammon A, et al. Role of rapid sequence whole-body MRI screening in SDH-associated hereditary paraganglioma. Fam Cancer 2014;13(2):257–65.

25. Changchien CR, Wu MC, Tasi WS, et al. Evaluation of prognosis for malignant rectal gastrointestinal stromal tumor by clinical parameters and immunohistochemical staining. Dis Colon Rectum 2004;47(11):1922–9.

26. Hellan M, Maker VK. Transvaginal excision of a large rectal stromal tumor: an alternative. Am J Surg 2006;191(1):121–3.

27. Dong C, Jun-Hui C, Xiao-Jun Y, et al. Gastrointestinal stromal tumors of the rectum: clinical, pathologic, immunohistochemical characteristics and prognostic analysis. Scand J Gastroenterol 2007;42(10):1221–9.

28. Otani Y, Kitajima M. Laparoscopic surgery: too soon to decide. Gastric Cancer 2005;8:135–6.

29. Novitsky YW, Kercher KW, Sing RF, et al. Long-term outcomes of laparoscopic resection of gastric gastrointestinal stromal tumors. Ann Surg 2006;243(6): 738–45.

30. Otani Y, Furukawa T, Yoshida M, et al. Operative indications for relatively small (2–5 cm) gastrointestinal stromal tumor of the stomach based on analysis of 60 operated cases. Surgery 2006;139(4):484–92.

31. Nishimura J, Zheng ZC, Zhang JJ, et al. Surgical strategy for gastric gastrointestinal stromal tumors: laparoscopic versus open resection. Surg Endosc 2007; 21(6):875–8.

32. Nakamori M, Iwahashi M, Nakamura M, et al. Laparoscopic resection for gastrointestinal stromal tumors of the stomach. Am J Surg 2008;196(3):425–9.

33. Nguyen SQ, Divino CM, Wang JL, et al. Laparoscopic management of gastrointestinal stromal tumors. Surg Endosc 2006;20(5):713–6.

34. Pappo AS, Janeway K, Laquaglia M, et al. Special considerations in pediatric gastrointestinal tumors. J Surg Oncol 2011;104(8):928–32.

35. McCarter MD, Antonescu CR, Ballman KV, et al. Microscopically positive margins for primary gastrointestinal stromal tumors: analysis of risk factors and tumor recurrence. J Am Coll Surg 2012;215(1):53–9.

36. Eisenberg BL, Harris J, Blanke CD, et al. Phase II trial of neoadjuvant/adjuvant imatinib mesylate (IM) for advanced primary and metastatic/recurrent operable gastrointestinal stromal tumor (GIST): early results of RTOG 0132/ACRIN 6665. J Surg Oncol 2009;99(1):42–7.

37. Wilkinson MJ, Fitzgerald JE, Strauss DC, et al. Surgical treatment of gastrointestinal stromal tumour of the rectum in the era of imatinib. Br J Surg 2015;102(8): 965–71.

38. DeMatteo RP, Lewis JJ, Leung D, et al. Two hundred gastrointestinal stromal tumors: recurrence patterns and prognostic factors for survival. Ann Surg 2000; 231(1):51–8.

39. DeMatteo RP, Ballman KV, Antonescu CR, et al. Long term results of adjuvant imatinib mesylate in localized high-risk primary gastrointestinal stromal tumor (GIST): ACOSOG Z9000 (ALLIANCE) intergroup phase 2 trial. Ann Surg 2013; 258(3):322–429.

40. DeMatteo RP, Ballman KV, Antonescu CR, et al. Adjuvant imatinib mesylate after resection of localised, primary gastrointestinal stromal tumour: A randomised, double-blind, placebo-controlled trial. Lancet 2009;373:1097–104.

41. Zhan SW, Wang PZ, Shao YF, et al. Efficacy and safety of adjuvant post-surgical therapy with imatinib in patients with high risk of relapsing GIST. J Clin Oncol 2007;25(No 18S):10045.

42. Joensuu H, Eriksson M, Sundby Hall K, et al. One vs three years of adjuvant imatinib for operable gastrointestinal stromal tumor: a randomized trial. JAMA 2012; 307(12):1265–72.

43. Casali PG, Le Cesne A, Poveda Velasco A, et al. Time to Definitive Failure to the First Tyrosine Kinase Inhibitor in Localized GI Stromal Tumors Treated With Imatinib As an Adjuvant: A European Organisation for Research and Treatment of Cancer Soft Tissue and Bone Sarcoma Group Intergroup Randomized Trial in Collaboration With the Australasian Gastro-Intestinal Trials Group, UNICANCER,

French Sarcoma Group, Italian Sarcoma Group, and Spanish Group for Research on Sarcomas. J Clin Oncol 2015;33(36):4276–83.

44. Kang KY, Kang BW, Im SA, et al. Two-year adjuvant imatinib mesylate after complete resection of localized, high-risk GIST with KIT exon 11 mutation. Cancer Chemother Pharmacol 2013;71(1):43–51.

45. Coreless CW, Ballman KV, Antonescu CR, et al. Pathologic and molecular features correlate with long-term outcome after adjuvant therapy of resected primary GI stromal tumor: the ACOSOG Z9001 trial. J Clin Oncol 2014;32:1563–70.

46. Joensuu H, Eriksson M, Hall KS, et al. Risk factors for gastrointestinal stromal tumor recurrence in patients treated with adjuvant imatinib. Cancer 2014;120(15): 2325–33.

47. Joenssu H, Vehtari A, Riihimäki J, et al. Risk of recurrence of gastrointestinal stromal tumour after surgery: an analysis of pooled population-based cohorts. Lancet Oncol 2012;13(3):265–74.

48. Rutkowski P, Bylina E, Wozniak A, et al. Validation of the Joensuu risk criteria for primary resectable gastrointestinal stromal tumour - the impact of tumour rupture on patient outcomes. Eur J Surg Oncol 2011;37(10):890–6.

49. Gold JS, Gönen M, Gutiérrez A, et al. Development and validation of a prognostic nomogram for recurrence-free survival after complete surgical resection of localised primary gastrointestinal stromal tumour: a retrospective analysis. Lancet Oncol 2009;10(11):1045–52.

50. Martín J, Poveda A, Llombart-Bosch A, et al. Deletions affecting codons 557-558 of the c-KIT gene indicate a poor prognosis in patients with completely resected gastrointestinal stromal tumors: a study by the Spanish Group for Sarcoma Research (GEIS). J Clin Oncol 2005;23(25):6190–8.

51. Van Oosterom A, Judson I, Verweij J, et al. Safety and efficacy of imatinib (STI571) in meta-static gastrointestinal stromal tumours: a phase I study. Lancet 2001;358:1421–3.

52. Van Oosterom A, Judson IR, Verweij J, et al. Update of phase I study of imatinib (STI571) in advanced soft tissue sarcomas and gastrointestinal stromal tumors: a report of the EORTC Soft Tissue and Bone Sarcoma Group. Eur J Cancer 2002; 38(Suppl 5):S83–7.

53. Demetri G, von Mehren M, Blanke CD, et al. Efficacy and safety of imatinib mesylate in advanced gastrointestinal stromal tumors. N Engl J Med 2002;347: 472–80.

54. Verweij J, van Oosterom A, Blay JY, et al. Imatinib mesylate is an active agent for GIST but does not yield responses in other soft tissue sarcomas that are unselected for a molecular target. Eur J Cancer 2003;39:2006–11.

55. Verweij J, Casali PG, Zalcberg J, et al. Progression-free survival in gastrointestinal stromal tumours with high-dose imatinib: randomized trial. Lancet 2004; 364(9440):1127–34.

56. Blanke CD, Rankin C, Demetri GD, et al. Phase III randomized, intergroup trial assessing imatinib mesylate at two dose levels in patients with unresectable or metastatic gastrointestinal stromal tumors expressing the KIT receptor tyrosine kinase: S0033. J Clin Oncol 2008;26:620–5.

57. Gastrointestinal Stromal Tumor Meta-Analysis Group. Comparison of two doses of imatinib for the treatment of unresectable or metastatic gastrointestinal stromal tumors: a meta-analysis of 1,640 patients. J Clin Oncol 2010;28(7):1247–53.

58. Blanke CD, Demetri GD, von Mehren M, et al. Long-Term Results From a Randomized Phase II Trial of Standard- Versus Higher-Dose Imatinib Mesylate for

Patients With Unresectable or Metastatic Gastrointestinal Stromal Tumors Expressing KIT. J Clin Oncol 2009;28(4):620–5.

59. von Mehren M, Heinrich MC, Joensuu H, et al. Follow-up results after 9 years (yrs) of the ongoing, phase II B2222 trial of imatinib mesylate (IM) in patients (pts) with meta-static or unresectable KIT + gastrointestinal stromal tumors (GIST). J Clin Oncol 2011;29(Suppl) [abstract: 10016].

60. Heinrich MC, Corless CL, Blanke CD, et al. Molecular correlates of imatinib resistance in gastrointestinal stromal tumors. J Clin Oncol 2006;24(29):4764–74.

61. Heinrich MC, Owzar K, Corless CL, et al. Correlation of kinase genotype and clinical outcome in the North American Inter-Group Phase III Trial of imatinib mesylate for treatment of advanced GI stromal tumor (CALGB 150105). J Clin Oncol 2008;26(33):5352–9.

62. Cassier PA, Fumagalli E, Rutkowski P, et al. Outcome of patients with platelet-derived growth factor receptor alpha-mutated gastrointestinal stromal tumors in the tyrosine kinase inhibitor era. Clin Cancer Res 2012;18(16):4458–64.

63. Demetri DG, van Oosterom AT, Garrett CR, et al. Efficacy and safety of sunitinib in patients with advanced gastrointestinal stromal tumour after failure of imatinib: a randomized controlled trial. Lancet 2006;368(9544):1329–38.

64. George S, Blay JY, Casali PG, et al. Clinical evaluation of continuous daily dosing of sunitinib malate in patients with advanced gastrointestinal stromal tumour after imatinib failure. Eur J Cancer 2009;45(11):1959–68.

65. Heinrich MC, Maki RG, Corless CL, et al. Primary and secondary kinase genotypes correlate with the biological and clinical activity of sunitinib in imatinib-resistant gastrointestinal stromal tumor. J Clin Oncol 2008;26(33):5352–9.

66. Gajiwala KS, Wu JC, Christensen J, et al. KIT kinase mutants show unique mechanisms of drug resistance to imatinib and sunitinib in gastrointestinal stromal tumor patients. Proc Natl Acad Sci U S A 2009;106(5):1542–7.

67. Demetri G, Reichardt P, Kang YK, et al. Efficacy and safety of regorafenib for advanced gastrointestinal stromal tumours after failure of imatinib and sunitinib (GRID): an international, multicentre, randomised, placebo-controlled, phase 3 trial. Lancet 2013;381(9863):295–302.

68. George S, Wang Q, Heinrich MC, et al. Efficacy and safety of regorafenib in patients with metastatic and/or unresectable GI stromal tumor after failure of imatinib and sunitinib: a multicenter phase II trial. J Clin Oncol 2012;30(19):2401–7.

69. Antonescu CR, Besmer P, Guo T, et al. Acquired resistance to imatinib in gastrointestinal stromal tumor occurs through secondary gene mutation. Clin Cancer Res 2005;11:4182–90.

70. Wardelmann E, Thomas N, Merkelbach-Bruse S, et al. Acquired resistance to imatinib in gastrointestinal stromal tumours caused by multiple KIT mutations. Lancet Oncol 2005;6(4):249–51.

71. Demetri G, Jeffers M, Reichardt P, et al. Mutational analysis of plasma DNA from patients (pts) in the phase III GRID study of regorafenib (REG) versus placebo (PL) in tyrosine kinase inhibitor (TKI)-refractory GIST: Correlating genotype with clinical outcomes. J Clin Oncol 2013;31(No 15 Suppl):10503.

72. Coreless CL, Ballman KV, Antonescu CR, et al. Pathologic and molecular features correlate with long-term outcome after adjuvant therapy of resected primary GI stromal tumor: the ACOSOG Z9001 trial. J Clin Oncol 2014;32(15):1563–70.

73. Bauer S, Rutkowski P, Hohenberger P, et al. Long-term follow-up of patients with GIST undergoing metastasectomy in the era of imatinib – analysis of prognostic factors (EORTC-STBSG collaborative study). Eur J Surg Oncol 2014;40(4):412–9.

74. Choi H. Critical issues in response evaluation on computed tomography: lessons from the gastrointestinal stromal tumor model. Curr Oncol Rep 2005;7(4):307–11.
75. Raut CP, Posner M, Desai J, et al. Surgical management of advanced gastrointestinal stromal tumors after treatment with targeted systemic therapy using kinase inhibitors. J Clin Oncol 2006;24(15):2325–31.
76. DeMatteo RP, Maki RG, Singer S, et al. Results of tyrosine kinase inhibitor therapy followed by surgical resection for metastatic gastrointestinal stromal tumor. Ann Surg 2007;245(3):347–52.
77. Gronchi A, Fiore M, Miselli F, et al. Surgery of residual disease following molecular-targeted therapy with imatinib mesylate in advanced/metastatic GIST. Ann Surg 2007;245(3):341–6.
78. Raut CP, Wang Q, Manola J, et al. Cytoreductive surgery in patients with metastatic gastrointestinal stromal tumor treated with sunitinib malate. Ann Surg Oncol 2010;17(2):407–15.
79. Tielen R, Verhoef C, van Coevorden F, et al. Surgery after treatment with imatinib and/or sunitinib in patients with metastasized gastrointestinal stromal tumors: is it worthwhile? World J Surg Oncol 2012;10:111.
80. Rajan DK, Soulen MC, Clark TW, et al. Sarcomas metastatic to the liver: response and survival after cisplatin, doxorubicin, mitomycin-C, ethiodol, and polyvinyl alcohol chemoembolization. J Vasc Interv Radiol 2001;12(2):187–93.
81. Mavligit GM, Zukwiski AA, Ellis LM, et al. Gastrointestinal leiomyosarcoma metastatic to the liver. Durable tumor regression by hepatic chemoembolization infusion with cisplatin and vinblastine. Cancer 1995;75(8):2083–8.
82. Pawlik TM, Vauthey JN, Abdalla EK, et al. Results of a single-center experience with resection and ablation for sarcoma metastatic to the liver. Arch Surg 2006;141(6):537–43.
83. Joensuu H, Eriksson M, Collan J, et al. Radiotherapy for GIST progressing during or after tyrosine kinase inhibitor therapy: A prospective study. Radiother Oncol 2015;116(2):233–8.
84. Seralta AS, Sanjuan FR, Moya AH, et al. Combined liver transplantation plus imatinib for unresectable metastases of gastrointestinal stromal tumours. Eur J Gastroenterol Hepatol 2004;16(11):1237–9.

Management of Bone Sarcoma

Christina J. Gutowski, MD[a], Atrayee Basu-Mallick, MD[b], John A. Abraham, MD[c,d,*]

KEYWORDS

- Bone sarcoma • Osteosarcoma • Ewing sarcoma • Chondrosarcoma
- Endoprosthetic reconstruction

KEY POINTS

- Advancements in chemotherapy have been the primary reason for improvements in survival from bone sarcoma in the past 20 years.
- There are currently no chemotherapy agents effective against conventional chondrosarcoma.
- Local recurrence of bone sarcoma is likely related to aggressive tumor biology, but relationship with survival is not fully understood.
- Multiple methods of reconstruction after bone sarcoma resection are available, each with its own benefits and drawbacks.
- Emerging technologies, such as computer-aided surgery, improved imaging, and improved implant design, have potential to improve results of treatment even further in the future.

INTRODUCTION
Incidence and Epidemiology

Bone sarcomas account for approximately 0.2% of new cancer cases in the United States each year. The vast majority of these are either osteosarcoma, Ewing sarcoma, or chondrosarcoma. In 2016, it is estimated that 3300 new cases will be diagnosed; this incidence has been rising on average 0.4% annually over the past decade.[1] More than 27% of new diagnoses are made in patients younger than 20 years; osteosarcoma specifically is reported to be the third most common cancer in adolescence, and eighth

We have no funding sources, or commercial/financial conflicts of interest to disclose.
[a] Department of Orthopedic Surgery, Sidney Kimmel Medical College at Thomas Jefferson University, 1025 Walnut Street, Room 516 College, Philadelphia, PA 19107, USA; [b] Department of Medical Oncology, Sarcoma and Bone Tumor Center at Sidney Kimmel Cancer Center, Thomas Jefferson University Hospital, 1025 Walnut Street, Suite 700, Philadelphia, PA 19107; [c] Department of Orthopedic Surgery, Rothman Institute at Jefferson University Hospital, 925 Chestnut Street, Philadelphia, PA 19107, USA; [d] Department of Surgical Oncology, Fox Chase Cancer Center, 333 Cottman Ave, Philadelphia, PA 19111, USA
* Corresponding author.
E-mail address: john.abraham@rothmaninstitute.com

Surg Clin N Am 96 (2016) 1077–1106
http://dx.doi.org/10.1016/j.suc.2016.06.002
0039-6109/16/$ – see front matter © 2016 Elsevier Inc. All rights reserved.

surgical.theclinics.com

most common cancer in children overall.[2] Unlike osteosarcoma and Ewing sarcoma, which peak in adolescent age groups, chondrosarcoma incidence increases with age.[3]

It is estimated that 1490 patients will die of bone sarcoma in 2016, representing 0.3% of all cancer deaths.[1] For osteosarcoma, the implementation of multimodal treatment with chemotherapy and surgery has led to a considerable improvement in overall survival, but since that time, survival rates have remained relatively stable. In 2015, cause-specific 10-year survival for patients with localized disease at the time of osteosarcoma diagnosis was 65.8%.[4] Metastatic disease at presentation, which is seen in approximately 24% of patients, lowers this survival rate to 24%.[4,5] Despite improvement in survival of localized disease with modern management, patients with recurrence or metastasis after initial treatment is still associated with a poor prognosis.

Pretreatment Evaluation and Staging

The goal of the preoperative evaluation is to determine the extent of the disease, and allow for optimum treatment planning. Local imaging usually includes orthogonal plain radiographs and MRI of the affected area (**Figs. 1** and **2**). Computed tomography (CT) scan may be helpful in identifying cortical involvement. Imaging of the entire affected bone should be included to identify any skip metastases, the presence of which worsens prognosis.[6]

Evaluation of distant disease is done by using chest CT scan to evaluate for pulmonary metastasis, and Technicium-99 whole-body bone scan and/or PET with fludeoxyglucose F 18 (F[18]-FDG PET)/CT to evaluate for bony metastases[7,8] (**Fig. 3**). Recent studies have demonstrated that PET/CT is more sensitive than bone scan for detecting metastatic bone lesions, while specificity and diagnostic accuracy were similar. The combination of bone scan and PET/CT provides the highest sensitivity, specificity, and diagnostic accuracy, but this must be balanced with the additional cost. PET/CT scan may have the additional benefit of demonstrating correlation with the aggressiveness of a bone lesion, although is not completely reliable for this purpose.[9,10]

Once biopsy is completed, various staging systems exist. The American Joint Committee on Cancer (AJCC) is most commonly used. For bone sarcoma specifically, an alternative system frequently used is the Musculoskeletal Tumor Society (MSTS) system, described by Enneking in 1980[11] (**Tables 1** and **2**).

Biopsy

When performed appropriately, diagnostic accuracy of surgical incisional biopsy has been shown to be 98%,[12] and as such, surgical biopsy is the preferred method of

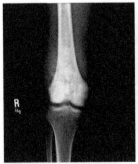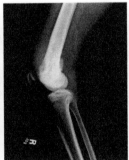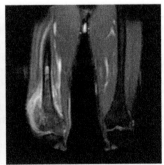

Fig. 1. Orthogonal radiographs and coronal short tau inversion recovery (STIR) MRI scan of conventional osteosarcoma of the right distal femur.

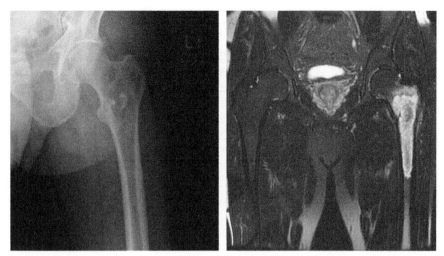

Fig. 2. Anteroposterior radiograph and coronal STIR MRI scan of chondrosarcoma of the left proximal femur.

obtaining tissue by most surgical pathologists. However, from a technical standpoint, open biopsy is associated with a complication rate of 16% and therefore must be performed by an experienced center. Mankin and colleagues[13,14] demonstrated that biopsy-related problems occurred with 3 to 5 times greater frequency at centers inexperienced with sarcoma treatment, when compared with sarcoma treatment centers. Several principles to minimize risk of contamination and complication while maintaining adequate yield and accuracy have been described (**Box 1**). Currently, percutaneous needle biopsy has replaced open surgical biopsy in most experienced centers as the primary method of biopsy due to low complication rate and a high level

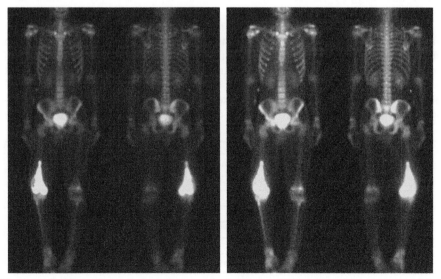

Fig. 3. Technicium-99 whole-body bone scan of patient with localized osteosarcoma of the right distal femur.

Table 1
American Joint Committee on Cancer staging system for bone sarcomas

Stage	Tumor Size	Lymph Involvement	Grade
IA	<8 cm	No lymph node involvement or metastasis	Low
IB	≥8 cm	No lymph node involvement or metastasis	Low
IIA	<8 cm	No lymph node involvement or metastasis	High
IIB	>8 cm	No lymph node involvement or metastasis	High
III	Skip metastasis	No lymph node involvement or metastasis	Any
IVA	Any size	No lymph node involvement, metastasis to the lung	Any
IVB	Any size	Any lymph node involvement or any metastasis to site other than the lung	Any

Adapted from Edge SB, Byrd DR, Compton CC, eds. AJCC Cancer Staging Manual. 7th ed. New York: Springer, 2010.

of accuracy, but relies heavily on the acumen of the bone pathologist given the low yield of tissue from this procedure.

Percutaneous needle biopsy

With complication rates of approximately 1%, percutaneous needle biopsy with or without image guidance represents a safe, cost-effective, minimally invasive alternative to surgical biopsy.[16–19] Diagnostic accuracy rates range from 74% to 93% when imaging modalities are used.[19–21] Major disadvantages of needle biopsies, in general, relate to the small amount of tissue obtained, and the potential for sampling error. For these reasons, fine needle aspirate (FNA) is usually insufficient for primary bone sarcoma. However, core needle biopsy (CNB) has consistently been shown to facilitate accurate histopathologic interpretation and achieve favorable patient outcomes.[17,19,22] The difference in hospital charges associated with percutaneous biopsies and open biopsies was found to be approximately $6000.[23] Furthermore, recent data suggest that seeding of the needle biopsy tract may not occur as it does in open surgical biopsy.[24]

Many studies have attempted to identify risk factors for poor diagnostic capability or patient outcome after CNB. Increased sensitivity, diagnostic accuracy, and ability to differentiate between benign and malignant lesions are seen in needle biopsy of bone sarcomas compared with soft tissue sarcomas.[17,21,23] In general, malignant bone tumors are associated with higher diagnostic yield than benign lesions.[24,25] Biopsies of necrotic areas of a tumor are likely to produce nondiagnostic tissue, so image guidance is critical in determining the optimal target of the biopsy needle. Highly

Table 2
Musculoskeletal Tumor Society staging system for bone sarcomas

Stage	Grade	Site
IA	Low	Intracompartmental
IB	Low	Extracompartmental
IIA	High	Intracompartmental
IIB	High	Extracompartmental
III	Any regional/distal metastases	Any

From Enneking WF, Spanier SS, Goodman MA. A system for the surgical staging of musculoskeletal sarcoma. Clin Orthop 1980;153:106–20.

> **Box 1**
> **Principles of safe and effective surgical biopsy of musculoskeletal lesions**
>
> *Principles of surgical biopsy*
>
> Plan the biopsy as carefully as the definitive resection procedure
>
> Carry out procedure with minimal contamination of normal tissues
>
> Drain tract must be clearly marked and close to and in line with surgical biopsy incision, to be resected at definitive procedure
>
> Pay careful attention to antiseptic technique, skin sterilization, hemostasis, and wound closure
>
> Avoid transverse incisions, and place skin incision in such a matter so as to not compromise subsequent definitive surgery
>
> Ensure adequate amount of representative tissue is obtained, communicate confirmation with pathologist
>
> Details must be provided to pathologist, including site of tumor, age, and radiologic differential diagnosis
>
> If pathologist is unable to make diagnosis, urge him or her to seek consultation promptly
>
> If the orthopedist or institution is not equipped to perform appropriate diagnostic studies, the definitive surgical resection, or adjuvant treatment, the patient should be referred to a treating center before biopsy performance
>
> Core needle biopsies under imaging control are often appropriate alternatives to surgical biopsy
>
> *Data from* Refs.[13–15]

vascularized tumors risk excessive blood in the core sample. In each case, the treatment team should weigh the advantages and disadvantages of open versus percutaneous biopsy; while using a core needle has many advantages and is proven safe and accurate, in certain circumstances the appropriate course remains an open surgical biopsy.

Although image guidance is usually by CT or ultrasound, MRI is becoming more readily available as a guidance modality for needle biopsy. In one large study, MRI-guided biopsy of bone lesions achieved 92% diagnostic sensitivity, 100% specificity, 100% positive predictive value, and 86% negative predictive value.[26] MRI detects areas of highest yield better than other modalities, allowing for optimal needle placement without ionizing radiation exposure. Disadvantages of MRI-guided needle biopsy are cost, need for MRI-compatible biopsy needles, and patient-specific contraindications to MRI, such as pacemakers, aneurysmal clips, or cochlear implants.[27]

For palpable lesions not in close proximity to neurovascular structures, office biopsy procedures have proven clinically effective, safe, and cost-efficient.[28] No differences have been found in accuracy of specific diagnosis, malignancy status, grade, or histologic type between biopsy samples obtained by surgical procedure or percutaneously without image assistance in the clinic setting for appropriate tumors.[29]

Treatment Overview

A multidisciplinary sarcoma team consisting of an orthopedic oncologic surgeon, medical oncologist, radiation oncologist, bone pathologist, and musculoskeletal radiologist is critical in optimizing outcomes in the treatment of bone sarcoma. Overall treatment strategy should depend on a multitude of factors (**Box 2**). A hierarchy of

---

Box 2
Criteria in surgical decision-making

Patient factors

Patient age

Personal/family/cultural considerations

Oncologic factors

Cancer stage

Anatomic location

Histologic subtype

Histologic grade

Treatment factors

Response to induction chemotherapy

Capabilities/biases of surgical team

Data from DeVita VT, Lawrence TS, Rosenberg SA. Cancer. Principles and practices of oncology. 10th edition. Philadelphia: Wolters Kluwer Health; 2015.

---

priorities exists when caring for a patient with sarcoma of bone: life, limb, limb function, limb length equality, and cosmesis (in that order).[30]

Local control is generally achieved with surgical resection, and for histologies in which chemotherapy is appropriate, systemic control is achieved with chemotherapy. A shift away from amputation in favor of limb salvage surgery has been observed, in an attempt to improve limb function without sacrifice of long-term survival.[31–33] In the vast majority of extremity bone sarcoma, limb salvage can be performed. In some cases, radiation therapy can be used for local control in Ewing sarcoma. Aside from Ewing sarcoma, however, radiation therapy alone is not adequate for local control of bone sarcoma.[34–36]

After the primary tumor has been addressed, resection of all metastatic lesions that are technically feasible is recommended for osteosarcoma. Long-term survival has been shown to increase fivefold with complete resection of the primary tumor as well as the metastatic sites, compared with primary tumor resection alone.[37] Survival can be as high as 75% in patients with a solitary lung metastasis that is resected along with the primary tumor, demonstrating the benefit of surgical treatment of all lesions when possible.[38] For Ewing sarcoma and chondrosarcoma, metastasectomy may have similar benefit.[39,40]

TREATMENT MODALITIES
Chemotherapy

Before the 1970s, before the emergence of chemotherapy, more than 80% of patients diagnosed with osteosarcoma or Ewing sarcoma developed distant metastases and eventually died, even with adequate surgical treatment. Several large, randomized prospective trials have since demonstrated dramatic improvements in prognosis secondary to chemotherapeutics: Eilber and colleagues[41] showed a 17% rate of relapse-free survival at 2 years for patients with nonmetastatic osteosarcoma treated without chemotherapy, compared with a 66% rate in similar patients treated with chemotherapy. These data illustrate the value of systemic therapy in conjunction with local control with the intent to reduce rate of future distant relapse.

Although this is true for most aggressive tumors like conventional osteosarcoma and Ewing sarcoma, there is still no effective chemotherapy for certain bone tumors like chondrosarcoma. These rare tumors with complex management are generally treated in tertiary sarcoma centers in the context of a clinical trial or through well-established individualized treatment protocol based on multidisciplinary evaluation. In general, nonmetastatic high-grade osteosarcoma, Ewing sarcoma, and spindle cell sarcoma of bone are treated with neoadjuvant chemotherapy followed by definitive local therapy and then adjuvant chemotherapy.[15]

Chemotherapy for osteosarcoma

The Multi-Institutional Osteosarcoma Study (MIOS) established the value that chemotherapy contributes to the treatment of high-grade osteosarcoma. Patients with newly diagnosed localized osteosarcoma of the extremity were randomized to resection followed by observation or followed by adjuvant chemotherapy. Sixty-six percent of the chemotherapy group were relapse-free compared with only 17% in the observation group at 2-year follow-up.[42,43] Eilber and colleagues[41] demonstrated similar findings, discontinuing their prospective randomized trial after 2 years due to the dramatically improved outcomes in the adjuvant chemotherapy group (55% vs 20% disease-free survival, and 80% vs 48% in improved patient survival).

A similarly designed study explored the role of neoadjuvant chemotherapy in osteosarcoma with the POG-8651 trial. Patients were prospectively randomized to immediate surgery followed by 42 weeks of adjuvant chemotherapy, or 10 weeks of neoadjuvant chemotherapy followed by surgery then 32 weeks of adjuvant chemotherapy. The timing of surgery did not impact outcomes, as both cohorts fared equally well. With these results, the utilization of neoadjuvant chemotherapy became more widespread, as it allows for more time for surgical planning and for the assessment of histologic necrosis in response to neoadjuvant treatment.[41] It also attempts to treat detectable metastases or presumed micrometastases as quickly as possible, and may also decrease the size of the primary tumor as well as promote tumor demarcation from surrounding tissues by decreasing neovascularity.[44] It is estimated that approximately half of patients with localized disease display greater than 90% response to preoperative chemotherapy.[45] In these responders, 5-year survival rates are more than 60%. For poor responders, this rate drops to 37% to 52%.[46]

The consensus standard chemotherapy regimen for high-grade osteosarcoma has become high-dose methotrexate, cisplatin, and doxorubicin. However, the type of chemotherapy should be based on age, comorbidities, tumor type and stage, and treatment expectations, with an understanding of the toxicities associated with various agents.[47] Combining multiple drugs avoids chemoresistance and increases necrosis rate.[48] In poor responders to the 3-drug regimen, the addition of ifosfamide to the postoperative regimen can lead to improvement in outcomes and cellular response similar to that of a good initial responder.[49] Interestingly, though, trials adding ifosfamide to the neoadjuvant chemotherapy regimen from treatment onset did not improve overall survival or event-free survival[50]; for this reason, it is not consistently included in the traditional regimen for classic osteosarcoma. Moreover, results from EURAMOS trial presented in the 2014 October Connective Tissue Oncology Society meeting showed that adding ifosfamide and etoposide to poor responders does not improve overall survival.[51]

The optimal chemotherapy regimen for adults with osteosarcoma have not been determined, as most trials included patients younger than 40 years. However, in one trial that had patients up to 65 years of age there was no clear benefit seen from addition of high-dose methotrexate.[52] Adults older than 40 years are generally treated with a doxorubicin and cisplatin-based treatment.

Future directions in the systemic treatment of osteosarcoma involve target-selective chemotherapeutic drugs, such as mammalian target of rapamycin (MTOR) inhibitors, have shown activity in the metastatic setting.[53] Additionally, liposomal muramyl tripeptide phosphatidylethanolamine (L-MTP-PE) is being studied, which modifies the patient's own immune system, stimulating the formation of tumoricidal macrophages. This agent has shown improved survivability in patients without clinically detectable metastases on presentation, through a mechanism unique to that of conventional chemotherapy.[54]

Chemotherapy for Ewing sarcoma

Ewing sarcoma is the third most common primary malignant neoplasm of bone, with an annual incidence of 2.9 cases per million.[55] It is more frequent in children and adolescents, and is the second most common bone malignancy in this age group.[56] Median age at diagnosis is 15 years, but it is occasionally seen in adults. It is most common in whites and is very uncommon in African and Asian populations. Treatment for Ewing sarcoma is multimodal, involving chemotherapy for systemic control as well as either surgical resection or radiation therapy to achieve local control. Before introduction of multidrug chemotherapy protocols in the 1970s, 5-year survival for patients was less than 25%.[57,58] Today, patients with localized disease experience 5-year survival rates that exceed 60%.[59] Worse prognosis is associated with metastatic disease at presentation, tumor size greater than 10 cm, patient age 20 years or older, and axial tumor location.[60] With isolated lung metastases on presentation, 5-year relapse-free survival is 29%. However, with bone metastases, this rate drops to 19%, and with metastases to both locations, the rate is 8%.[61]

One of the earliest clinical trials involving chemotherapy for Ewing sarcoma was the North American Intergroup Ewing Sarcoma Study (IESS-1), which showed success of a combination regimen abbreviated "VACA" or "VDCA": vincristine, doxorubicin, actinomycin-D, and cyclophosphamide. It showed an improved 5-year relapse-free survival: 60% versus 24% versus 44% when compared with VAC (vincristine, Actinomycin-D, cyclophosphamide) or VAC with bilateral lung irradiation, respectively. It also showed that larger size and pelvic location tumors did worse.[62] The optimal mode of VACA administration was clarified by the second Intergroup study, which demonstrated that early high-dose intermittent doxorubicin achieved better outcomes than the IESS-1 dose with relapse free survival in 5 years as high as 73% for nonpelvic tumors. It also showed better survival for large pelvic tumors compared with IESS-1.[63]

A further improvement in 5-year relapse-free survival was noted in nonmetastatic Ewing sarcoma with the addition of alternating ifosfamide and etoposide to the VDCA regimen versus VDCA alone (69% as opposed to 54%, respectively).[64] Based on the previously described studies, the trend is to treat with 6-agent chemotherapy with 3 to 6 cycles upfront followed by local therapy followed by an additional 6 to 10 cycles of chemotherapy.

High-dose chemotherapy with autologous stem cell transplantation for high-risk localized disease should be done only under a clinical trial at present times given lack of data for definite benefit.[65] Given high response rates with alkylating agents that show a steep dose response curve dose intense regimens have been investigated; however, these have not shown to be clearly beneficial when compared with standard dosing and have increased toxicity.[66]

Another approach investigated was to give the same multidrug regimen every 2 weeks instead of every 3 weeks (ie, dose-dense). It was found to have similar toxicity as compared with the standard 3-week regimen; however, had a better event-free survival (73% vs 42%) in children.[67,68] The benefit of a similar approach in adults seems to be unclear and appears to be limited to children younger than 17 years.[69]

Patients with the metastatic disease are treated with a similar approach to localized disease; however, they have a worse prognosis. High-dose chemotherapy followed by autologous hematopoietic transplantation has been studied in a nonrandomized setting and given mixed results from different trials; this approach is still considered investigational and should be done only under a clinical trial.[70–72] The final results from Euro Ewing Trial will likely shed more light on the specific subset of patients who will benefit from this approach.[73]

Chemotherapy for chondrosarcoma

Traditional chemotherapy plays a minimal role in the treatment of conventional chondrosarcoma.[74,75] It may convey some benefit in select cases of dedifferentiated chondrosarcoma, but the literature to support this is controversial.[76–79] However, exciting research into the molecular genetics of this disease may illuminate specific molecular targets to focus on. One effort is based on the genes coding for isocitrate dehydrogenase (IDH-1 and IDH-2), as up to 70% of conventional chondrosarcomas carry a mutation at these gene loci. Animal models have demonstrated 50% to 60% growth inhibition of tumor cells after administration of a tool compound that overrides this pathologic IDH1/2 pathway.[80] Another potential treatment involves many chondrosarcomas' upregulation of hypoxia inducible factor-1 alpha (HIF1-α), which is associated with increased vascular endothelial growth factor (VEGF) production, increased cellular proliferation, and resistance to chemotherapy and radiation.[81] Tyrosine kinase inhibitors target VEGF, and clear cell chondrosarcoma has shown good response to the tyrosine kinase inhibitor sunitinib in a case report.[82] Approximately 96% of central conventional chondrosarcomas have mutations in the retinoblastoma (Rb) pathway, a well-known tumor suppressor gene.[83] Trials are currently ongoing involving pemetrexed disodium, a multitargeted antifolate that prevents formation of precursor nucleotides, thought to stop uncontrolled proliferation though interaction with the pathologic Rb mechanism.[84,85] Last, MTOR inhibitors like sirolimus with cyclophosphamide have shown modest clinical activity in chondrosarcoma, making them another agent of interest for this mostly chemo-resistant disease.[86]

Radiation Therapy

The role of radiation therapy in the treatment of primary localized bone sarcomas is limited. With the exception of Ewing sarcoma, radiation is not an effective standalone modality for local control. The use of radiation may be considered as an adjunct therapy in the case of a margin-positive resection, for palliation in the case of unresectable tumors, or for palliation in symptomatic primary tumors in the setting of widespread metastatic disease.

In the setting of Ewing sarcoma, radiation alone has been shown to be an effective means of local control, although local recurrence rates are higher than with surgical resection. Radiation can be used in place of resection in cases of Ewing sarcoma when surgery would be associated with significant functional loss, such as in difficult locations of the pelvis, spine, or chest wall. A Children's Oncology Group retrospective study of 465 patients with Ewing sarcoma treated with either surgery or radiation for local control, demonstrated similar event-free survival, overall survival, and distant failure rates on multivariate analysis comparing resection with radiation.[87] The risk of local failure, however, was greater for the radiation group compared with the surgical resection group. This finding is corroborated by pooled analyses of the Cooperative

Ewing Sarcoma Study (CESS) data, which found that patients who received definitive radiotherapy had lower event-free survival rates than surgical patients, whereas overall rate of distant failure did not differ.[88,89] In 2006, Bacci and colleagues[90] demonstrated that for appendicular Ewing sarcoma, surgery led to significantly improved 5-year event-free survival compared with radiation (68% vs 49%, respectively), whereas for patients with central tumors, which have higher rates of local recurrence at baseline, there was no significant difference found in event-free survival or local recurrence rates between those treated with radiation or surgery.

Advanced radiotherapy techniques have been studied extensively in Ewing sarcoma, such as proton beam radiation,[91] brachytherapy,[92] and intraoperative radiation.[93] In a 2012 report of initial results of 30 pediatric patients with Ewing sarcoma treated with proton beam therapy, Rombi and colleagues[94] demonstrated the low toxicity profile of this technique with an 86% rate of local control for an average of 38.4 months. Overall survival was found to be 89%. Hoekstra and colleagues[95] suggested a positive effect on local recurrence with intraoperative radiotherapy (IORT) in a pilot study on 5 patients with pelvic girdle sarcomas; 80% of patients remained locally free of tumor with follow-ups of 8 to 53 months, in comparison with the 27% rate observed in historic controls. In 2015, a 20-year follow-up study on 71 patients treated with intraoperative electron beam radiotherapy found a 74% 10-year local control, 57% disease-free survival rate, and 68% overall survival rate in patients undergoing intraoperative radiotherapy for Ewing sarcoma (37 patients) or rhabdomyosarcoma (34 patients), arguing in support of this technique as a well-tolerated strategy to improve local recurrence rates.[93]

A role for proton beam radiation in combination with surgery is being established in the treatment of chordoma, particularly localized to the skull base or axial skeleton. Data from a prospective study examining the outcome of proton therapy as either adjuvant or definitive treatment for nonmetastatic chordoma or chondrosarcoma demonstrated local recurrence-free survival of 92%, with disease-free survival of 87%.[91] Longer-term studies have corroborated these findings, reporting local recurrence to be 7.8% at mean follow-up of 69.2 months, for a cohort of 77 patients with skull-base chondrosarcoma.[96]

Carbon ion beam radiotherapy, which delivers a larger mean energy per unit length of trajectory than photon or proton beams, has shown positive results in the treatment of certain bone sarcomas.[97] This method has been studied primarily in unresectable bone tumors[98] and in patients refusing surgery.[99] A local recurrence rate of 62% and 5-year overall survival rate of 33% was demonstrated in a study of 78 patients with medically inoperable osteosarcoma of the trunk who received carbon ion beam radiotherapy.[100] Results are more favorable in patients with medically unresectable sacral chordomas: Imai and colleagues[101] reported an overall survival rate at 5 years of 86% in their 95-patient cohort, with local control rate at 5 years of 88%. In their more recent report, the same group observed 5-year and 10-year local control rates of 77.2% and 52%, respectively, in 188 cases of unresectable sacral chordomas after carbon ion therapy alone.[98] This is comparable, if not favorable, to the accepted local recurrence rate after surgery being approximately 45% to 78%.[102,103] Five-year and 10-year survival rates were 81.1% and 66.8%, respectively. Nishida and colleagues[104] demonstrated that the functional outcomes reported after surgical resection were 55% according to the Musculoskeletal Tumor Society scoring system, whereas they were 75% after carbon ion beam radiotherapy, and that definitive radiation treatment was associated with significantly improved emotional acceptance scores.

The most common complications of radiation therapy are wound complications, limb-length discrepancies, joint contractures, pathologic fractures, and secondary malignancy. Even relatively low doses have been associated with the development of radiation-induced sarcomas within the field,[105] and there is evidence that radiation-associated soft tissue sarcomas carry a worse prognosis than those not related to radiation exposure.[106] As the population of long-term cancer survivors grows, these long-term sequelae will become increasingly concerning, and must be reconciled with the improvements in oncologic outcomes associated with advanced radiotherapy techniques.[107]

Surgical Resection

The primary goal of surgical treatment of bone sarcoma is to achieve complete resection of the primary tumor with negative margins, with a secondary goal being preservation of as functional a limb as is possible. Sarcoma growth has been described as "centrifugal," or from the inside outward, and as tumor growth progresses, a pseudocapsule develops at the interface of tumor and normal tissue. Pseudopods of tumor extend into this reactive zone; resection through this zone will leave tumor cells behind.[11] Adequate resection is critical, as margin status is the most important determinant of recurrence.[7,108,109] National Comprehensive Cancer Network guidelines recommend wide local excision of bone sarcomas[7]; however, "wide resection" is not easily defined (**Table 3**). In poor responders to preoperative chemotherapy, a wider margin may be needed to achieve a definitive resection.[110] In the pelvis and spine, complete resection is often more challenging than it is in the extremities due to anatomic complexity.[111,112] In a recent study of 52 patients with pelvic bone sarcomas, Farfalli and colleagues[113] found that 15% of resections resulted in intralesional margins, 63% with marginal margins, and only 21% wide margins; intralesional resection was found to be a significant risk factor for local recurrence in this and other series. In a report of 1121 patients with extremity sarcomas, the same institution reported that only 9% of resections resulted in inadequate margins, highlighting the importance of anatomic location of the tumor when planning surgical resection.[108]

Resection: amputation versus limb salvage

Before the popularization of limb salvage surgery (LSS) in the 1970s, amputation was the standard of care for malignant bone tumors. Improvements in chemotherapy protocols have been the primary advancement that supported a paradigm shift away from amputation and toward LSS for sarcoma of the extremities. Additional advancements in endoprosthetic design, musculoskeletal imaging, and surgical technique have all contributed to the success of LSS in most cases. With modern treatment, it is estimated that limb salvage surgery is a reasonable option in 85% of appendicular osteosarcomas.[114] In some cases, however, amputation still remains the best surgical option, most commonly in the setting of critical nerve involvement.

No prospective randomized study exists comparing oncological outcomes of LSS with those after amputation. Nonrandomized comparative studies have shown no statistically significant difference in overall survival.[32,115,116] In 2015, Reddy and

Table 3	
Margins in surgical tumor resection	
Type of Margin	**Plane of Dissection**
Intralesional	Within diseased tissue of tumor
Marginal	Within reactive zone
Wide	Through normal tissue, beyond reactive zone
Radical	Extracompartmental

colleagues[117] reported that amputation in patients with osteosarcoma conferred no clear survival benefit over LSS, even in the subset of patients with close margins during LSS and poor response to neoadjuvant chemotherapy.

Quality of life after amputation and LSS has been shown to be similar by many studies.[118,119] In a recent survey of 250 patients who received amputation for pelvic/lower extremity tumors, 84% of patients who had undergone hemipelvectomy, hip disarticulation, or transfemoral amputation required use of a walking aid and reported significantly higher pain levels than those who did not. The average Toronto Extremity Salvage Score (TESS) in all responders in this study (all amputation levels: hemipelvectomy to foot) was 56.4%,[120] as compared with the 85% TESS achieved by patients treated with LSS in a separate report.[121] Up to 83% of patients treated with LSS for Ewing sarcoma were found to participate in sports on a regular basis.[122] Physiologic cost index, a measure of energy consumption, was also found to be greater after above-knee amputation than LSS.[121] Job satisfaction, occupational relations, material well-being, and reintegration into normal daily living activity are higher among patients treated with LSS than those undergoing above-knee amputation.[121,123] Financially, external prosthetic fitting costs for amputees have been shown to surpass the cost of limb salvage in the long term: most active young patients will require a sophisticated artificial limb that will be replaced many times, and will opt for a second prosthesis for sports and swimming.[124]

Although functional results may be better in some cases after limb salvage than amputation, complications unique to reconstruction occur 3 times more commonly after LSS, and 4 times more commonly after endoprosthetic reconstructions, compared with ablative procedures.[125] Return to the operating room is more frequent in patients undergoing LSS compared with amputees.[124] Complications after LSS have been classified into "mechanical," "nonmechanical," and "pediatric" modes of failure.[126] Soft tissue failure, aseptic loosening, and breakage/fracture/dislocation of the implant comprise the "mechanical failure" category. Infection and tumor progression are included in the "nonmechanical" category, and pediatric complications, such as growth arrest and joint dysplasia, comprise the third. In cases of amputation, the risk of many of these complications is nonexistent; instead, amputees most often suffer from wound breakdown, infection, and phantom limb pain. Rates of wound infection have been reported to be as high as 45% in patients undergoing hindquarter amputation,[127] but are generally much lower when the amputation occurs more distally.[119,125,128]

Wound complication rates as high as 38%, and infection rates of 11%, have been reported after LSS.[129,130] Risk factors for infection include pelvic reconstruction (with allograft or endoprosthesis), tibial endoprosthetic reconstruction, radiation therapy, and pediatric expandable implants.[113,130,131] Most deep infections occur within the initial 2-year postoperative period, or within 2 years of the most recent surgical intervention. In a study of patients with infected endoprosthetic reconstructions, local surgical debridement with or without placement of antibiotic implants was successful only 6% of the time; 37% ultimately underwent amputation to treat their infection.[130] In patients who underwent allograft reconstructions, greater risk of infection was associated with tibial allografts, male patients, procedures performed in a conventional operating room, and prolonged utilization of postoperative antibiotics. In 82% of cases of allograft infection, local debridement failed and removal with antibiotic cement spacer placement was required.[132]

Local recurrence

Local recurrence after bone sarcoma resection remains incompletely understood. The literature is inconclusive on whether LSS in the era of chemotherapy is associated with an increased risk of local recurrence compared with amputation.[108,116,133] Classically, a close link between margin status and local recurrence has been shown, and the emergence of LSS has been suggested to increase the incidence of inadequate margins.[108] However, the definition of an adequate margin in this context is unknown. In a recent study, Li and colleagues[134] examined the impact of a close margin (<5 mm) on local recurrence in patients with osteosarcoma receiving chemotherapy and found no increase in local recurrence rate compared with wider margins. A similar finding was obtained in a large analysis of 1355 patients with osteosarcoma receiving surgery and chemotherapy: although surgical margin width was not a risk factor for local recurrence, a poor response to neoadjuvant chemotherapy and an inability to complete the chemotherapy protocol were significantly associated with local recurrence.[135] In an investigation of local recurrence of chondrosarcoma, a notably chemotherapy-insensitive tumor, amputation versus limb salvage was not found to be a significant risk factor for local recurrence; tumor size and margin status were.[109] These data support the current prevailing concept that local recurrence is a function of tumor biology as well as margin status.

The prognostic significance of local recurrence in the absence of distant metastases on overall survival is not fully understood.[136–138] Local recurrence was found to be a significant and independent predictor of poor overall survival in chondrosarcoma, imparting a hazard ratio of 3.4 according to one study.[109] Although distant osteosarcoma metastases confer a poor prognosis,[139] one study showed 31% of those with local recurrence alone were cured by further treatment.[140] Another study found 5-year postrecurrence survival in patients with osteosarcoma with local recurrence without distant metastasis to be 42%, and 58% of these patients eventually developed distant metastases despite local treatment of their relapse.[141] In a recent case-control study, Kong and colleagues[142] showed local recurrence to have very little impact on overall survival in patients with high-risk osteosarcoma; instead, initial tumor volume and enlargement after chemotherapy were significant predictors of poor survival. Through a multivariate analysis, they suggest that poor histologic response and enlargement after chemotherapy are drivers of both local recurrence and poor overall prognosis individually, and that these 2 outcomes are not themselves causally associated. Findings such as these introduce questions regarding surgical treatment for local recurrence; for example, is repeat limb-sparing surgery adequate? In their 2006 study of 44 patients, Bacci and colleagues[143] found that amputation for local recurrence did confer a longer postrecurrence survival than a second limb-sparing procedure. In 2014, Loh and colleagues[144] reported that in 18 pediatric patients with locally recurring osteosarcoma in the absence of metastases at time of relapse, postrecurrence survival was significantly longer in patients in whom surgical margins of more than 1 cm were achieved during resection of the local recurrence. Takeuchi and colleagues[141] reviewed 45 patients with localized recurrence of high-grade osteosarcoma and found that independent predictors of worse overall survival were recurrent tumor size greater than 5 cm and concurrent metastasis. The relationship between local recurrence and survival is therefore complex, and is likely a function of both adequacy of surgery and aggressiveness of the tumor.

RECONSTRUCTIVE CONSIDERATIONS

Resection of tumors in "expendable bones," such as the fibula, patella, scapula, or radius/ulna, is often successful without reconstruction. In other weight-bearing locations, structural integrity must be restored through reconstruction to optimize postoperative function. Options for reconstruction include allograft, allograft-prosthetic composite, endoprosthesis, and extracorporeal irradiated autograft. Emerging technologies promise future improvements in implant design, fixation and function, operative technique, and mitigation of complications.

Allograft Reconstruction

Advantages of this allograft reconstruction include restoration of bone stock, potential sparing of uninvolved adjacent joints in intercalary reconstructions, and anatomic soft tissue attachment sites.[145] Disadvantages include the requirement for weight-bearing protection until allograft-host healing, potential for osteoarthritis development (in osteoarticular grafts), risk of disease transmission or graft rejection, and risk of operative complications of allografts: nonunion, fracture, and infection.[145,146]

Up to 20% of initial allograft reconstructions fail, and up to 54% of patients may have a complication that requires additional surgery.[147–149] Success rates vary with type of graft reconstruction used. Intercalary allografts have been associated with acceptable long-term functional outcomes in 82% to 84% of patients,[150,151] and limb survival as high as 97%.[149] Osteoarticular allografts have shown slightly worse success rates (61% and 63% good or excellent results at long-term follow-up, respectively, according to one study of femoral reconstruction).[145] In a recent report of 87 patients who underwent intercalary allograft reconstruction with at least 24 months of follow-up, Bus and colleagues[146] reported that up to 76% of their patients experienced 1 or more complications, most often nonunion (40%). Risk factors for failure and complications included age of 18 years or older, allograft length greater than or equal to 15 cm, intramedullary nail-only fixation, and diaphyseal localization, and these findings were consistent with those previously reported.[150,152] There is general consensus regarding age, length, lack of rigid fixation, and diaphyseal location as risk factors for complications after this procedure.

Graft fracture and nonunion are thought to possibly result from the avascular nature of the bulk allograft.[153,154] To address this challenge, the implantation of massive allograft encasing an intercalary vascularized fibula autograft was described in the literature in 1993, and has come to be known as the "Capanna technique."[155] In the 2007 report of their long-term results, Capanna and colleagues[156] reported a significant improvement in fracture risk: 13% in their series compared with baseline allograft fracture rates in of 17% to 34%; and nonunion rate of 8.8% in their series compared with the 12% to 63% rate established in the literature on allografts alone. Their overall success rate was reported as 93.5%, with 73.0% of their patients healing after the first operation and not requiring additional surgery, and this is in contrast to the large subset of patients treated with allograft who require a second procedure.[151] In their 2016 study of 18 pediatric/adolescent patients undergoing the Capanna technique, Houdek and colleagues[154] were unable to recreate the initially reported results; a 33% nonunion rate and 39% allograft fracture rate were observed. Although this technique is technically challenging and time-consuming, it may represent a step toward improvement in outcome of allograft reconstruction that can be achieved as our understanding of the technique's failure mechanisms continues to advance.

Allograft-Prosthetic Composites

One of the challenges of using osteoarticular allografts for joint reconstruction is the inability to adequately cryopreserve chondrocytes in the graft. This, combined with the instability that often occurs after suboptimal graft fixation, leads to accelerated cartilage degeneration.[157,158] Allograft-prosthetic composite (APC) reconstructions (**Figs. 4** and **5**) offer the durability of a prosthetic articular surface reconstruction, combined with the enhanced soft tissue attachment capability of an allograft.[159] APC reconstructions have been found to provide better stability in certain anatomic locations for an arthroplasty component than a stemmed endoprosthetic implant, potentially due to enhancement of soft tissue attachment sites.[160,161] Once healing has occurred between the graft and host bone, the stress transfer from the implant to the host bone resembles that of a standard arthroplasty as compared with the stress concentration at the stem-body junction that occurs with megaprostheses.[159]

The technique is most often used in lower extremity joints[162] but has also been described in conjunction with reverse total shoulder arthroplasty with good results.[163] Weight-bearing restriction is still required postoperatively to allow for allograft incorporation, which is delayed by chemotherapy. Nonunion is the most common complication facing this procedure, reported at nearly 23% in one study.[164]

Endoprosthetic Reconstruction

Endoprosthetic replacement is the most common method of limb salvage reconstruction after bone tumor resection in the adult population.[165] This strategy provides near-immediate stability of the limb and allows for earlier weight bearing than biologic reconstructive options, and the technology involved has advanced considerably over recent years. In 1993, one report showed event-free prosthetic survival at 5 years to be 88% for the proximal femur, 59% for the distal femur, and only 54% for the proximal tibia.[166] More recently, 5-year implant survival has been reported to have improved to as high as 78.0% for lower extremity and 89.7% for upper extremity reconstructions.[33,167] A 2016 report of distal femoral endoprosthetic reconstruction showed a 93% rate of limb salvage over a 25-year period at one institution.[168] Revision rates, however, are high, with one study reporting a 34% overall revision rate at an average of 15 years of follow-up, due to mechanical failure (15%), infection (10%), and local disease recurrence (5%).[169]

In 2006, Farid and colleagues[160] published a head-to-head comparison of endoprosthetic and APC reconstruction of the proximal femur. They found similar rates of complications in both groups: in the endoprosthetic group, the most common

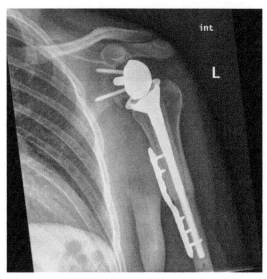

Fig. 4. Left proximal humerus reconstruction with allograft-prosthetic composite reverse total shoulder arthroplasty.

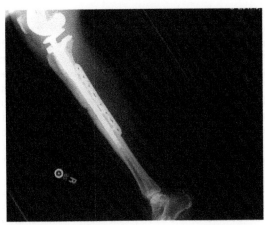

Fig. 5. Right proximal tibia reconstruction with allograft-prosthetic composite hinged total knee arthroplasty.

adverse outcome was aseptic loosening, which occurred 10% of the time. In the APC group, a 10% rate of graft nonunion was encountered. Musculoskeletal Tumor Society scores were similar for both groups, as was implant survivorship at 10 years. The greatest difference found was that the patients with APC regained significantly greater hip abductor strength, which may have imparted improved ambulatory function.

Regarding distal femur resections, AlGeshyan and colleagues[170] compared gait parameters in patients undergoing allograft reconstruction versus metallic endoprosthetic reconstruction. They found that although all patients exhibited decreased range of motion at the knee postoperatively, the allograft-reconstructed knees demonstrated normal patterns of rotation, whereas the patients with endoprosthetic reconstruction had abnormal patterns of rotation and differences in rotational moments. A study conducted by Benedetti and colleagues[171] found significant decrease in knee extension strength after metallic distal femoral replacement. They also observed a stiff-knee gait pattern in their patients who required much of the vastus medialis and intermedius to be resected before endoprosthetic reconstruction. These data suggest that although massive endoprosthetic replacement is the most popular reconstructive option, recreation of normal joint kinematics and optimization of soft tissue reattachment to these metal implants remains a challenge.

Extracorporeal-Irradiated Autografts

Extracorporeal irradiation of a bone tumor resection specimen, followed by reimplantation of the autograft bone was first described by Spira and Lubin in 1968.[172] This technique facilitates reconstruction of defects with an inexpensive, anatomically identical graft that restores bone stock, and obviates the risk of disease transmission and graft rejection.[173,174] Puri and colleagues[174] described optimization of the technique in 2012, beginning with transverse osteotomies at either end of the resection segment after indicator marks are created to facilitate rotational alignment at reimplantation.[175] Soft tissue and periosteum are then sterilely stripped from the bone, before the bone is wrapped in vancomycin-soaked gauze for transport from the operating room. A single 50-Gy dose of radiation is administered to the resected segment using 6-MV photons or 60 cobalt gamma rays with parallel opposing portals. The marrow contents are reamed out and bone cement is injected into the medullary cavity, and then the specimen is reimplanted in appropriate rotational alignment and secured with internal fixation. In a report of 31 patients, the osteotomy sites united primarily in 88% of cases. This rate is higher than most union rates reported after cadaveric allograft fixation,[151] and may be due to the precise geometric matching of the osteotomized ends. A 13.0% infection rate and 9.6% local recurrence rate were observed; all recurrences were associated with disseminated disease in the soft tissue, noncontiguous with the irradiated graft. Other studies have shown the rate of fracture for irradiated grafts to be as high as 20%.[173,176] Use of a vascularized fibula autograft in conjunction with the irradiated host autograft bone has been described, associated with 88% good or excellent functional outcome.[177]

Emerging Surgical and Implant Technology

As the number of young, active sarcoma survivors continues to rise, it is expected that rates of aseptic mechanical loosening will rise in parallel.[178] One implant strategy to combat this is an alternative implant fixation device, the Compress prosthesis, which is designed to apply compression at the bone-implant interface, resulting in hypertrophic bone growth in accordance with the Wolff law[179] (**Fig. 6**). This relatively new device has a published survival rate as high as 89% at 5 years and 80% at 10 years when used for primary oncologic reconstruction,[180–182] and comparison studies have shown it to achieve equal or higher survival rates than cemented and press-fit stemmed implants.[183,184] The device may have a role in the revision settings as well, after endoprosthetic failure with standard stem fixation has occurred.

Radiolucent intramedullary nails made of carbon fiber–reinforced polyetheretherketone (CFR-PEEK) as an alternative to metal implants have recently been shown to minimize implant artifact on MRI or CT in patients who underwent long-bone fixation requiring postoperative cross-sectional imaging surveillance. In comparison with titanium nails, a statistically significant superiority of the percentage of visualized cortex, corticomedullary junction, and muscle-bone interface on MRI images of CFR-PEEK nails was observed, which suggests potential benefit of this material in the setting of oncologic reconstructions.[185] Additionally, biomechanical testing has found the 4-point bending strength, torsional stiffness, and bending fatigue of these implants to be comparable to titanium nails, with an inert biochemical profile and similar elastic modulus to bone.[186] The CFR-PEEK nail was not associated with increased risk of superficial or deep infection, painful or symptomatic hardware, or completion of an impending pathologic fracture.

Computer-Aided Surgery

Navigation technology has been used in orthopedic spine surgery, trauma surgery, and arthroplasty for many years, and has been shown to improve the precision and reproducibility of hardware placement.[187–189] In orthopedic oncology, initial reports of intraoperative navigation focused on the safety and improved visualization achieved during pelvic mass excision.[190] Over time, additional advantages of computer-aided surgery beyond surgical navigation alone have been realized that are applicable to the resection and reconstruction of bone sarcoma.

In a simulation study by Cartiaux and colleagues,[191] it was found that experienced surgeons achieved negative margins only 52% of the time when performing complex musculoskeletal resections on plastic models; the addition of computer-aided surgery to these simulations improved negative margin achievement significantly. In vivo, these findings have been supported by studies that have shown the intralesional resection rate of pelvic tumors improving from 29.0% to 8.7%, with addition of computer-aided surgery to traditional resection techniques,[192] and accuracy of pelvic/sacral tumor resection within an average of 2.82 mm of planned osteotomies

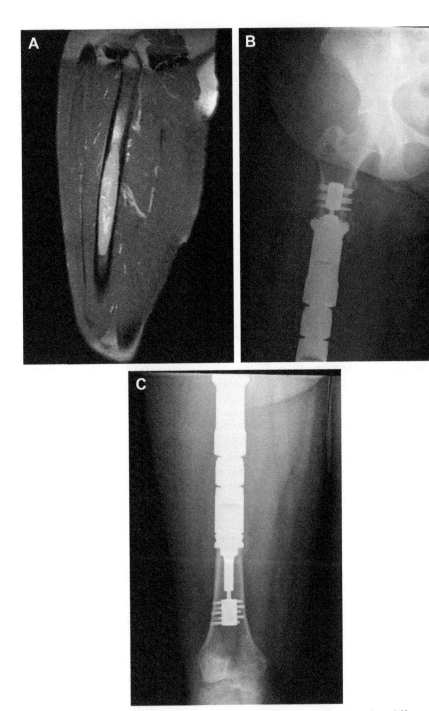

Fig. 6. (*A*) Preoperative STIR coronal MRI scan of right femur diaphyseal undifferentiated pleomorphic sarcoma of bone. (*B, C*) Intercalary prosthetic reconstruction with Compress device after resection.

when performed with navigation.[193] Cho and colleagues[194] suggested a decrease in local recurrence rates as a result of improved margin status. For resection of bone sarcomas in anatomically challenging areas such as the pelvis, sacrum, or spine, the ability of navigation to preoperatively map a tumor's extent and couple it to enhanced 3-dimensional intraoperative visualization offers great promise. In the case of epiphyseal or metaphyseal long-bone sarcomas, computer-aided surgery allows for precise periarticular resection that can be used to preserve the whole or partial epiphysis.[195]

The improvement in precision of hardware placement using computer-aided surgery has been shown in the trauma and spine literature, particularly with the placement of dangerous screws across the sacroiliac joint, acetabular region, and pedicles.[196–198] In oncology applications, computer-aided design and computer-aided modeling cutting jigs, patient-specific instrumentation, and a custom-designed prostheses can achieve accurate and precise reconstruction of a large bony defect in addition to aiding with hardware placement.[199] Advanced preoperative planning using computer-aided surgical techniques can allow 2 surgical teams to work simultaneously, one performing the resection and the other creating an allograft identical to the resection specimen to be used for reconstruction.[200] A similar technique can be applied to custom-made metallic implants, in which the implant manufacturer and surgeon work on the same preoperative plan to create an implant that precisely matches the resection.

SUMMARY

Treatment of bone sarcoma requires careful planning and involvement of an experienced multidisciplinary team. Significant advancements in systemic therapy, radiation, and surgery in recent years have contributed to improved functional and survival outcomes for patients with these difficult tumors, and emerging technologies hold promise for further advancement.

REFERENCES

1. SEER Stat Fact Sheet: Bone and Joint Cancer. National Institutes of Health Surveillance, Epidemiology, and End Results Program. Available at: http://seer.cancer.gov/statfacts/html/bones.html. Accessed February 16, 2016.
2. Ottaviani G, Jaffe N. The epidemiology of osteosarcoma. Cancer Treat Res 2010;152:3–13.
3. Arora RS, Alston RD, Eden TOB, et al. The contrasting age-incidence patterns of bone tumours in teenagers and young adults: implications for aetiology. Int J Cancer 2012;131(7):1678–85.
4. Duchman KR, Gao Y, Miller BJ. Prognostic factors for survival in patients with high-grade osteosarcoma using the Surveillance, Epidemiology, and End Results (SEER) Program database. Cancer Epidemiol 2015;39(4):593–9.
5. Jawad MU, Cheung MC, Clarke J, et al. Osteosarcoma: improvement in survival limited to high-grade patients only. J Cancer Res Clin Oncol 2011;137:597–607.
6. Sajadi KR, Heck RK, Neel MD, et al. The incidence and prognosis of osteosarcoma skip metastases. Clin Orthop Relat Res 2004;426:92–6.
7. American Joint Committee on Cancer: Bone. In: Edge SB, Byrd DR, Compton CC, et al, editors. AJCC Staging Manual. ed 7. New York: Springer; 2010. p. 281–90.
8. Meyer JS, Nadel HR, Marina N, et al. Imaging guidelines for children with Ewing sarcoma and osteosarcoma: a report from the Children's Oncology Group Bone Tumor Committee. Pediatr Blood Cancer 2008;51(2):163.

9. Costelloe CM, Chuang HH, Madewell JE. FDG PET/CT of primary bone tumors. Am J Roentgenol 2014;202:W521–31.

10. Dimitrakopoulou-Strauss A, Strauss LG, Heichel T, et al. The role of quantitative F^{18}-FDG PET studies for the differentiation of malignant and benign bone lesions. J Nucl Med 2002;43:510–8.

11. Enneking WF, Spanier SS, Goodman MA. A system for the surgical staging of musculoskeletal sarcoma. Clin Orthop 1980;153:106–20.

12. deHeeten GJ, Oldhoff J, Oosterhuis JW, et al. Biopsy of bone tumours. J Surg Oncol 1985;28(4):247–51.

13. Mankin HJ, Lange TA, Spanier SS. The hazards of biopsy in patients with malignant primary bone and soft-tissue tumors. J Bone Joint Surg Am 1982;64-A(8): 1121–7.

14. Mankin HJ, Mankin CJ, Simon MA. The hazards of biopsy, revisited. For the members of the Musculoskeletal Tumor Society. J Bone Joint Surg Am 1996; 78-A(5):656–63.

15. European Sarcoma Network Working Group. Bone sarcomas: ESMO clinical practice guidelines for diagnosis, treatment, and follow-up. Ann Oncol 2012; 23(S7):vii100–9.

16. Dupuy DE, Rosenberg AE, Punyaratabandhu T, et al. Accuracy of CT-guided needle biopsy of musculoskeletal neoplasms. Am J Roentgenol 1998;171(3): 759–62.

17. Pohlig F, Kirchhoff C, Lenze U, et al. Percutaneous core needle biopsy versus open biopsy in diagnostics of bone and soft tissue sarcoma: a retrospective study. Eur J Med Res 2012;17:29.

18. Ogilvie CM, Torbert JT, Finstein JL, et al. Clinical utility of percutaneous biopsies of musculoskeletal tumors. Clin Orthop Relat Res 2006;450:95–100.

19. Welker JA, Henshaw RM, Jelinek J, et al. The percutaneous needle biopsy is safe and recommended in the diagnosis of musculoskeletal masses. Cancer 2000;89(12):2677–86.

20. Hau A, Kim I, Kattapuram S, et al. Accuracy of CT-guided biopsies in 359 patients with musculoskeletal lesions. Skeletal Radiol 2002;31(6):349–53.

21. Kiatisevi P, Thanakit V, Sukunthanak B, et al. Computed tomography-guided core needle biopsy versus incisional biopsy in diagnosing musculoskeletal lesions. Skeletal Radiol 2002;31(6):349–53.

22. Mitsuyoshi G, Naito N, Kawai A, et al. Accurate diagnosis of musculoskeletal lesions by core needle biopsy. J Surg Oncol 2006;94(1):21–7.

23. Skrzynski MC, Biermann S, Montag A, et al. Diagnostic accuracy and charge-savings of outpatient core needle biopsy compared with open biopsy of musculoskeletal tumors. J Bone Joint Surg Am 1996;78A(5):644–9.

24. UyBico SJ, Motamedia K, Omura MC, et al. Relevance of compartmental anatomic guidelines for biopsy of musculoskeletal tumors. J Vasc Interv Radiol 2012 Apr;23(4):511–8.

25. Didolkar MM, Anderson ME, Hochman MG, et al. Image guided core needle biopsy of musculoskeletal lesions: are nondiagnostic results clinically useful? Clin Orthop Relat Res 2013;471:3601–9.

26. Carrino JA, Khurana B, Ready JE, et al. Magnetic resonance imaging-guided percutaneous biopsy of musculoskeletal lesions. J Bone Joint Surg Am 2007; 89:2179–87.

27. Alanen J, Keski-Nisula L, Blanco-Sequeiros R, et al. Cost comparison analysis of low-field (0.23T) MRI- and CT-guided bone biopsies. Eur Radiol 2004;14(1): 123–8.

28. Adams SC, Potter BK, Pitcher DJ, et al. Office-based core needle biopsy of bone and soft tissue malignancies. Clin Orthop Relat Res 2010;468:2774–80.

29. Srisawat P, Verraphun P, Punyaratabandhu T, et al. Comparative study of diagnostic accuracy between office-based closed needle biopsy and open incisional biopsy in patients with musculoskeletal sarcomas. J Med Assoc Thai 2014;97(S-2):S30–8.

30. DeVita VT, Lawrence TS, Rosenberg SA. Cancer. Principles and practices of oncology. 10th edition. Philadelphia: Wolters Kluwer Health; 2015.

31. Rosen G, Murphy ML, Huvos AG, et al. Chemotherapy, en bloc resection, and prosthetic bone replacement in the treatment of osteogenic sarcoma. Cancer 1976;37:1–11.

32. Eillber FR, Eckhardt J, Morton DL. Advance in the treatment of sarcomas of the extremity: current status of limb salvage surgery. Cancer 1984;54:2695–701.

33. Goshenger G, Gebert C, Ahrens H, et al. Endoprosthetic reconstruction in 250 patients with sarcoma. Clin Orthop Relat Res 2006;450:164–71.

34. Schwarz R, Bruland O, Cassoni A, et al. The role of radiotherapy in osteosarcoma. Cancer Treat Res 2009;152:147–64.

35. Errani C, Longhi A, Rossi G, et al. Palliative therapy for osteosarcoma. Expert Rev Anticancer Ther 2011;11:217–27.

36. Mahajan A, Woo SY, Kornguth DG, et al. Multimodality treatment of osteosarcoma: radiation in a high-risk cohort. Pediatr Blood Cancer 2008;50:976–82.

37. Kager L, Zoubek A, Potschger U, et al. Primary metastatic osteosarcoma: presentation and outcome of patients treated on neoadjuvant Cooperative Osteosarcoma Study Group protocols. J Clin Oncol 2003;21(10):2011–8.

38. Harris MB, Gieser P, Goorin AM, et al. Treatment of metastatic osteosarcoma at diagnosis: a Pediatric Oncology Group Study. J Clin Oncol 1998;16:3641–8.

39. Letourneau PA, Shackett B, Xiao L, et al. Resection of pulmonary metastases in pediatric patients with Ewing sarcoma improves survival. J Pediatr Surg 2011; 46(2):332–5.

40. Italiano A, Mir O, Cioffi A, et al. Advanced chondrosarcomas: role of chemotherapy and survival. Ann Oncol 2013;24(11):2916–22.

41. Eilber F, Giuliano A, Eckardt J, et al. Adjuvant chemotherapy for osteosarcoma: a randomized prospective trial. J Clin Oncol 1987;5(1):21–6.

42. Link MP, Goorin AM, Miser AW, et al. The effect of adjuvant chemotherapy on relapse-free survival in patients with osteosarcoma of the extremity. N Engl J Med 1986;314(25):1600–6.

43. Goorin AM, Schwartzentruber DJ, Devidas M, et al. Presurgical chemotherapy compared with immediate surgery and adjuvant chemotherapy for nonmetastatic osteosarcoma: Pediatric Oncology Group Study POG-8651. J Clin Oncol 2003;21:1574–80.

44. Smith J, Heelan RT, Huvos AG, et al. Radiographic changes in primary osteogenic sarcoma following intensive chemotherapy: radiological-pathological correlation in 63 patients. Radiology 1982;143:355–60.

45. Meyers PA, Schwartz CL, Krailo M, et al. Osteosarcoma: a randomized, prospective trial of the addition of ifosfamide and/or muramyl tripeptide to cisplatin, doxorubicin, and high-dose methotrexate. J Clin Oncol 2005;23:2004–11.

46. Bacci G, Bertoni F, Longhi A, et al. Neoadjuvant chemotherapy for high-grade central osteosarcoma of the extremity: histologic response to preoperative chemotherapy correlates with histologic subtype of the tumor. Cancer 2003; 97:3068–75.

47. Walczak BE, Irwin RB. Sarcoma chemotherapy. J Am Acad Orthop Surg 2013; 21:480–91.

48. Bacci G, Ferrari S, Bertoni F, et al. Histologic response of high-grade nonmetastatic osteosarcoma of the extremity to chemotherapy. Clin Orthop Relat Res 2001;386:186–96.

49. Bacci G, Ferrari S, Bertoni F, et al. Long-term outcome for patients with nonmetastatic osteosarcoma of the extremity treated at the Instituto Ortopedico Rizzoli according to the Instituto Ortopedico Rizzoli/osteosarcoma-2 protocol: an updated report. J Clin Oncol 2000;18(24):4016–27.

50. Maki RG. Ifosfamide in the neoadjuvant treatment of osteogenic sarcoma. J Clin Oncol 2012;30(17):2033–5.

51. Bielack SS, Smeland S, Whelan JS, et al. Methotrexate, Doxorubicin, and Cisplatin (MAP) Plus Maintenance Pegylated Interferon Alfa-2b Versus MAP Alone in Patients With Resectable High-Grade Osteosarcoma and Good Histologic Response to Preoperative MAP: First Results of the EURAMOS-1 Good Response Randomized Controlled Trial. J Clin Oncol 2015;33(20): 2279–87.

52. Bramwell VH, Burgers M, Sneath R, et al. A comparison of two short intensive adjuvant chemotherapy regimens in operable osteosarcoma of limbs in children and young adults: the first study of the European Osteosarcoma Intergroup. J Clin Oncol 1992;10:1579.

53. Chawla SP, Sankhala KK, Chua V, et al. A phase II study of AP23573 (an mTOR inhibitor) in patients (pts) with advanced sarcomas (abstract). J Clin Oncol 2005;24:833s.

54. Meyers PA, Schwartz CL, Krailo M, et al. Osteosarcoma: the addition of muramyl tripeptide to chemotherapy improves overall survival: a report from the Children's Oncology Group. J Clin Oncol 2008;26:633–8.

55. Arndt CA, Rose PS, Folpe AL, et al. Common musculoskeletal tumors of childhood and adolescence. Mayo Clin Proc 2012;87(5):475–87.

56. Gibbs CP Jr, Weber K, Scarborough MT. Malignant bone tumors. Instr Course Lect 2002;51:413–28.

57. Ewing J. Diffuse endothelioma of bone. CA Cancer J Clin 1972;22:95–8.

58. Phillips RF, Higinbotham NL. The curability of Ewing's endothelioma of bone in children. J Pediatr 1967;70:391–7.

59. Bacci G, Picci P, Gitelis S, et al. The treatment of localized Ewing's sarcoma: the experience at the Instituto Rizzoli in 163 cases treated with and without adjuvant chemotherapy. Cancer 1982;49:1561–70.

60. Lee J, Hoang BH, Ziogas A, et al. Analysis of prognostic factors in Ewing sarcoma using a population-based cancer registry. Cancer 2010;116:1964–73.

61. Cotterill SJ, Ahrens S, Paulussen M, et al. Prognostic factors in Ewing's tumor of bone: analysis of 975 patients from the European Intergroup Cooperative Ewing's Sarcoma Study Group. J Clin Oncol 2000;18(17):3108–14.

62. Newbit ME, Gehan EA, Burgert EO, et al. Multimodal therapy for management of primary, nonmetastatic Ewing's sarcoma of bone: a long-term follow-up for the First Intergroup study. J Clin Oncol 1990;8:1664–74.

63. Burgert EO, Nesbit ME, Garnsey LA, et al. Multimodal therapy for the management of nonpelvic, localized Ewing's sarcoma of bone: intergroup Study IESS-II. J Clin Oncol 1990;8:1514–24.

64. Grier HE, Krailo MD, Tarbell NJ, et al. Addition of ifosfamide and etoposide to standard chemotherapy for Ewing's sarcoma and primitive neuroectodermal tumor of bone. N Engl J Med 2003;348:694–701.

65. Ferrari S, Sundby Hall K, Luksch R, et al. Nonmetastatic Ewing family tumors: high-dose chemotherapy with stem cell rescue in poor responder patients. Results of the Italian Sarcoma Group/Scandinavian Sarcoma Group III protocol. Ann Oncol 2011;22:1221–7.

66. Granowetter L, Womer R, Devidas M, et al. Dose-intensified compared with standard chemotherapy for nonmetastatic Ewing sarcoma family of tumors: a Children's Oncology Group Study. J Clin Oncol 2009;27:2536.

67. Womer RB, Daller RT, Fenton JG, et al. Granulocyte colony stimulating factor permits dose intensification by interval compression in the treatment of Ewing's sarcomas and soft tissue sarcomas in children. Eur J Cancer 2000;36:87.

68. Womer RB, West DC, Krailo MD, et al. Randomized controlled trial of interval-compressed chemotherapy for the treatment of localized Ewing sarcoma: a report from the Children's Oncology Group. J Clin Oncol 2012;30:4148.

69. Womer RB, West DC, Krailo MD, et al. Chemotherapy intensification by interval compression in localized Ewing sarcoma family of tumors (ESFT) (abstract 855). Data presented at the 13th annual meeting of the Connective Tissue Oncology Society (CTOS). Seattle, Washington, October 31-November 2, 2007. Abstract 855. Available at: http://www.ctos.org/meeting/2007/program.asp. Accessed December 11, 2012.

70. Oberlin O, Rey A, Desfachelles AS, et al. Impact of high-dose busulfan plus melphalan as consolidation in metastatic Ewing tumors: a study by the Société Française des Cancers de l'Enfant. J Clin Oncol 2006;24:3997.

71. Meyers PA, Krailo MD, Ladanyi M, et al. High-dose melphalan, etoposide, total-body irradiation, and autologous stem-cell reconstitution as consolidation therapy for high-risk Ewing's sarcoma does not improve prognosis. J Clin Oncol 2001;19:2812.

72. Ladenstein R, Lasset C, Pinkerton R, et al. Impact of megatherapy in children with high-risk Ewing's tumours in complete remission: a report from the EBMT Solid Tumour Registry. Bone Marrow Transplant 1995;15:697.

73. Juergens C, Weston C, Lewis I, et al. Safety assessment of intensive induction with vincristine, ifosfamide, doxorubicin, and etoposide (VIDE) in the treatment of Ewing tumors in the EURO-E.W.I.N.G. 99 clinical trial. Pediatr Blood Cancer 2006;47:22.

74. Eriksson AI, Schiller A, Mankin JH. The management of chondrosarcoma of bone. Clin Orthop 1980;153:44–66.

75. Gelderblom H, Hogendoorn PCW, Dijkstra SD, et al. The clinical approach towards chondrosarcoma. Oncologist 2008;13:320–9.

76. Mitchell AD, Ayoub K, Mangham DC, et al. Experience in the treatment of dedifferentiated chondrosarcoma. J Bone Joint Surg Br 2000;82:55–61.

77. Staals EL, Bacchini P, Mercuri M, et al. Dedifferentiated chondrosarcoma arising in preexisting osteochondromas. J Bone Joint Surg Am 2007;89:987–93.

78. Grimer RJ, Gosheger G, Taminiau A, et al. Dedifferentiated chondrosarcoma: prognostic factors and outcome from a European group. Eur J Cancer 2007; 43(14):2060–5.

79. Dickey ID, Rose PS, Fucks B, et al. Dedifferentiated chondrosarcoma: the role of chemotherapy with updated outcomes. J Bone Joint Surg Am 2004;86(11): 2412–8.

80. Rohle D, Popvici-Muller J, Palaskas N, et al. An inhibitor of mutant IDH-1 delays growth and promotes differentiation in glioma cells. Science 2013;340:626–30.

81. Lin C, McGough R, Aswad B, et al. Hypoxia induces HIF-1alpha and VEGF expression in chondrosarcoma cells and chondrocytes. J Orthop Res 2004; 22(6):1175–81.

82. Dallas J, Imanirad I, Rajani R, et al. Response to sunitinib in combination with proton beam radiation in a patient with chondrosarcoma: a case report. J Med Case Rep 2012;6:41.

83. Schrage YM, Lam S, Jochemsen AG, et al. Central chondrosarcoma progression is associated with pRb pathway alterations; CDK4 downregulation and p16 overexpression inhibit cell growth in vitro. J Cell Mol Med 2008;13(9A): 2843–52.

84. Bertino JR, Waud WR, Parker WB, et al. Targeting tumors that lack methylthioadenosine phosphorylase (MTAP) activity: current strategies. Cancer Biol Ther 2011;11(7):627–32.

85. Van Oosterwijk JG, Anninga JK, Gelderblom H, et al. Update on targets and novel treatment options for high grade osteosarcoma and chondrosarcoma. Hematol Oncol Clin North Am 2013;27(5):1021–48.

86. Bernstein-Molho R, Kollender Y, Issakov J, et al. Clinical activity of mTOR inhibition in combination with cyclophosphamide in the treatment of recurrent unresectable chondrosarcomas. Cancer Chemother Pharmacol 2012;70:855.

87. DuBois SG, Krailo MD, Gebhardt MC, et al. Comparative evaluation of local control strategies in localized Ewing sarcoma of bone. Cancer 2015;121:467–75.

88. Schuck A, Ahrens S, Paulussen M, et al. Local therapy in localized Ewing tumors: results of 1058 patients treated in the CESS 81, CESS 86, and EICESS 92 trials. Int J Radiat Oncol Biol Phys 2003;55:168–77.

89. Ozaki T, Hillmann A, Hoffmann C, et al. Significance of surgical margin on the prognosis of patients with Ewing's sarcoma. A report from the Cooperative Ewing's Sarcoma Study. Cancer 1996;78:892–900.

90. Bacci G, Longhi A, Briccoli A, et al. The role of surgical margins in the treatment of Ewing's sarcoma family tumors: experience of a single institution with 512 patients treated with adjuvant and neoadjuvant chemotherapy. Int J Radiat Oncol Biol Phys 2006;65(3):766–72.

91. Baumann BC, Lustig RA, Mazzoni S, et al. A prospective clinical trial of proton therapy for chordoma and chondrosarcoma. Int J Radiat Oncol Biol Phys 2015; 93(3-S):E641.

92. Ozaki T, Hillmann A, Rube C, et al. The impact of intraoperative brachytherapy on surgery of Ewing's sarcoma. J Cancer Res Clin Oncol 1997;123(1):53–6.

93. Sole CV, Calvo FA, Polo A, et al. Intraoperative electron-beam radiation therapy for pediatric Ewing sarcomas and rhabdomyosarcomas: long-term outcomes. Int J Radiat Oncol Biol Phys 2015;92(5):1069–76.

94. Rombi B, DeLaney TF, MacDonald SM, et al. Proton radiotherapy for pediatric Ewing's sarcoma: initial clinical outcomes. Int J Radiat Oncol Biol Phys 2012; 82(3):1142–8.

95. Hoekstra HJ, Sindelar WF, Kinsella TJ. Surgery with intraoperative radiotherapy for sarcomas of the pelvic girdle: a pilot experience. Int J Radiat Oncol Biol Phys 1988;15:1013–6.

96. Weber DC, Badiyan S, Malyapa R, et al. Long-term outcomes of and prognostic factors of skull-base chondrosarcoma patients treated with pencil-beam scanning proton therapy at the Paul Scherrer Institute. Neuro Oncol 2015;18(2): 236–43.

97. Kamada T, Tsujii H, Tsuji H, et al. Efficacy and safety of carbon ion radiotherapy in bone and soft tissue sarcomas. J Clin Oncol 2002;20:4466–71.

98. Imai R, Kamada T, Araki N, Working Group for Bone and Soft Tissue Sarcomas. Carbon ion radiotherapy for unresectable sacral chordoma: an analysis of 188 cases. Int J Radiat Oncol Biol Phys 2016;95(1):322–7.

99. Sugahara S, Kamada T, Imai R, et al, Working Group for the Bone and Soft Tissue Sarcomas. Carbon ion radiotherapy for localized primary sarcoma of the extremities: results of a phase I/II trial. Radiother Oncol 2012;105(2):226–31.

100. Matsunobu A, Imai R, Kamada T, et al. Impact of carbon ion radiotherapy for unresectable osteosarcoma of the trunk. Cancer 2012;118(18):4555–63.

101. Imai R, Kamada T, Sugahara S, et al. Carbon ion radiotherapy for sacral chordoma. Br J Radiol 2011;84(S-1):S48–54.

102. Ruggieri P, Angelini A, Ussia G, et al. Surgical margins and local control in resection of sacral chordomas. Clin Orthop Relat Res 2010;468(10):2939–47.

103. Hulen CA, Temple T, Fox WP, et al. Oncologic and functional outcome following sacrectomy for sacral chordoma. J Bone Joint Surg Am 2006;88(7):1532–9.

104. Nishida Y, Kamada T, Imai R, et al. Clinical outcome of sacral chordoma with carbon ion radiotherapy compared with surgery. Int J Radiat Oncol Biol Phys 2011; 79:110–6.

105. Berrington de Gonzalez A, Kutsenko A, Rajaraman P. Sarcoma risk after radiation exposure. Clin Sarcoma Res 2012;2(1):18.

106. Gladdy RA, Qin LX, Moraco N, et al. Do radiation-associated soft tissue sarcomas have the same prognosis as sporadic soft tissue sarcomas? J Clin Oncol 2010;28(12):2064–9.

107. Paulino AC. Late effects of radiotherapy for pediatric extremity sarcomas. Int J Radiat Oncol Biol Phys 2004;60(1):265–74.

108. Bacci G, Forni C, Longhi A, et al. Local recurrence and local control of non-metastatic osteosarcoma of the extremities: a 27-year experience in a single institution. J Surg Oncol 2007;96:118–23.

109. Fiorenza F, Abudu A, Grimer RJ, et al. Risk factors for survival and local control in chondrosarcoma of bone. J Bone Joint Surg Br 2002;84:93–9.

110. Kawaguchi N, Ahmed AR, Matsumoto S, et al. The concept of curative margin in surgery for bone and soft tissue sarcoma. Clin Orthop Relat Res 2004;419: 165–72.

111. Ozaki T, Flege S, Liljenqvist U, et al. Osteosarcoma of the spine: experience of the Cooperative Osteosarcoma Study Group. Cancer 2002;94(4):1069.

112. Schoenfeld AJ, Hornicek FJ, Pedlow FX, et al. Osteosarcoma of the spine: experience in 26 patients treated at the Massachusetts General Hospital. Spine J 2010;10(8):708–14.

113. Farfalli GL, Albergo JI, Ritacco LE, et al. Oncologic and clinical outcomes in pelvic primary bone sarcomas treated with limb salvage surgery. Musculoskelet Surg 2015;99(3):237–42.

114. Grimer RJ. Surgical options for children with osteosarcoma. Lancet Oncol 2005; 6:85–92.

115. Rosenberg SA, Tepper J, Glatstein E, et al. The treatment of soft tissue sarcomas of the extremities: prospective randomized evaluations of (1) limb-sparing surgery plus radiation therapy compared with amputation and (2) the role of adjuvant chemotherapy. Ann Surg 1982;196:305–15.

116. Bacci G, Ferrari S, Lari S, et al. Osteosarcoma of the limb: amputation or lib salvage in patients treated with neoadjuvant chemotherapy. J Bone Joint Surg Br 2002;84:88–92.

117. Reddy KIA, Wafa H, Gaston CL, et al. Does amputation offer any survival benefit over limb salvage in osteosarcoma patients with poor chemonecrosis and close margins? Bone Joint J 2015;97-B:115–20.

118. Rougraff BT, Simon MA, Kneisl JS, et al. Limb salvage compared with amputation for osteosarcoma of the distal end of the femur: a long-term oncological, functional, and quality of life study. J Bone Joint Surg Am 1994;76:649–56.

119. Nagarajan R, Neglia JP, Clohisy DR, et al. Limb salvage and amputation in survivors of pediatric lower-extremity bone tumors: what are the long-term implications? J Clin Oncol 2002;20(22):4493.

120. Furtado S, Grimer RJ, Cool P, et al. Physical functioning, pain, and quality of life after amputation for musculoskeletal tumours. A national survey. Bone Joint J 2015;97-B:1284–90.

121. Malek F, Somerson JS, Mitchel S, et al. Does limb-salvage surgery offer patients better quality of life and functional capacity than amputation? Clin Orthop Relat Res 2012;470:2000–6.

122. Hobusch GM, Lang N, Schuh R, et al. Do patients with Ewing's sarcoma continue with sports activities after limb salvage surgery of the lower extremity? Clin Orthop Relat Res 2015;473(3):839–46.

123. Mason GE, Aung L, Gall S, et al. Quality of life following amputation or limb preservation in patients with lower extremity bone sarcoma. Front Oncol 2013; 3(210):1–6.

124. Grimer RJ, Carter SR, Pynsent PB. The cost-effectiveness of limb salvage for bone tumors. J Bone Joint Surg Br 1997;79-B(4):558–61.

125. Renard AJ, Veth RP, Schreuder HWB, et al. Function and complications after ablative and limb-salvage therapy in lower extremity sarcoma of bone. J Surg Oncol 2000;73(4):198–205.

126. Henderson ER, O'Connor MI, Ruggieri P, et al. Classification of failure of limb salvage after reconstructive surgery for bone tumors. Bone Joint J 2014;96-B: 1436–40.

127. Grimer RJ, Chandrasekar CR, Carter SR, et al. Hindquarter amputation. Is it still needed and what are the outcomes? Bone Joint J 2013;95-B:127–31.

128. Bacci G, Picci P, Ferrari S, et al. Primary chemotherapy and delayed surgery for nonmetastatic osteosarcoma of the extremities: results in 164 patients preoperatively treated with high doses of methotrexate followed by cisplatin and doxorubicin. Cancer 1993;72:3227–38.

129. Nichter S, Menendez LR. Reconstructive considerations for limb salvage surgery. Orthop Clin North Am 1993;24:511–21.

130. Jeys LM, Grimer RJ, Carter SR, et al. Periprosthetic infection in patients treated for an orthopaedic oncological condition. J Bone Joint Surg Am 2005;87:842–9.

131. Angelini A, Drago G, Trovarelli G, et al. Infection after surgical resection for pelvic bone tumors: an analysis of 270 patients from one institution. Clin Orthop Relat Res 2014;472:349–59.

132. Aponte-Tinao LA, Ayerza MA, Muscolo DL, et al. What are the risk factors and management options for infection after reconstruction with massive bone allografts? Clin Orthop Relat Res 2016;474:669–73.

133. Brosojo O. Surgical procedure and local recurrence in 223 patients treated 1982-1997 according to two osteosarcoma chemotherapy protocols. The Scandinavian Sarcoma Group experience. Acta Orthop Scand Suppl 1999;285: 58–61.

134. Li X, Moretti VM, Ashana AO, et al. Impact of close surgical margin on local recurrence and survival in osteosarcoma. Int Orthop 2012;36:131–7.

135. Andreou D, Bielack SS, Carrle D, et al. The influence of tumor- and treatment-related factors on the development of local recurrence in osteosarcoma after adequate surgery. An analysis of 1355 patients treated on neoadjuvant Cooperative Osteosarcoma Study Group protocols. Ann Oncol 2011;22(5):1228–35.

136. Grimer RJ, Sommerville S, Warnock D, et al. Management and outcome after local recurrence of osteosarcoma. Eur J Cancer 2005;41:578–83.

137. Rodriguez-Galindo C, Shah N, McCarville MB, et al. Outcome after local recurrence in osteosarcoma: the St. Jude Children's Research Hospital experience (1970-2000). Cancer 2004;100:1928–35.

138. Weeden S, Grimer RJ, Cannon SR, et al. The effect of local recurrence on survival in resected osteosarcoma. Eur J Cancer 2001;37:39–46.

139. Kempf-Bielack B, Bielack SS, Jurgens H, et al. Osteosarcoma relapse after combined modality therapy: an analysis of unselected patients in the Cooperative Osteosarcoma Study Group (COSS). J Clin Oncol 2005;23:559–68.

140. Grimer RJ, Taminiau AM, Cannon SR. Surgical subcommittee of the European Osteosarcoma Intergroup. Surgical outcomes in osteosarcoma. J Bone Joint Surg Br 2002;84:395–400.

141. Takeuchi A, Lewis VO, Satcher RL, et al. What are the factors that affect survival and relapse after local recurrence of osteosarcoma? Clin Orthop Relat Res 2014;472(1):3188–95.

142. Kong CB, Song WS, Cho WH, et al. Local recurrence has only small effect on survival in high-risk extremity osteosarcoma. Clin Orthop Relat Res 2012; 470(5):1482–90.

143. Bacci G, Longhi A, Cesari M, et al. Influence of local recurrence on survival in patients with extremity osteosarcoma treated with neoadjuvant chemotherapy: the experience of a single institution with 44 patients. Cancer 2006;106:2701–6.

144. Loh AHP, Navid F, Wang C, et al. Management of local recurrence of pediatric osteosarcoma following limb-sparing surgery. Ann Surg Oncol 2014;21: 1948–55.

145. Fox EJ, Anwar M, Gebhardt MC, et al. Long-term followup of proximal femoral allografts. Clin Orthop Relat Res 2002;397:106–13.

146. Bus MPA, Dijkstra PDS, van de Sande MA, et al. Intercalary allograft reconstructions following resection of primary bone tumors. J Bone Joint Surg Am 2014; 19(96):e26.

147. Sorger JI, Hornicek FJ, Zavatta M, et al. Allograft fractures revisited. Clin Orthop Relat Res 2001;382:66–74.

148. Mankin HJ, Springfield DS, Gebhardt MC, et al. Current status of allografting for bone tumors. Orthopedics 1992;15:1147–54.

149. Aponte-Tinao L, Ayerza MA, Muscolo DL, et al. Survival, recurrence, and function after epiphyseal preservation and allograft reconstruction in osteosarcoma of the knee. Clin Orthop Relat Res 2015;473:1789–96.

150. Aponte-Tinao L, Farfalli GL, Ritacco LE, et al. Intercalary femur allografts are an acceptable alternative after tumor resection. Clin Orthop Relat Res 2012;470(3): 728–34.

151. Ortiz-Cruz E, Gebhardt MC, Jennings LC, et al. The results of transplantation of intercalary allografts after resection of tumors. A long-term follow-up study. J Bone Joint Surg Am 1997;79(1):97–106.

152. Frisoni T, Cevolani L, Giorgini A, et al. Factors affecting outcome of massive intercalary bone allografts in the treatment of tumours of the femur. J Bone Joint Surg Br 2012;94(6):836–41.

153. Berrey BH Jr, Lord CF, Gebhardt MC, et al. Fractures of allografts. Frequency, treatment, and end results. J Bone Joint Surg Am 1990;72:825–33.

154. Houdek MT, Wagner ER, Stans AA, et al. What is the outcome of allograft and intramedullary free fibula (Capanna Technique) in pediatric and adolescent patients with bone tumors? Clin Orthop Relat Res 2016;474:660–8.

155. Capanna RB, Campanacci M. A new technique for reconstructions of large metadiaphyseal bone defects. Orthop Traumatol 1993;3:159–77.

156. Capanna R, Campanacci DA, Belot N, et al. A new reconstructive technique for intercalary defects of long bones: the association of massive allograft with vascularized fibular autograft. Long-term results and comparison with alternative techniques. Orthop Clin North Am 2007;38:51–60.

157. Enneking WF, Campanacci DA. Retrieved human allografts. A clinicopathological study. J Bone Joint Surg Am 2001;83A:971–86.

158. Aponte-Tinao LA, Ritacco LE, Albergo JI, et al. The principles and applications of fresh frozen allografts to bone and joint reconstruction. Orthop Clin North Am 2014;45(2):257–69.

159. Gitelis S, Rasecki P. Allograft prosthetic composite arthroplasty for osteosarcoma and other aggressive bone tumors. Clin Orthop Relat Res 1991;270:197–201.

160. Farid Y, Lin PP, Lewis VO, et al. Endoprosthetic and allograft-prosthetic composite reconstruction of the proximal femur for bone neoplasms. Clin Orthop Relat Res 2006;442:223–9.

161. Benedetti MG, Bonatti E, Malfitano C, et al. Comparison of allograft-prosthetic composite reconstruction and modular prosthetic replacement in proximal femur bone tumors: functional assessment by gait analysis in 20 patients. Acta Orthop 2013;84(2):218–23.

162. Gitelis S, Heligman D, Quill G, et al. The use of large allografts for tumor reconstruction and salvage of the failed total hip arthroplasty. Clin Orthop 1988;231:62.

163. King JJ, Nystrom LM, Grimer NB, et al. Allograft-prosthetic composite reverse total shoulder arthroplasty for reconstruction of proximal humerus tumor resections. J Shoulder Elbow Surg 2016;25:45–54.

164. Hejna MJ, Gitelis S. Allograft prosthetic composite replacement for bone tumors. Semin Surg Oncol 1997;13:18–24.

165. Racano A, Pazionis T, Farrokhyar F, et al. High infection rate outcomes in long-bone tumor surgery with endoprosthetic reconstruction in adults: a systematic review. Clin Orthop Relat Res 2013;471:2017–27.

166. Horowitz SM, Glasser DB, Lane JM, et al. Prosthetic and extremity survivorship after limb salvage for sarcoma. How long do the reconstructions last? Clin Orthop Relat Res 1993;293:280–6.

167. Ahlmann ER, Menendez LR, Kermani C, et al. Survivorship and clinical outcome of modular endoprosthetic reconstruction for neoplastic disease of the lower limb. J Bone Joint Surg Br 2006;88-B:790–5.

168. Houdek MT, Wagner ER, Wilke BK, et al. Long term outcomes of cemented endoprosthetic reconstruction for periarticular tumors of the distal femur. Knee 2016;23(1):167–72.

169. Jeys LM, Kulkarni A, Grimer RJ, et al. Endoprosthetic reconstruction for the treatment of musculoskeletal tumors of the appendicular skeleton and pelvis. J Bone Joint Surg Am 2008;90:1265–71.

170. AlGheshyan F, Eltoukhy M, Zakaria K, et al. Comparison of gait parameters in distal femoral replacement using a metallic endoprosthesis versus allograft reconstruction. J Orthop 2015;12(S1):S25–30.

171. Benedetti MG, Catani F, Donati D, et al. Muscle performance about the knee joint in patients who had distal femoral replacement after resection of a bone tumor. J Bone Joint Surg Am 2000;82(11):1619.

172. Spira E, Lubin E. Extracorporeal irradiation of bone tumors: a preliminary report. Isr J Med Sci 1968;4:1015–9.

173. Chen TH, Chen WM, Huang CK. Reconstruction after intercalary resection of malignant bone tumors: comparison between segmental allograft and extracorporeally-irradiated autograft. J Bone Joint Surg Br 2005;87-B:704–9.

174. Puri A, Gulia A, Jambhekar N, et al. The outcome of the treatment of diaphyseal primary bone sarcoma by resection, irradiation, and re-implantation of the host bone. J Bone Joint Surg Br 2012;94-B:982–8.

175. Cascio BM, Thomas KA, Wilson SC. A mechanical comparison and review of transverse, step-cut, and sigmoid osteotomies. Clin Orthop Relat Res 2003; 411:296–304.

176. Currey JD, Foreman J, Laketic I, et al. Effects of ionizing radiation on the mechanical properties of human bone. J Orthop Res 1997;15:111–7.

177. Krieg AH, Davidson AW, Stalley PD. Intercalary femoral reconstruction with extracorporeal irradiated autogenous bone graft in limb salvage surgery. J Bone Joint Surg Br 2007;89-B:366–71.

178. Zimel MN, Farfalli GL, Zindman AM, et al. Revision distal femoral arthroplasty with the Compress ® prosthesis has low rate of mechanical failure at 10 years. Clin Orthop Relat Res 2016;474(2):528–36.

179. Cristofolini L, Bini S, Toni A. In vitro testing of a novel limb salvage prosthesis for the distal femur. Clin Biomech 1998;13:608–15.

180. Monument MJ, Bernthal NM, Bowles AJ, et al. What are the 5-year survivorship outcomes of compressive endoprosthetic osseointegration fixation of the femur? Clin Orthop Relat Res 2015;473:883–90.

181. Healey JH, Morris CD, Athanasian EA, et al. Compress knee arthroplasty has 80% 10-year survivorship and novel forms of bone failure. Clin Orthop Relat Res 2013;471:774–83.

182. Pedtke AC, Wustrack RL, Fang AS, et al. Aseptic failure: how does the Compress® implant compare to cemented stems? Clin Orthop Relat Res 2012;470:735–42.

183. Farfalli GL, Boland PJ, Morris CD, et al. Early equivalence of uncemented press-fit and compress femoral fixation. Clin Orthop Relat Res 2009;467:2792–9.

184. Bhangu AA, Kramer MJ, Grimer RJ, et al. Early distal femoral endoprosthetic survival: cemented stems versus the compress implant. Int Orthop 2006;30: 465–72.

185. Zimel MN, Hwang S, Riedel ER, et al. Carbon fiber intramedullary nails reduce artifact in postoperative advanced imaging. Skeletal Radiol 2015;44:1317–25.

186. Steinberg EL, Rath E, Shlaifer A, et al. Carbon fiber reinforced PEEK optima—a composite material biomechanical properties and wear/debris characteristic of CF-PEEK composites for orthopedic trauma implants. J Mech Behav Biomed Mater 2013;17:221–8.

187. Leung KS, Tang N, Cheung LWH, et al. Image-guided navigation in orthopaedic trauma. J Bone Joint Surg Br 2010;92-B:1332–7.

188. Jolles BM, Genoud P, Hoffmeyer P. Computer assisted cup placement techniques in total hip arthroplasty improves accuracy of placement. Clin Orthop Relat Res 2004;426:174–9.

189. Richter M, Cakir B, Schmidt R. Cervical pedicle screws: conventional versus computer-assisted placement of cannulated screws. Spine 2005;30:2280–7.

190. Hufner T, Kfuri M Jr, Galanski M, et al. New indications for computer-assisted surgery: tumor resection in the pelvis. Clin Orthop Relat Res 2004;426:219–25.
191. Cartiaux O, Banse X, Paul L, et al. Computer-assisted planning and navigation improves cutting accuracy during simulated bone tumor surgery of the pelvis. Comput Aided Surg 2013;18:19–26.
192. Jeys L, Matharu GS, Nandra RS, et al. Can computer navigation-assisted surgery reduce the risk of an intralesional margin and reduce the rate of local recurrence in patients with a tumour of the pelvis or sacrum? Bone Joint J 2013; 95-B(10):1417–24.
193. Ritacco LE, Milano FE, Farfalli GL, et al. Accuracy of 3-D planning and navigation in bone tumor resection. Orthopedics 2013;36(7):e942–50.
194. Cho HS, Oh JH, Han I, et al. The outcomes of navigation-assisted bone tumour surgery: minimum three-year follow-up. J Bone Joint Surg Br 2012;94(10): 1414–20.
195. Muscolo DL, Ayerza MA, Aponte-Tinao LA, et al. Partial epiphyseal preservation and intercalary allograft reconstruction in high-grade metaphyseal osteosarcoma of the knee. J Bone Joint Surg Am 2004;86-A(12):2686–93.
196. Hinsche AF, Giannoudis PV, Smith RM. Fluoroscopy-based multiplanar image guidance for insertion of sacroiliac screws. Clin Orthop 2002;395:135–44.
197. Amiot LP, Lang K, Putzier M, et al. Comparative results between conventional and computer-assisted pedicle screw installation in the thoracic, lumbar, and sacral spine. Spine 2000;25(5):606–14.
198. Zura RD, Kahler DM. A transverse acetabular nonunion treated with computer-assisted percutaneous internal fixation: a case report. J Bone Joint Surg Am 2000;82A:219–24.
199. Wong KC, Kumta SM, Sze KY, et al. Use of a patient-specific CAD/CAM surgical jig in extremity bone tumor resection and custom prosthetic reconstruction. Comput Aided Surg 2012;17(6):284–93.
200. Docquier PL, Paul L, Cartiaux O, et al. Computer-assisted resection and reconstruction of pelvic tumor sarcoma. Sarcoma 2010;2010:125162.

Pediatric Sarcomas

Regan F. Williams, MD[a],*, Israel Fernandez-Pineda, MD[b],
Ankush Gosain, MD, PhD[a]

KEYWORDS

- Rhabdomyosarcoma • Osteosarcoma • Ewing's sarcoma
- Nonrhabdomyosarcoma soft tissue sarcoma

KEY POINTS

- Pediatric sarcomas are best treated with a multidisciplinary team to include surgery, radiation, and oncology.
- Rhabdomyosarcomas (RMS) often occur in young children, whereas nonrhabdomyosarcomas occur in infants and teenagers.
- All patients with RMS receive chemotherapy.
- Low-grade osteosarcomas and low risk nonrhabdomyosarcomas are treated with surgery alone.

Pediatric sarcomas are a heterogeneous group of tumors and account for approximately 10% of childhood solid tumors.[1] Treatment is focused on multimodality therapy, which has improved the prognosis over the past 2 decades. Current regimens focus on decreasing treatment for low-risk patients to decrease the long-term side effects of chemotherapy and radiation while maximizing therapy for patients with metastatic disease in an attempt to improve survival. Pediatric sarcomas can be divided into soft tissue sarcomas and osseous tumors. Soft tissue sarcomas are further delineated into rhabdomyosarcoma (RMS), which affect young children and nonrhabdomyosarcoma, which are most common in adolescents. The most common bone sarcomas are osteosarcoma (OS) and Ewing sarcoma (ES).

RHABDOMYOSARCOMA
Epidemiology

RMS is the most common soft tissue sarcoma in children and adolescents, accounting for nearly 250 cases of childhood cancer in the United States each year.[2] RMS is a

The authors have nothing to disclose.
[a] Department of Surgery, University of Tennessee Health Science Center, 49 North Dunlap Avenue, Second Floor, Memphis, TN 38105, USA; [b] Department of Surgery, St Jude Children's Research Hospital, MS133, Room B3019, 262 Danny Thomas Place, Memphis, TN 38105-3678, USA
* Corresponding author.
E-mail address: rfwillia@uthsc.edu

malignant soft tissue tumor of mesenchymal origin, accounting for approximately 3.5% of cancers among children aged 0 to 14 years and 2% of the cases among adolescents aged 15 to 19 years.[3] The incidence of RMS is 4.5 per million children, with one-half of cases seen in the first decade of life.[4] During the course of 4 consecutive Intergroup Rhabdomyosarcoma Study Group clinical trials, our understanding of RMS tumor biology has advanced, and the outcome for children and adolescents with RMS has improved significantly.[5–8] Five-year survival for RMS has increased, from 53% to 67% for children younger than 15 years and from 30% to 51% for adolescents aged 15 to 19 years.[9]

The incidence of RMS varies depending on histologic subtype.[2] Embryonal RMS patients are predominantly male (male = 1.5 × female), with a peak incidence in the 0- to 4-year age group (approximately 4 cases per million). Adolescents have a lower incidence, with approximately 1.5 cases per million. The incidence of alveolar RMS is relatively constant through childhood (1 case per million) and does not show a gender predilection.[9] Undifferentiated sarcoma is more common in infants less than 1 year of age, with increased numbers found in the trunk and abdomen and fewer in the parameningeal site as compared with noninfants.[10]

The most common primary tumor sites for RMS are the head, the genitourinary (GU) tract, and the extremities.[11] Extremity tumors are more commonly found in the hand and foot of older patients, and are more likely to display alveolar histology and metastatic spread.[12] Less frequently seen primary tumor sites include the trunk, chest wall, perineal/anal region, and abdomen (including retroperitoneum and biliary tract).

The majority of RMS cases are sporadic, with no identifiable risk factors.[2] Embryonal RMS is associated with high birth weight and infants that are large for gestational age.[13] The Li-Fraumeni syndrome (germline *p53* mutations),[14] pleuropulmonary blastoma (*DICER1* mutations),[15] neurofibromatosis type I,[16] Costello syndrome (germline *HRAS* mutations),[17,18] Beckwith-Wiedemann syndrome,[19] and Noonan syndrome are all associated with RMS.[20]

Prognosis

The prognosis for children with RMS depends on age, primary tumor site, tumor size, resectability, presence or absence of metastases, number of metastatic sites, presence or absence of regional lymph node involvement, histopathologic subtype (alveolar vs embryonal), and, in some cases, delivery of radiation therapy.[5–8,11,21,22]

In children with localized disease who receive combined-modality therapy, there is greater than 70% survival at 3 years.[8] Relapses are uncommon after this point, with a less than 10% late event rate through 10 years. However, children with gross residual disease in unfavorable sites after initial surgery and those who have metastatic disease at diagnosis are more likely to experience relapse.[23]

Patient- and tumor-specific factors with prognostic implications include the following:

- Age: Children aged 1 to 9 years have improved prognosis, whereas those less than 1 year and greater than 9 years have worse prognosis (5-year survival is 76% for patients <1 year, 87% for patients 1–9 years, and 76% for patients >10 years).[10] It is unclear if infants have poorer outcomes because of disease-specific factors or owing to adjustments that are made to therapy owing to their small size (eg, less chemotherapy because of intolerant bone marrow, less use of radiation therapy).[8,24] Additionally, adolescent patients seem to present with unfavorable tumor-specific factors, such as alveolar histology, regional lymph node involvement, and metastatic disease.[25] Finally, 5-year survival rates for adults are markedly worse than those for children.[26]

- Primary tumor site: Sites with favorable prognosis include the orbit and nonparameningeal head and neck, paratesticular, vulva, vagina, uterus (nonbladder, nonprostate GU tract), and biliary tract.[5,7]
- Tumor size: Smaller tumors ($\leq$5 cm) have improved survival; however, it is unclear if this relationship is true across all ages, because tumor volume versus body surface area may be of importance.[7]
- Metastatic disease: Children who present with metastatic disease have a worse prognosis and outcome, although this varies by primary tumor histology and site/number of metastases.[27] Additionally, regional lymph node involvement portends a worse prognosis.[28]
- Tumor resectability: The extent of remaining disease after the primary surgical resection correlates with outcome. In the Intergroup Rhabdomyosarcoma Study III (IRS-III) study, patients without residual tumor after surgery (group I) experienced greater than 90% survival at 5 years, those with microscopic disease (group II) had approximately 80% survival at 5 years, and those with gross residual disease (localized, group III) had approximately 70% survival at 5 years.[7]
- Tumor histology: Alveolar histology is associated with a worse outcome than embryonal histology. Alveolar histology is more common amongst patients with other unfavorable features, including age less than 1 year, age greater than 10 years, extremity primary tumor site, and metastatic disease. Alveolar histology has been associated with a less favorable outcome even in patients whose primary tumor was completely resected.[5] In the IRS-III study, the outcome for patients with completely resected alveolar tumors was similar to that for other group I tumors, but patients with alveolar histology received more intensive therapy.[7]

Classification

RMS is divided into 3 histologic subtypes: embryonal, alveolar, and pleomorphic. Embryonal RMS has embryonal, botryoid, and spindle cell subtypes.[2] Additionally, embryonal and alveolar histologies have distinct molecular profiles that are used in diagnosis and treatment planning.[29–31]

Embryonal RMS is the most frequently observed subtype in children, accounting for approximately 60% to 70% of cases.[2] These tumors may occur in any location, although the typically arise in the head and neck region or in the GU tract. Embryonal tumors often show loss of heterozygosity at 11p15 and gains on chromosome 8. One-third of cases show mutations of genes in the RAS signaling pathway (NRAS, KRAS, HRAS, and NF1). Less frequently observed mutations include FGFR4, PIK3CA, CTNNB1, FBXW7, and BCOR.[18,32]

Botryoid tumors are embryonal tumors that arise under the mucosal surface of body orifices such as the vagina, bladder, nasopharynx, and biliary tract, accounting for approximately 10% of all RMS cases. The spindle cell variant of embryonal RMS is most frequently observed at the paratesticular site.[2] Botryoid and spindle cell subtypes are associated with very favorable outcomes.[2]

Alveolar RMS accounts for approximately 20% of pediatric cases, with a higher frequency seen in children greater than 10 years and in extremities, trunk, and perineum/perianal primary sites.[2] To be designated as alveolar, the tumor must have greater than 50% alveolar elements. The majority (approximately 75%) of alveolar tumors carry a PAX-FOXO1 fusion between the FOXO1 gene (chromosome 13) and either PAX3 (chromosome 2, approximately 60%) (t(2;13) (q35;q14)) or PAX7 (chromosome 1, approximately 20%) (t(1;13) (p36;q14)).[33] Less frequently, other fusions involving

PAX3 are seen. Cases associated with the PAX7 fusion tend to occur in younger patients and may be associated with longer event-free survival versus PAX3 fusions.[18,33]

Pleomorphic RMS occurs predominantly in adults over age 30 and is rarely seen in children.[26] In children, these tumors are referred to as anaplastic and may not carry a worse prognosis.[34]

Staging and Risk Stratification

Once the diagnosis of RMS is established, evaluation then focuses on determining the extent of disease for treatment planning. Evaluation includes chest radiography, computed tomography (CT) scan of the chest, bilateral bone marrow aspirates and biopsies, and bone scan. For lower extremity or GU tract tumors, a CT scan of the abdomen and pelvis is included. For parameningeal tumors, MRI of the base of the skull and brain and lumbar puncture are included. In general, cross-sectional imaging (CT or MRI) of regional lymph node basins should be considered and concerning lymph nodes biopsied. Two modalities that are under investigation for metastatic evaluation include sentinel lymph node biopsy and fluorodeoxyglucose-PET imaging.[35,36]

Tumors are segregated into those occurring in favorable sites (orbit, nonparameningeal head/neck, GU tract other than bladder/prostate, biliary tract) versus unfavorable sites (all others). After this, TNM (tumor/node/metastasis) classification is determined (**Table 1**). Together, these determine the pretreatment tumor stage (**Table 2**). Next, the surgical–pathologic group is assigned based on surgical findings (**Table 3**). Finally, these factors are combined with histology to determine the risk group (**Table 4**), which determines treatment.

Treatment

Multimodality therapy, consisting of systemic chemotherapy and either surgery or radiation therapy (or both) for local control, is employed in all children with RMS.[37]

Surgical resection consists of wide and complete resection of the primary tumor with a surrounding envelope of normal tissue.[38] This is performed at diagnosis (prechemotherapy), unless it involves sacrifice of normal tissue that either cannot be resected or would result in an unacceptable loss of function, or is not technically feasible.

Table 1 TNM staging of RMS	
Tumor (T)	**Definition**
T1a	Confined to anatomic site of origin, ≤5 cm diameter
T1b	Confined to anatomic site of origin, >5 cm diameter
T2a	Extension or fixation to surrounding tissue, ≤5 cm diameter
T2b	Extension or fixation to surrounding tissue, >5 cm diameter
Nodal Status (N)	**Definition**
N0	No clinical regional lymph node involvement
N1	Clinical regional lymph node involvement
Nx	Unknown
Metastasis (M)	**Definition**
M0	No metastatic disease
M1	Metastatic disease

From National Institutes of Health. National Cancer Institute Physician Data Query. Available at: http://www.cancer.gov/publications/pdq.

Table 2
Pretreatment tumor stage of rhabdomyosarcoma

Stage	Primary Site	T	Tumor Size	N	M
1	Favorable	T1 or T2	Any	Any	M0
2	Unfavorable	T1 or T2	a	N0 or Nx	M0
3	Unfavorable	T1 or T2	a	N1	M0
			b	Any	
4	Any	T1 or T2	Any	Any	M1

From National Institutes of Health. National Cancer Institute Physician Data Query. Available at: http://www.cancer.gov/publications/pdq.

Exceptions to the operative approach include primaries in the orbit and possibly some GU sites. Resection of RMS that arises from muscle (particularly in the extremities) does not require excision of the entire muscle of origin or the entire compartment. However, adequate margins of normal tissue are preferable to leaving gross or microscopic tumor. Reexcision for positive margins may limit adjuvant therapy and decrease long-term side effects from therapy. Surgical guidelines vary by specific primary sites (eg, head/neck, extremity, trunk, GU) and are beyond the scope of this review.[39]

In the majority of cases, upfront surgical resection is not feasible, and a biopsy is performed. The majority of patients have group III (gross residual) disease and receive definitive radiation therapy for control of the primary tumor after chemotherapy. Selected patients may undergo delayed primary excision to remove residual tumor if the delayed excision is deemed feasible with acceptable functional/cosmetic outcome and if a dose reduction in radiation therapy is expected to reduce significantly the risk of long-term adverse effects. Radiation therapy is given to clinically or radiologically suspicious lymph nodes unless the suspicious lymph nodes are biopsied and shown to be histologically tumor free. Retroperitoneal lymph node dissection is limited to children greater than 10 years of age with paratesticular RMS owing to the high rate of lymph node involvement and decreased survival when these patients are understaged.[40]

The intensity and duration of chemotherapy for RMS is dependent on Risk Group (see **Table 4**). Currently, low-risk patients are treated with triple drug chemotherapy consisting of vincristine, dactinomycin, and low-dose cyclophosphamide. Intermediate risk patients receive similar therapy with higher doses of cyclophosphamide,

Table 3
Surgical–Pathological Group of rhabdomyosarcoma

Group	Definition
I	Localized disease, completely resected, no lymph node involvement
II	Total gross resection with evidence of regional spread: grossly resected tumor with microscopic residual disease; regional disease with involved nodes, completely resected with no microscopic residual; regional disease with involved nodes, grossly resected but with evidence of microscopic residual disease or histologic involvement of most distal lymph node from the primary site
III	Incomplete resection with gross residual disease: localized tumor, incompletely removed with gross residual disease (biopsy of primary tumor only or resection of primary tumor >50%)
IV	Distant metastasis at diagnosis

From National Institutes of Health. National Cancer Institute Physician Data Query. Available at: http://www.cancer.gov/publications/pdq.

Table 4
Risk group classification of rhabdomyosarcoma

Risk Group	Stage	Group	Histology
Low	1	I, II, III	Embryonal
	2, 3	I, II	Embryonal
Intermediate	2, 3	III	Embryonal
	1, 2, 3	I, II, III	Alveolar
High	4	IV	Any

with additional agents (additional courses) being tested for efficacy in prolonging event-free and overall survival. High-risk patients also receive vincristine, dactinomycin, and low-dose cyclophosphamide therapy plus irinotecan, etoposide, and doxorubicin, with studies to date failing to demonstrate increased efficacy with additional or alternative agents. Biologic agents are currently being studied in high-risk patients.

Summary

RMS is the most common soft tissue sarcoma in children. Before the use of multimodal therapy including surgery, chemotherapy, and radiotherapy, fewer than one-third of children with RMS survived. The use of intensive combination chemotherapy, better staging, more effective local therapy with surgery and radiation, and improved supportive care have resulted in marked advances. Currently, more than 70% of children with localized RMS and more than 50% of selected children with metastatic disease (those who are younger than 10 years and have embryonal histology) can be cured of their disease. After completion of therapy, patients should have radiographic imaging every 3 months looking for recurrence. Imaging is spread out over time with follow-up imaging ending 5 years after completion of therapy. The diversity of primary tumor sites, the unique surgical and radiation therapy considerations for these primary sites, and the need for ongoing trials to improve outcomes, particularly intermediate- and high-risk disease, underscore the importance of treating children with RMS in medical centers with appropriate experience in all diagnostic and therapeutic modalities.

NONRHABDOMYOSARCOMA SOFT TISSUE SARCOMAS
Epidemiology

Nonrhabodmyosarcoma soft tissue sarcomas (NRSTS) are a heterogeneous group of tumors that are most common in adolescents and young adults. They comprise 60% of soft tissue sarcomas over all ages in the Surveillance, Epidemiology and End Results database from 1975 to 2012.[41] The most common subtypes only account for 10% of pediatric soft tissue sarcomas. A small proportion occur in infants such as infantile fibrosarcoma (**Fig. 1**), hemangiopericytoma, and malignant rhabdoid tumors.

Most NRSTS are owing to sporadic mutations but a few can be associated with genetic syndromes, such as Li–Fraumeni syndrome, hereditary retinoblastoma, neurofibromatosis type 1, Gorlin syndrome, and Werner syndrome.[42]

Histology

NRSTS derive from cells similar to mesenchymal cells (fibroblasts, smooth muscle cells and perineural cells). They are classified into 4 groups by the International Classification of Childhood Cancers: (1) fibrosarcomas, (2) Kaposi's sarcoma, (3) the "other specified" soft tissue sarcomas (synovial sarcoma, angiosarcoma, hemangiopericytoma, leiomyosarcoma, liposarcoma, and extraosseous Ewing sarcoma [ES]), and

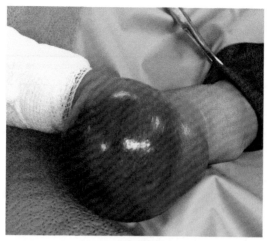

Fig. 1. Infantile fibrosarcoma in a 4-month-old boy.

(4) unspecified soft tissue sarcomas.[41] These classifications have no bearing on treatment and prognosis, which is mostly based on risk assessment. Most have characteristic chromosomal translocations that aid in diagnosis (**Table 5**).

Grading of tumors is based on adult systems, the National Cancer Institute-based Pediatric Oncology group system and the Federation Nationale des Centers de lute Contre le Cancer system. Both systems have been shown to predict prognosis in children.[43]

Prognostic Factors

Several studies have demonstrated common themes with regard to prognosis of patients with NRSTS: extent of disease (local vs metastatic), extent of tumor resection (resectable vs unresectable), maximal tumor diameter (<5 vs >5 cm), and tumor grade (low vs high).[44–46] Using these factors, 3 distinct risk groups were proposed (**Table 6**):

- Low risk
  - Patients with grossly resected nonmetastatic tumors except those patients with high grade and greater than 5 cm in maximal diameter tumors.
  - A 5-year survival estimate of 90%.
  - Comprise about 50% of the population of NRSTS.

Table 5	
Cytogenetics in nonrhabdomyosarcoma soft tissue sarcomas	
Diagnosis	**Translocation**
Alveolar soft part sarcoma	t(X;17)
Dermatofibrosarcoma protuberans	t(17;22)
Infantile fibrosarcoma	t(12;15)
Liposarcoma	t(12;16)
Myxoid chondrosarcoma	t(9;22)
Synovial Sarcoma	t(X;18)

Table 6
Risk classification for nonrhabdomyosarcoma soft tissue sarcomas

Level	Description
Low risk	Grossly resected nonmetastatic tumors except high grade or >5 cm in diameter
Intermediate risk	High grade and/or tumors >5 cm Initially unresectable tumors
High risk	Metastatic tumors

- Intermediate risk
  - Patients with both high-grade and greater than 5-cm tumors.
  - Patients with initially unresectable nonmetastatic tumors, regardless of grade or size.
  - A 5-year survival estimate of 50%.
  - Comprise approximately 35% of NRSTS patients.
- High risk
  - Patients with metastatic tumors, including those with regional lymph node metastasis.
  - A 5-year survival estimate of 15%.
  - Comprise 15% of NRSTS tumors.

These risk groups were validated using Surveillance, Epidemiology and End Results data from 1988 to 2007 and were used in the most recent Children's Oncology Group protocol, which recently closed for accrual.[47] On multivariate analysis, malignant peripheral nerve sheath histology, chemotherapy-resistant histology, and higher risk group were significantly poor prognostic factors for overall and cancer-specific survival. Chemoresistant histologies include fibrohistiocytic tumors, fibroblastic/myofibroblastic tumors, tumors of uncertain differentiation, extraskeletal OS, pericyte tumor, nerve sheath tumors, and undifferentiated sarcomas.

Staging

Diagnosis is made with imaging and confirmed with biopsy. Imaging modalities depend on the location of the tumor and include ultrasonography, CT, and MRI. The most common site of metastasis is the lung and all workups should chest imaging.[48] Lymph nodes should be investigated in patient with lymphadenopathy and tumors with propensity for nodal metastasis (epithelioid, synovial, clear cell and vascular sarcomas).[49,50] Brain and bone imaging are reserved for patients with symptoms.

Treatment

Treatment for NRSTS includes surgical excision with 1-cm margins if possible, radiation for positive margins or unresectable disease, and adjuvant chemotherapy for high-risk tumors. These modalities vary depending on the risk classification and are now focused on adaptive therapy, which limits adjuvant therapy in low-risk patients to decrease long-term side effects and increases therapy in high-risk patients to improve survival.

Low risk
Patients with low-risk tumors can be classified into 4 cohorts.

1. Low-grade tumor completely excised with negative microscopic margins. These patients do not require radiation or chemotherapy. Close observation occurs after surgical resection and relapse is usually salvaged with multimodality therapy.
2. Small (<5 cm), high-grade tumor completely excised with negative microscopic margins. Recent adult trials have shown these patients can be managed safely without radiotherapy.[51–53] Close observation is necessary to allow for rescue therapy if local recurrence occurs.
3. Low-grade tumor excised with positive microscopic margins. These patients only require surgical excision with close follow-up for recurrence.
4. Small (<5 cm), high-grade tumor excised with positive microscopic margins. Owing to the high grade of the tumor, these patients do need adjuvant radiotherapy for adequate local control.

Intermediate risk

1. Large (>5 cm), high-grade tumors completely excised. These patients have significant risk for local recurrence and metastatic disease; therefore, they should receive radiation for local control[54] and chemotherapy for systemic control. Doxorubicin and ifosfamide are common chemotherapeutic agents, which have shown effectiveness, particularly in adult studies.[55]
2. Unresectable tumors. These patients need both radiation and chemotherapy before attempt at resection.

High risk

1. These patients should receive intensive combined chemoradiotherapy before resection of the primary tumor.
2. After completion of therapy, all metastatic sites should be excised if possible.
3. Bone marrow transplant after intensive chemotherapy has been conducted as part of a clinical trial and did not show a benefit to traditional chemotherapy.[56]

Summary

Nonrhabdomyosarcoma soft tissue sarcomas are a diverse group of tumors with variable and the prognosis depends on the extent of disease, size and grade of tumor, and extent of resection. Children with NRSTS have a good prognosis if tumor resection is possible. Lymph node or distant metastasis portends a dismal survival (<15%) warranting aggressive multimodality therapy to improve overall survival.

BONE SARCOMAS
Osteosarcoma

Epidemiology
OS is the most common primary malignant bone tumor in children and adolescents, with an estimate of 4.8 per million new cases each year in children younger 20 years in the United States. This results in an incidence of roughly 450 cases per year in this age group, accounting for approximately 3% to 5% of childhood tumors.[57] OS is more common in males and African Americans. Children younger than 5 years are rarely affected; after age 5, the incidence increases with a peak at age 15 years. A second peak occurs in the sixth to seventh decade. This second peak has been associated with Paget disease and prior radiation therapy, although one-half of older OS patients have neither condition. The adolescent peak occurs at a younger age in girls (13 years) compared with boys (15–17 years), and this corresponds with the age of greatest bone growth. More than 50% of these tumors

arise from the long bones around the knee and distal femur, followed by the proximal tibia.[58]

Chemotherapy has played a role in the increased overall survival obtained through different clinical trials over the last decades leading to dramatic prognostic improvements in young patients with localized extremity disease, with relapse-free survival rates of approximately 50% to 80%; before 1970, the estimated overall survival for patients treated with surgery alone was approximately 20%.[59]

Clinical presentation

The most common clinical presentation of OS is pain that becomes continuous and severe with time. This pain is often attributed to recent trauma or bone growth. In some patients, a mass may be palpable and the progressive swelling will affect adjacent joints. Pathologic fractures may occur in OS patients either spontaneously or as a result of minimal trauma. Respiratory symptoms from metastatic lung involvement is rare and require extensive bilateral lung disease.

Systemic symptoms such as fever and malaise are uncommon.[60] The time between onset of symptoms and diagnosis ranges from 2 to 4 months in developed countries.[61] Some genetic conditions, including Rothmund–Thomson syndrome, Li–Fraumeni syndrome, Paget disease, and some tumors such as retinoblastoma, predispose to develop OS.[62]

Prognostic factors

Several prognostic factors affecting overall survival have been identified in patients with OS, but these have not been helpful in identifying patients who might benefit from treatment intensification.[63] Some of these prognostic factors include tumor location, tumor size, localized versus metastatic disease, surgical resectability, and degree of tumor necrosis after neoadjuvant chemotherapy. Other possible prognostic factors identified in localized high-grade OS include age at diagnosis, serum lactate dehydrogenase level at diagnosis, alkaline phosphatase level, histologic subtype, and body mass index at initial presentation. Older patients are considered to do worse secondary to the increased proportion of unfavorable axial lesions with increasing age.

Tumor location Axial skeleton primary tumors (particularly the pelvis or the spine) are associated with a worse prognosis related to the inability to achieve a complete surgical resection and maintain local control. This tumor location is more likely to present with metastatic disease at diagnosis, which could be secondary to a prolonged latency period before obtaining the diagnosis. Within an extremity, a distal tumor location has a more favorable prognosis than a proximal location, secondary to the ability to completely remove the tumor with negative margins. A better prognosis has been documented in patients with head and neck OS when compared with extremity tumors, and this may be related to the relatively smaller size of tumors in this anatomic area and a higher proportion of low-grade tumors. Extraskeletal OS is rare in childhood and the outcomes seem to be similar to that for patients with primary bone tumors. The proximal tibia is considered to be a prognostically favorable site when compared with the distal femur, but conclusions are not consistent. An earlier growth spurt of the humerus has been associated with an earlier development of OS at this site, but this is also controversial.[60,64]

Tumor size Larger tumors have been associated with a worse prognosis, although no correlation between tumor size and response to chemotherapy has been documented. The worse overall survival in patients with large primary bone tumors must be associated with an increased macrometastatic and micrometastatic burden.

Interestingly, the proportion of large tumors is higher in proximity to the trunk. The reason proximal site represents an independent risk factor remains to be determined.[63,64]

Localized versus metastatic disease at diagnosis Radiographically detectable metastases at diagnosis are seen in 20% to 25% of patients with OS, with the lung being the most common site. Among patients with nonmetastatic disease at diagnosis, 20% to 25% will relapse, usually in the lungs. For patients with localized tumors, prognosis is better, with an overall event-free survival of 60% to 70%. This survival remains at about 20% to 30% for patients with metastatic disease at diagnosis. In this group, the prognosis seems to be determined by the site, the number of metastases, and their surgical resectability. Factors that predict a better outcome in patients with pulmonary metastatic disease include fewer pulmonary nodules, unilateral pulmonary metastases, and longer intervals between primary tumor resection and metastases.[65] Patients with skip metastases ($\geq$2 discontinuous neoplastic lesions in the same affected bone) have been reported to have a worse prognosis. Analysis of the German Cooperative Osteosarcoma Study experience, however, suggests that skip lesions in the same bone do not confer a worse prognosis if they are included in the definitive surgical resection. Skip lesions across a joint have a worse prognosis. Bone metastases in a bone other than the primary bone should be considered systemic disease.[66]

Surgical resectability Complete resection of the primary tumor and metastatic disease is required for cure in patients with OS. This goal is more often missed in individuals with axial tumors or those with widespread metastatic disease. The ability to achieve a complete resection of recurrent disease is the most important prognostic factor at first relapse, with a 5-year survival rate of 20% to 45% after complete resection of metastatic pulmonary disease. For patients with axial skeletal tumors who are not candidates for surgery or who undergo surgery resulting in positive margins, radiation therapy may improve survival.[67]

Degree of tumor necrosis after neoadjuvant chemotherapy Tumor response after neoadjuvant chemotherapy in the resected tumor represents an important prognostic factor in primary, localized extremity OS. Patients with 90% or greater necrosis have a better prognosis than those with less necrosis who are at a higher risk for recurrence within the first 2 years. In general, male sex, long clinical history, and axial location confer a higher risk of poor degree of tumor necrosis.[68,69]

Staging

For the purposes of treatment, high-grade OS is divided in patients without clinically detectable metastatic disease (localized OS) and patients with detectable metastases at the time of initial presentation by routine clinical studies (metastatic OS). These studies include conventional radiography, MRI of the primary tumor, CT scan of the chest, bone scintigraphy, and PET scan. Patients with skip lesions confined to the bone that includes the primary tumor should be considered to have localized disease if the skip lesions can be included in the definitive surgical resection.[70]

Treatment

Procurement of adequate diagnostic pathologic specimens is key to determining the correct diagnosis, whether collected from the primary tumor or a suspected metastatic site (most commonly the lung), which avoids the violation of the primary tumor. Improperly performed biopsies may make definitive resections difficult to perform. A biopsy of the primary tumor carries a higher risk of postoperative hematoma and tumor seeding. For open biopsies, a small longitudinal incision, which allows access to adequate tissue should be made. Once the diagnosis of high-grade OS is obtained, neoadjuvant multiagent chemotherapy based on cisplatin, methotrexate, doxorubicin, ifosfamide and etoposide is started.[71,72] Low-grade OS is treated with surgery alone. After the completion of neoadjuvant chemotherapy, local control with either a limb salvage procedure or an amputation is performed. If feasible, limb salvage surgery has become the standard of care with similar survival outcomes when properly performed. This procedure involves both the en bloc resection of the tumor and the reconstruction with synthetic materials, biologic materials, or a combination of both. Vascular and nerve reconstruction, muscle flaps, and skin grafts may be necessary. A multidisciplinary team that includes pediatric surgical oncologists, orthopedic surgeons, plastic surgeons, anesthesiologists with pain management skills, physical therapists, psychologists, occupational therapists, and wound care nurses should be involved in the care of the patients. Patients should receive radiographic follow-up every 3 months for the first year, every 6 months for the second year, and yearly thereafter for 5 years. After 5 years, the patients should be seen in a late effects clinic to monitor for toxicity from therapy.

Ewing Sarcoma

Epidemiology

The term "Ewing sarcoma" is the official World Health Organization term and includes ES of the bone, extraskeletal ES, Askin tumor of the thoracic wall, and peripheral primitive neuroectodermal tumor.[73] ES is the second most common primary malignant bone tumor in children and adolescents after OS, with an estimate of 2.9 per million new cases each year in younger than 20 years in the United States. ES is slightly more common in males and its incidence is 9 times greater in Caucasians than in African Americans. The median age at diagnosis is 15 years, and more than 50% of patients are adolescents. The most common osseous location is the lower extremity (41%), followed by pelvis (26%), chest wall (16%), upper extremity (9%), spine (6%), hand/foot (3%), and skull (2%). Extraosseous ES may be seen in the trunk, extremities, head/neck, and retroperitoneum. Patients with extraosseous ES are more likely to be older, female, nonwhite, and have axial primary tumors.[74,75] ES belongs to the group of neoplasms commonly referred to as small, round, blue cell tumors of childhood. A reciprocal chromosomal translocation involving the *EWSR1* gene between chromosome 11 and 22 [t(11;22) (q24;q12)] is present in about 85% of ES and represents the key feature in the diagnosis.[76] Before the era of chemotherapy, only 10% of ES patients treated with radiation alone survived. With multiagent chemotherapy regimens, surgery, and radiation, cure rates of greater than 60% can be achieved in patients with localized disease.

Clinical presentation

The most common presenting symptoms in patients with ES are a palpable mass or local pain, which can be intermittent and less severe at night. The pain is often mistaken for bone growth or from injuries.[77] Median duration of symptoms before diagnosis varies from 2 to 9 months.[78] Systemic symptoms are more common in patients with metastatic disease, which accounts for 25% of patients at diagnosis. Tumor location within the chest or pelvis may preclude an early diagnosis. Most malignant chest wall tumors in children are ES, although other histologies, including RMS, OS, and chondrosarcoma, can occur.

Prognostic factors

In addition to stage (localized vs metastatic), other prognostic factors including tumor location, tumor size, age, gender, serum lactate dehydrogenase level at diagnosis, and others (complex karyotype, detectable fusion transcripts in morphologically normal marrow and biological factors) have been investigated.[79–81]

Localized versus metastatic disease The presence or absence of metastatic disease is the single most powerful prognostic factor of outcome in ES. Patients with metastatic disease confined to the lung have a better prognosis than patients with extrapulmonary metastatic disease. In general, patients with unilateral lung involvement do better than patients with bilateral lung involvement. Patients with metastasis to bone only seem to have a better outcome than patients with metastases to both bone and lung. Regional lymph node involvement is associated with an inferior overall outcome.[80,81]

Degree of response to neoadjuvant chemotherapy Minimal or no residual viable tumor after neoadjuvant chemotherapy have a significantly better event-free survival compared with patients with a large amount of residual viable tumor. Patients with poor response to neoadjuvant chemotherapy have an increased risk for local recurrence.[82]

Tumor location A better prognosis is seen in patients with ES in the distal part of the extremities, followed by patients with proximal extremity tumors. Patients with central or pelvic tumors have the worst prognosis.

Tumor size Larger tumors (>8 cm) have been associated with a worse prognosis and tend to occur in unfavorable sites.

Age Patients younger than 15 years have a better prognosis than adolescents aged 15 years or older, young adults, or adults.

Gender Girls with ES have a better prognosis than boys.

Lactate dehydrogenase Increased serum lactate dehydrogenase levels before treatment are associated with a poorer prognosis.

Staging
Pretreatment staging studies in patients with ES should include conventional radiography, MRI and/or CT scan of the primary tumor, bone scan or PET scan, CT scan of the chest, and bone marrow aspiration and biopsy, which differs from the OS metastatic pattern.[83] Tumors are considered localized when, by clinical and imaging techniques, there is no spread beyond the primary location or regional lymph node involvement. If there is a question of regional lymph node involvement, an excisional biopsy may be required. Microscopically detectable bone marrow metastases occur in fewer than 10% of patients and are associated with a poor prognosis.

Treatment
Cure for patients with ES requires systemic chemotherapy in conjunction with either surgery, radiation therapy, or both modalities for local tumor control.[84] The best approach for local control remains a matter of discussion. In general, radiation therapy has been associated with a higher rate of local recurrence and a significant risk for second radio-induced malignancies, whereas surgery has been associated with more functional defects.[85,86] For tumors located in the extremities, the same surgical principles applied to OS are valid, with the possibility of adding radiation therapy in case the resection margin is positive for tumor.[87] For tumors located in the pelvis or spine, radiation therapy plays an important role for local control. Patients who are selected to receive radiation therapy alone usually represent a group of patients

with an unfavorable prognosis.[88] For chest wall ES, an initial tumor biopsy followed by neoadjuvant chemotherapy and delayed surgical resection lead to high rates of cure and minimized morbidity. Complete surgical resection also avoids the need for adjuvant radiotherapy to the chest with its associated morbidities, such as scoliosis, second malignancies, and growth discrepancies.

Multiagent chemotherapy includes vincristine, cyclophosphamide, actinomycin-D, and doxorubicin with neoadjuvant therapy necessary for unresectable disease. For patients with metastatic disease at initial presentation, adjuvant radiation therapy to the metastatic sites is recommended. The use of whole lung irradiation in this group of patients have been shown to improve outcomes. Also, radiation therapy may be indicated for bone metastases if limited in number.[89]

SUMMARY

Pediatric sarcomas are a diverse group of tumors that are best managed with multidisciplinary care. The combination of chemotherapy, surgery and radiation has improved survival. Patients should be seen long term in a late effects clinic to monitor for signs and symptoms of toxicity or secondary malignancies.

REFERENCES

1. National Cancer Institute. Homepage on the Internet. Available at: http://www.cancer.gov. Accessed February 1, 2016.
2. Pappo AS, Shapiro DN, Crist WM, et al. Biology and therapy of pediatric rhabdomyosarcoma. J Clin Oncol 1995;13(8):2123–39.
3. Gurney JG, Severson RK, Davis S, et al. Incidence of cancer in children in the United States. Sex-, race-, and 1-year age-specific rates by histologic type. Cancer 1995;75(8):2186–95.
4. Ognjanovic S, Linabery AM, Charbonneau B, et al. Trends in childhood rhabdomyosarcoma incidence and survival in the United States, 1975-2005. Cancer 2009;115(18):4218–26.
5. Maurer HM, Beltangady M, Gehan EA, et al. The Intergroup Rhabdomyosarcoma Study-I. A final report. Cancer 1988;61(2):209–20.
6. Maurer HM, Gehan EA, Beltangady M, et al. The Intergroup Rhabdomyosarcoma Study-II. Cancer 1993;71(5):1904–22.
7. Crist W, Gehan EA, Ragab AH, et al. The Third Intergroup Rhabdomyosarcoma Study. J Clin Oncol 1995;13(3):610–30.
8. Crist WM, Anderson JR, Meza JL, et al. Intergroup Rhabdomyosarcoma Study-IV: results for patients with nonmetastatic disease. J Clin Oncol 2001;19(12):3091–102.
9. Smith MA, Altekruse SF, Adamson PC, et al. Declining childhood and adolescent cancer mortality. Cancer 2014;120(16):2497–506.
10. Malempati S, Rodeberg DA, Donaldson SS, et al. Rhabdomyosarcoma in infants younger than 1 year: a report from the Children's Oncology Group. Cancer 2011;117(15):3493–501.
11. Raney RB, Maurer HM, Anderson JR, et al. The Intergroup Rhabdomyosarcoma Study Group (IRSG): Major Lessons From the IRS-I Through IRS-IV Studies as Background for the Current IRS-V Treatment Protocols. Sarcoma 2001;5(1):9–15.
12. Lawrence W, Hays DM, Heyn R, et al. Surgical lessons from the Intergroup Rhabdomyosarcoma Study (IRS) pertaining to extremity tumors. World J Surg 1988;12(5):676–84.

13. Ognjanovic S, Carozza SE, Chow EJ, et al. Birth characteristics and the risk of childhood rhabdomyosarcoma based on histological subtype. Br J Cancer 2010;102(1):227–31.

14. Diller L, Sexsmith E, Gottlieb A, et al. Germline p53 mutations are frequently detected in young children with rhabdomyosarcoma. J Clin Invest 1995;95(4):1606–11.

15. Doros L, Yang J, Dehner L, et al. DICER1 mutations in embryonal rhabdomyosarcomas from children with and without familial PPB-tumor predisposition syndrome. Pediatr Blood Cancer 2012;59(3):558–60.

16. Crucis A, Richer W, Brugières L, et al. Rhabdomyosarcomas in children with neurofibromatosis type I: a national historical cohort. Pediatr Blood Cancer 2015;62(10):1733–8.

17. Martinelli S, McDowell HP, Vigne SD, et al. RAS signaling dysregulation in human embryonal Rhabdomyosarcoma. Genes Chromosomes Cancer 2009;48(11):975–82.

18. Shern JF, Chen L, Chmielecki J, et al. Comprehensive genomic analysis of rhabdomyosarcoma reveals a landscape of alterations affecting a common genetic axis in fusion-positive and fusion-negative tumors. Cancer Discov 2014;4(2):216–31.

19. Cohen MM. Beckwith-Wiedemann syndrome: historical, clinicopathological, and etiopathogenetic perspectives. Pediatr Dev Pathol 2005;8(3):287–304.

20. Kratz CP, Franke L, Peters H, et al. Cancer spectrum and frequency among children with Noonan, Costello, and cardio-facio-cutaneous syndromes. Br J Cancer 2015;112(8):1392–7.

21. Sorensen PHB, Lynch JC, Qualman SJ, et al. PAX3-FKHR and PAX7-FKHR gene fusions are prognostic indicators in alveolar rhabdomyosarcoma: a report from the children's oncology group. J Clin Oncol 2002;20(11):2672–9.

22. Punyko JA, Mertens AC, Baker KS, et al. Long-term survival probabilities for childhood rhabdomyosarcoma. A population-based evaluation. Cancer 2005;103(7):1475–83.

23. Sung L, Anderson JR, Donaldson SS, et al. Late events occurring five years or more after successful therapy for childhood rhabdomyosarcoma: a report from the Soft Tissue Sarcoma Committee of the Children's Oncology Group. Eur J Cancer 2004;40(12):1878–85.

24. Joshi D, Anderson JR, Paidas C, et al. Age is an independent prognostic factor in rhabdomyosarcoma: a report from the Soft Tissue Sarcoma Committee of the Children's Oncology Group. Pediatr Blood Cancer 2004;42(1):64–73.

25. Egas-Bejar D, Huh WW. Rhabdomyosarcoma in adolescent and young adult patients: current perspectives. Adolesc Health Med Ther 2014;5:115–25.

26. Sultan I, Qaddoumi I, Yaser S, et al. Comparing adult and pediatric rhabdomyosarcoma in the Surveillance, Epidemiology and End Results program, 1973 to 2005: an analysis of 2,600 patients. J Clin Oncol 2009;27(20):3391–7.

27. Breneman JC, Lyden E, Pappo AS, et al. Prognostic factors and clinical outcomes in children and adolescents with metastatic rhabdomyosarcoma–a report from the Intergroup Rhabdomyosarcoma Study IV. J Clin Oncol 2003;21(1):78–84.

28. Rodeberg DA, Garcia-Henriquez N, Lyden ER, et al. Prognostic significance and tumor biology of regional lymph node disease in patients with rhabdomyosarcoma: a report from the Children's Oncology Group. J Clin Oncol 2011;29(10):1304–11.

29. Alaggio R, Coffin CM. The evolution of pediatric soft tissue sarcoma classification in the last 50 years. Pediatr Dev Pathol 2015;18(6):481–94.

30. Vroobel K, Gonzalez D, Wren D, et al. Ancillary molecular analysis in the diagnosis of soft tissue tumours: reassessment of its utility at a specialist centre. J Clin Pathol 2015;69(6):505–10.

31. Harel M, Ferrer FA, Shapiro LH, et al. Future directions in risk stratification and therapy for advanced pediatric genitourinary rhabdomyosarcoma. Urol Oncol 2016;34(2):103–15.

32. Zhu B, Davie JK. New insights into signalling-pathway alterations in rhabdomyosarcoma. Br J Cancer 2015;112(2):227–31.

33. Missiaglia E, Williamson D, Chisholm J, et al. PAX3/FOXO1 fusion gene status is the key prognostic molecular marker in rhabdomyosarcoma and significantly improves current risk stratification. J Clin Oncol 2012;30(14):1670–7.

34. Qualman S, Lynch J, Bridge J, et al. Prevalence and clinical impact of anaplasia in childhood rhabdomyosarcoma: a report from the Soft Tissue Sarcoma Committee of the Children's Oncology Group. Cancer 2008;113(11):3242–7.

35. Eugene T, Corradini N, Carlier T, et al. ^{18}F-FDG-PET/CT in initial staging and assessment of early response to chemotherapy of pediatric rhabdomyosarcomas. Nucl Med Commun 2012;33(10):1089–95.

36. Alcorn KM, Deans KJ, Congeni A, et al. Sentinel lymph node biopsy in pediatric soft tissue sarcoma patients: utility and concordance with imaging. J Pediatr Surg 2013;48(9):1903–6.

37. Raney RB, Anderson JR, Barr FG, et al. Rhabdomyosarcoma and undifferentiated sarcoma in the first two decades of life: a selective review of intergroup rhabdomyosarcoma study group experience and rationale for Intergroup Rhabdomyosarcoma Study V. J Pediatr Hematol Oncol 2001;23(4):215–20.

38. Leaphart C, Rodeberg D. Pediatric surgical oncology: management of rhabdomyosarcoma. Surg Oncol 2007;16(3):173–85.

39. Children's Oncology Group. Available at: http://www.childrensoncologygroup. org. Accessed February 6, 2016.

40. Wiener ED, Anderson JR, Ojimba JI, et al. Controversies in the management of paratesticular rhabdomyosarcoma: is staging retroperitoneal lymph node dissection necessary for adolescents with resected paratesticular rhabdomyosarcomas. Semin Pediatr Surg 2001;10(3):146–52.

41. National Cancer Institute. Surveillance, Epidemiology, and End Results program. Available at: http://seer.cancer.gov. Accessed February 6, 2016.

42. Spunt SL, Skapek SX, Coffin CM. Pediatric nonrhabdomyosarcoma soft tissue sarcomas. Oncologist 2008;13:668–78.

43. Khoury JD, Coffin CM, Spunt SL, et al. Grading of nonrhabdomyosarcoma soft tissue sarcoma in children and adolescents. Cancer 2010;116:2266–74.

44. Spunt SL, Hill DA, Motosue AM, et al. Clinical features and outcome of initially unresected nonmetastatic pediatric nonrhabdomyosarcoma soft tissue sarcoma. J Clin Oncol 2002;20:3225–35.

45. Spunt SL, Poquette CA, Hurt YS, et al. Prognostic factors for children and adolescents with surgically resected nonrhabdomyosarcoma soft tissue sarcoma: an analysis of 121 patients treated at St Jude Children's Research Hospital. J Clin Oncol 1999;17:3697–705.

46. Pappo AS, Rao BN, Jenkins JJ, et al. Metastatic nonrhabdomyosarcomatous soft-tissue sarcomas in children and adolescents: the St. Jude Children's Research Hospital experience. Med Pediatr Oncol 1999;33:76–82.

47. Waxweiler TV, Rusthoven CG, Proper MS, et al. Non-rhabdomyosarcoma soft tissue sarcomas in children: a Surveillance, Epidemiology and End Results analysis validating COG risk stratifications. Int J Radiat Oncol Biol Phys 2015;92(2): 339–48.

48. Fleming JB, Cantor SB, Varma DG, et al. Utility of chest computed tomography for staging in patients with T1 extremity soft tissue sarcomas. Cancer 2001;92:863–8.

49. Fong Y, Coit DG, Woodruff JM, et al. Lymph node metastasis from soft tissue sarcoma in adults. Analysis of data from a prospective database of 1772 sarcoma patients. Ann Surg 1993;217:72–7.

50. Blazer DG, Sabel MS, Sondak VK. Is there a role for sentinel lymph node biopsy in the management of sarcoma? Surg Oncol 2003;12(3):201–6.

51. Baldini EH, Goldberg J, Jenner C, et al. Long-term outcomes after function-sparing surgery without radiotherapy for soft tissue sarcoma of the extremities and trunk. J Clin Oncol 1999;17:3252–9.

52. Rydholm A, Gustafson P, Rooser B, et al. Limb-sparing surgery without radiotherapy based on anatomic location of soft tissue sarcoma. J Clin Oncol 1991; 9:1757–65.

53. Fabrizio PL, Stafford SL, Pritchard DJ. Extremity soft-tissue sarcomas selectively treated with surgery alone. Int J Radiat Oncol Biol Phys 2000;48:227–32.

54. Yang JC, Chang AE, Baker AR, et al. Randomized prospective study of the benefit of adjuvant radiation therapy in the treatment of soft tissue sarcomas of the extremity. J Clin Oncol 1998;16:197–203.

55. Demetri GD, Elias AD. Results of single-agent and combination chemotherapy for advanced soft tissue sarcomas. Implications for decision making in the clinic. Hematol Oncol Clin North Am 1995;9:765–85.

56. Peinemann F, Labeit AM. Autologous haematopoietic stem cell transplantation following high-dose chemotherapy for non-rhabdomyosarcoma soft tissue sarcomas: a Cochrane systematic review*. BMJ Open 2014;4(7):e005033.

57. Mirabello L, Troisi RJ, Savage SA. Osteosarcoma incidence and survival rates from 1973 to 2004: data from the Surveillance, Epidemiology, and End Results Program. Cancer 2009;115:1531–43.

58. Bacci G, Longhi A, Bertoni F, et al. Primary high-grade osteosarcoma: comparison between preadolescent and older patients. J Pediatr Hematol Oncol 2005; 27:129–34.

59. Bacci G, Balladelli A, Palmerini E, et al. Neoadjuvant chemotherapy for osteosarcoma of the extremities in preadolescent patients: the Rizzoli Institute experience. J Pediatr Hematol Oncol 2008;30:908–12.

60. Bielack SS, Kempf-Bielack B, Delling G, et al. Prognostic factors in high-grade osteosarcoma of the extremities or trunk: an analysis of 1,702 patients treated on neoadjuvant cooperative osteosarcoma study group protocols. J Clin Oncol 2002;20:776–90.

61. Goyal S, Roscoe J, Ryder WD, et al. Symptom interval in young people with bone cancer. Eur J Cancer 2004;40:2280–6.

62. Kansara M, Thomas DM. Molecular pathogenesis of osteosarcoma. DNA Cell Biol 2007;26:1–18.

63. Pakos EE, Nearchou AD, Grimer RJ, et al. Prognostic factors and outcomes for osteosarcoma: an international collaboration. Eur J Cancer 2009;45:2367–75.

64. Andreou D, Bielack SS, Carrle D, et al. The influence of tumor- and treatment-related factors on the development of local recurrence in osteosarcoma after adequate surgery. An analysis of 1355 patients treated on neoadjuvant Cooperative Osteosarcoma Study Group protocols. Ann Oncol 2011;22:1228–35.

65. Bacci G, Rocca M, Salone M, et al. High grade osteosarcoma of the extremities with lung metastases at presentation: treatment with neoadjuvant chemotherapy and simultaneous resection of primary and metastatic lesions. J Surg Oncol 2008;98:415–20.

66. Kager L, Zoubek A, Kastner U, et al. Skip metastases in osteosarcoma: experience of the Cooperative Osteosarcoma Study Group. J Clin Oncol 2006;24: 1535–41.

67. Bacci G, Fabbri N, Balladelli A, et al. Treatment and prognosis for synchronous multifocal osteosarcoma in 42 patients. J Bone Joint Surg Br 2006;88:1071–5.

68. Bacci G, Mercuri M, Longhi A, et al. Grade of chemotherapy-induced necrosis as a predictor of local and systemic control in 881 patients with non-metastatic osteosarcoma of the extremities treated with neoadjuvant chemotherapy in a single institution. Eur J Cancer 2005;41(14):2079–85.

69. Kim MS, Cho WH, Song WS, et al. Time dependency of prognostic factors in patients with stage II osteosarcomas. Clin Orthop Relat Res 2007;463:157–65.

70. Bielack S, Carrle D, Casali PG, ESMO Guidelines Working Group. Osteosarcoma: ESMO clinical recommendations for diagnosis, treatment and follow-up. Ann Oncol 2009;20(Suppl 4):137–9.

71. Bernthal NM, Federman N, Eilber FR, et al. Long-term results (>25 years) of a randomized, prospective clinical trial evaluating chemotherapy in patients with high-grade, operable osteosarcoma. Cancer 2012;118:5888–93.

72. Goorin AM, Schwartzentruber DJ, Devidas M, et al. Presurgical chemotherapy compared with immediate surgery and adjuvant chemotherapy for nonmetastatic osteosarcoma: Pediatric Oncology Group Study POG-8651. J Clin Oncol 2003; 21:1574–80.

73. de Alava E, Lessnick SL, Sorensen PH. Ewing sarcoma. In: Fletcher CDM, Bridge JA, Hogendoorn PCW, et al, editors. WHO classification of tumors of soft tissue and bone. 4th edition. Lyon (France): International Agency for Research on Cancer (IARC); 2013. p. 305–9.

74. Esiashvili N, Goodman M, Marcus RB Jr. Changes in incidence and survival of Ewing sarcoma patients over the past 3 decades: surveillance epidemiology and end results data. J Pediatr Hematol Oncol 2008;30:425–30.

75. Jawad MU, Cheung MC, Min ES, et al. Ewing sarcoma demonstrates racial disparities in incidence-related and sex-related differences in outcome: an analysis of 1631 cases from the SEER database, 1973-2005. Cancer 2009;115:3526–36.

76. Urano F, Umezawa A, Yabe H, et al. Molecular analysis of Ewing's sarcoma: another fusion gene, EWS-E1AF, available for diagnosis. Jpn J Cancer Res 1998;89:703–11.

77. Widhe B, Widhe T. Initial symptoms and clinical features in osteosarcoma and Ewing sarcoma. J Bone Joint Surg Am 2000;82:667–74.

78. Brasme JF, Chalumeau M, Oberlin O, et al. Time to diagnosis of Ewing tumors in children and adolescents is not associated with metastasis or survival: a prospective multicenter study of 436 patients. J Clin Oncol 2014;32:1935–40.

79. Cotterill SJ, Ahrens S, Paulussen M, et al. Prognostic factors in Ewing's tumor of bone: analysis of 975 patients from the European Intergroup Cooperative Ewing's Sarcoma Study Group. J Clin Oncol 2000;18:3108–14.

80. Bacci G, Longhi A, Ferrari S, et al. Prognostic factors in non-metastatic Ewing's sarcoma tumor of bone: an analysis of 579 patients treated at a single institution with adjuvant or neoadjuvant chemotherapy between 1972 and 1998. Acta Oncol 2006;45:469–75.

81. Rodríguez-Galindo C, Liu T, Krasin MJ, et al. Analysis of prognostic factors in Ewing sarcoma family of tumors: review of St. Jude Children's Research Hospital studies. Cancer 2007;110:375–84.
82. Ferrari S, Bertoni F, Palmerini E, et al. Predictive factors of histologic response to primary chemotherapy in patients with Ewing sarcoma. J Pediatr Hematol Oncol 2007;29:364–8.
83. Meyer JS, Nadel HR, Marina N, et al. Imaging guidelines for children with Ewing sarcoma and osteosarcoma: a report from the Children's Oncology Group Bone Tumor Committee. Pediatr Blood Cancer 2008;51:163–70.
84. Thacker MM, Temple HT, Scully SP. Current treatment for Ewing's sarcoma. Expert Rev Anticancer Ther 2005;5:319–31.
85. Juergens C, Weston C, Lewis I, et al. Safety assessment of intensive induction with vincristine, ifosfamide, doxorubicin, and etoposide (VIDE) in the treatment of Ewing tumors in the EURO-E.W.I.N.G. 99 clinical trial. Pediatr Blood Cancer 2006;47:22–9.
86. Dunst J, Schuck A. Role of radiotherapy in Ewing tumors. Pediatr Blood Cancer 2004;42:465–70.
87. Donaldson SS. Ewing sarcoma: radiation dose and target volume. Pediatr Blood Cancer 2004;42:471–6.
88. Bacci G, Ferrari S, Longhi A, et al. Role of surgery in local treatment of Ewing's sarcoma of the extremities in patients undergoing adjuvant and neoadjuvant chemotherapy. Oncol Rep 2004;11:111–20.
89. Krasin MJ, Rodriguez-Galindo C, Davidoff AM, et al. Efficacy of combined surgery and irradiation for localized Ewings sarcoma family of tumors. Pediatr Blood Cancer 2004;43:229–36.

The Role for Radiation Therapy in the Management of Sarcoma

Brooke K. Leachman, MD, Thomas J. Galloway, MD*

KEYWORDS

- External beam radiation therapy • IMRT • IGRT
- Preoperative versus postoperative radiation • Radiation treatment planning

KEY POINTS

- Radiation therapy is an integral component of limb-sparing therapy for extremity soft tissue sarcoma. The benefit of radiation is clearer for high- than low-grade tumors.
- Local recurrence after appropriately delivered radiation and surgery is expected to be less than 10%.
- Radiation therapy can be delivered either before or after definitive surgical resection. Although the decision regarding appropriate sequencing is unique to each case, many tumors are amenable to either schedule, and treatment decisions are subject to institutional bias.
- Image guidance and intensity-modulated radiotherapy has the potential to improve the therapeutic ratio, mainly through the reduction in treatment-related toxicity.
- Retroperitoneal sarcomas are rare tumors with a high propensity for local failure. Retrospective series suggest that the addition of radiation (generally delivered before resection) decreases the incidence of local failure.

INTRODUCTION

Sarcomas are rare tumors of connective tissue, with diverse histology and site of origin in the body. This article concentrates on the role of radiation in the management of sarcoma of the extremities and retroperitoneum, first with respect to timing and dose. Next the authors focus on practical aspects of treatment planning. Finally, patient set-up and toxicity, acute and late, are addressed.

AMPUTATION VERSUS LIMB-SPARING SURGERY WITH ADJUVANT RADIATION

Amputation was the standard of care in the management of soft tissue sarcoma (STS) for decades, with local recurrence (LR) rates of less than 20% compared with more

Disclosures: None.
Department of Radiation Oncology, Fox Chase Cancer Center, 333 Cottman Avenue, Philadelphia, PA 19111, USA
* Corresponding author.
E-mail address: Thomas.Galloway@fccc.edu

than 70% after local excision alone (**Table 1**).[1–4] The locally invasive nature of sarcomas along tissue planes and muscle fibers and around vasculature highlights the benefits of amputation over gross local resection alone.

Retrospective data published in the 1960s to 1970s suggested reduced risk of LR when limb-sparing surgery (LSS) was supplemented with adjuvant radiation, although it was not until prospective data were published that this treatment became widely practiced.[5,6]

Published in 1982, the landmark National Cancer Institute (NCI) trial randomized 43 patients to amputation or LSS (defined as resection of gross disease but preservation of neurovasculature necessary for function) followed by adjuvant radiation.[6] All patients received adjuvant chemotherapy (doxorubicin, cyclophosphamide, and methotrexate), delivered concurrently with radiation to 45 to 50 Gy to patients randomized to LSS. Disease-free survival and overall survival at 5 years were similar, 78% and 88% for patients treated with amputation alone versus 71% and 83% for LSS and adjuvant radiation (P = .75 and .99). There was a nonsignificant trend toward increased LR for LSS compared with amputation (P = .06), although there were only four LRs among patients who had LSS compared with distant-only failures among the amputation group. Distant metastases were found in 3 of 16 and 2 of 27 patients treated with amputation or LSS, respectively. Since that time, LSS essentially became the standard of care in the United States for patients with disease amenable to LSS; amputation rates fell to less than 10%.[7]

LIMB-SPARING SURGERY WITH OR WITHOUT ADJUVANT RADIATION

Once amputation fell out of favor, investigation of the benefit of radiation to LSS was necessary. There are two prospective randomized trials that evaluate LSS with or without adjuvant radiation. First, a follow-up trial at the NCI investigated the necessity of adjuvant radiation following LSS.[8] Ninety-one patients with high-grade and 50 patients with low-grade tumor histology received five cycles of adjuvant doxorubicin and cyclophosphamide, of which 44 and 26, respectively, were randomized to concurrent radiation (45 Gy to a wide field with 18 Gy boost to the tumor bed, defined by surgical clips). With median follow-up more than 9 years, only one patient with low-grade lesion treated with chemoradiation had an LR, compared with nine and eight incidents of LR among patients with high- and low-grade lesions who received chemotherapy alone (P<.05 for both groups). However, there was no difference in probability of distant metastases or overall survival at 10 years.

A second prospective trial investigated the necessity of radiation in 164 patients who underwent LSS for extremity STS (more than two-thirds high grade) through randomization of patients to intraoperative brachytherapy (BRT) or no further adjuvant local or systemic therapy.[9] BRT used after-loading catheters placed intraoperatively to

Table 1			
Local recurrence rates based on surgical intervention			
Author and Year	**% Local Excision**	**% Wide Excision**	**% Amputation**
Shieber & Graham,[1] 1962	87	39	—
Gerner et al,[2] 1975	93	60	8
Markhede et al,[4] 1982	74	8	0
Leibel et al,[3] 1982	30	28	13

Data from Refs.[1–4]

cover the tumor bed plus 2.0-cm margins at the superior and inferior borders and 1.5- to 2.0-cm margins at the medial and lateral borders. Beginning on postoperative Day 5 or 6, patients were treated with iridium-192 that delivered 45 Gy over 4 to 6 days. Among all patients, reduction in LR was not significant if patients with synchronous local and distant recurrences were excluded (P = .055) or among patients with low-grade lesions. However, for patients with high-grade histology, there were five LRs of 56 patients treated with BRT versus 19 LRs of 63 patients in the control arm (P = .0025). Actuarial local control rates were estimated at 89% and 66%, respectively. The local control benefit of BRT was sustained even among patients with negative margins (8 of 63 treated with BRT developed recurrence compared with 20 of 72 in the control group; P = .04) but there was no benefit in the presence of microscopically positive margins.

Although the previously cited trials[8,9] demonstrated the improved local control of LSS followed by adjuvant radiation, there was no benefit to overall survival or reduction in distant metastases. Tumor grade is known to be one of the most important prognostic factors reflecting tumor biology, yet the previously mentioned studies included patients with high- and low-grade lesions. Large databases suggest that a survival benefit may exist for patients with high-grade tumors. A large state registry analysis demonstrated a significant improvement in overall survival in patients with low compared with high-grade lesions regardless of therapy, 34% versus 15% at 5 years.[10] There was no significant different in overall survival for low-grade lesions treated with or without radiation, but there was a significant benefit to radiation therapy (RT) for high-grade lesions, namely 25 versus 16 months median survival with radiation. Paired analyses of the National Cancer Database examined practice patterns and outcomes for low- and high-grade sarcoma.[11,12] Findings revealed that well-differentiated, low-grade lesions were treated with radiation in 27% of cases, compared with high-grade lesions treated with radiation in 62% of cases. There was no overall survival benefit to radiation for low-grade lesions, even in the presence of positive margins or tumors larger than 5 cm, whereas high-grade lesions experienced significantly lower long-term survival when managed without external beam radiation.

These data suggest that low-grade lesions may be overtreated and high-grade lesions may be undertreated. Thus, although the two main prospective trials demonstrating the usefulness of radiation in the management of extremity sarcoma do not demonstrate a survival benefit, this may be related to the limited statistical power of the small, randomized trials. Modern analyses have attempted to determine which (if any patients) do not require radiation.

A prospective single-arm trial included 88 patients with primary T1 STS of the extremity and superficial trunk (75% intermediate- to high-grade) who underwent resection.[13] Seventy-four patients who had microscopically negative (R0) margins (defined as "no tumor on ink" as opposed to a minimum distance or achievement of a fascial margin) were treated with surgery alone compared with 14 who had microscopically positive (R1) margins and were treated with adjuvant radiation (64 Gy to the tumor bed and a 5- to-7.0-cm margin where possible). Of patients treated with surgery alone for R0 margin, five patients had LR and one had synchronous local and regional recurrence compared with six LRs among patients treated with surgery and radiation for R1 margins. The 5-year LR rate was 7.9% and 42.9% for R0 and R1 groups, respectively. None of the patients in the R0 surgery alone group required amputation for LR, whereas two patients in the R1 surgery plus radiation group underwent amputation. There was no difference in overall survival between the groups.

Thus appropriately selected T1a intermediate- to high-grade sarcomas treated with surgery alone can achieve an acceptably low rate of LR (5%–10%). However appropriate selection is key because R0 resections are dependent not only on tumor size but also tumor location. Management with surgery alone is only possible when the preoperative biopsy is done correctly and a negative margin is achieved. Patients should only be recommended for single modality management after rigorous multidisciplinary review with assessment of whether further local therapy would be possible in the event of LR.

To aid in the determination of which patient can be managed with surgery alone, a predictive nomogram to assess the risk of LR for individual patients treated with surgery alone has been created.[14] Retrospectively, a cohort was identified consisting of 684 patients who underwent surgery alone in the years 1982 to 2006 for definitive treatment of their STS. Multivariate analysis revealed five factors significantly predictive of LR, including age greater than 50 years, high grade, lesion size greater than 5 cm, close or positive margin status, and histology (not atypical lipoma or well-differentiated liposarcoma). The concordance index of the nomogram was 0.73, compared with American Joint Committee on Cancer staging alone with a concordance index of 0.61.

PREOPERATIVE VERSUS POSTOPERATIVE RADIOTHERAPY

The optimal timing of RT has been debated since the role for LSS was established. The benefits or preoperative radiation include delivery of a lower total dose (usually 50 Gy compared with 60–70 Gy after resection) to an intact gross lesion in a smaller field (because the postoperative field needs to cover the operative bed, surgical wound, and drain sites) and the potential for radiation to optimize resection margins and prevent tumor seeding. Additionally, an intact vascular supply preoperatively presents a more favorable environment for oxygen-free radical generation secondary to radiation, compared with the relative hypoxia of the postoperative tumor bed. Conversely, postoperative radiation is favored over preoperative if there is need for pathologic confirmation (complicated by preoperative radiation), concern for wound healing impairment especially for closure under tension, or the potential for radiation complications to delay definitive resection. Advantages and disadvantages are summarized in **Table 2**.

Table 2			
Summary of preoperative and postoperative radiation: advantages and disadvantages			
Preoperative Radiation		**Postoperative Radiation**	
Advantages	**Disadvantages**	**Advantages**	**Disadvantages**
Smaller target volume	Increased postoperative wound complications	Tailor treatment based on pathology	Larger target volume
Lower dose	Interval from radiation to surgery (3–6 wk)	Fewer postoperative wound complications	Higher dose
Improved tumor oxygenation	Psychological delay in surgery	Historical standard of care after LSS	Possible hypoxia of tumor bed
Reduced surgical seeding and possibly improves resectability	May need postoperative radiotherapy if positive margin		

Both retrospective and prospective experiences inform the decision regarding radiation timing. A small retrospective series from MD Anderson Cancer Center (MDACC) favored preoperative radiation to gross disease followed by surgical resection, showing reduced rate of positive margins (29% vs 9%, respectively) and superior local control compared with LSS and postoperative radiation (88% and 67%, respectively; $P = .02$) for patients who underwent first resection at their institution.[15]

A larger MDACC retrospective series included 517 patients treated with either postoperative radiation (n = 246) generally in the 1960s and 1970s or preoperative radiation (n = 271) generally in the 1980s and 1990s, according to the preference of the multidisciplinary team.[16] Not surprisingly, the groups varied considerably, with more patients undergoing adjuvant radiation who had locally recurrent disease, smaller lesions, positive margins, and certain pathologies. The authors found that the difference in LR was entirely explained by the difference in the patient characteristics between groups and not strictly the sequence of therapy. There was no difference in freedom from distant metastases (61% and 64% preoperative vs postoperative radiation), 10-year disease-free survival (54% and 46%), or 10-year disease-specific survival (64% and 54%).

A single randomized trial from the NCI Canada (NCIC) Clinical Trial Group, the NCIC SR2 trial, compared functional outcomes with preoperative (50 Gy) and postoperative (66 Gy) external beam RT among 190 patients with STS.[17] Patients were treated within 3 to 6 weeks of surgery. Preoperative patients received a boost of 16 to 20 Gy in the event of positive margins (occurred in 14 of 88 cases, of whom 10 received the adjuvant radiation boost). Local and locoregional recurrence, distant failure, and progression-free survival were no different between the groups. However, this trial was stopped early after planned analysis of the primary end point, wound complications (most severely in the thigh), showed an increased rate in patients who had preoperative compared with postoperative radiation (35% and 17%, respectively; $P = .01$). Patients treated neoadjuvantly more commonly required nonprimary wound closure. Preoperative RT, anatomic site, and gross tumor size were associated with wound complications based on logistic regression. Fibrosis was more common with postoperative radiation (48.2% compared with 31.5%; $P = .07$). Greater edema and joint stiffness rates associated with postoperative radiation were not statistically significant, and worse outcomes in these three measures were significantly associated with lower function scores. There was no difference in function by treatment arm at 2 years.[18] LR, regional recurrence, distant failure, and progression-free survival were similar among the groups, although there was a trend toward higher overall survival among patients who had preoperative radiation (78% vs 68%; $P = .048$).

A meta-analysis of five studies (the NCIC randomized controlled trial discussed previously and four retrospective cohort reports) included 1098 patients with STS, of whom 526 and 572 received preoperative and postoperative RT.[19] Preoperative radiation reduced the risk of LR, but was significant only based on analysis with fixed effects method versus a random effects method, thus the authors concluded that preoperative therapy might reduce LR. The analysis also found that delay in surgery for preoperative radiation does not seem to increase the risk of metastatic spread, which is more likely determined by tumor biology than timing of therapy.

In summary, a consideration of patient and treatment factors influences the choice sequence of RT and surgery. Generally, preoperative RT (dose of 50 Gy) is preferred for larger lesions especially involving critical structures. Surgery is generally performed 3 to 6 weeks after the completion of radiation and care must be taken to examine the pathologic specimen for positive margins, which may necessitate consideration of a postoperative boost (discussed later). In contrast, postoperative therapy (at least

60 Gy) is usually preferred after an unplanned excision or unexpectedly difficult resection, failure to obtain negative margins, or possibly when wound closure is expected to be under greater tension.

IMAGE GUIDANCE AND INTENSITY-MODULATED RADIOTHERAPY

Intensity-modulated RT (IMRT) with image guidance is a modern method of radiation delivery that allows for delivery of conformal, high-dose radiation to a target with reduced radiation dose to the uninvolved skin, subcutaneous, and connective tissue. Sophisticated dosimetry analysis suggests that local failure after conventional radiation of sarcoma is rare regardless of the timing of radiation (6.4%), and that marginal/out of field failures are rarer still (<2%).[20] Thus, it would seem that the application of IMRT in the management of extremity STS would result in similar oncologic outcomes, perhaps with an improved toxicity profile. The initial IMRT experience in the management of STS was designed to limit radiation dose to involved bone, given the known risk of fracture.[21]

The largest reported experience of IMRT in the management of extremity STS examined 165 patients treated over an 8-year time frame and entered into a prospective database. When compared with a previously treated cohort, the use of IMRT seemed to significantly decrease the edema ($P = .05$) and radiation dermatitis ($P = .002$) of treatment. In addition, a lower risk of LR at 5 years was observed for patients treated with IMRT compared with conventional external beam radiation (LR 7.6% vs 15.1%; $P = .05$), although it is unclear why a smaller field of radiation results in better oncologic outcomes.[22] Nonetheless, the LR rate in this IMRT series is consistent with what has been reported from large non-IMRT series.[20,23,24] Disease-free survival and overall survival at 5-year were similar.

More recently, prospective trials have been performed evaluating the efficacy and toxicity avoidance of IMRT. The NCIC prospective phase II study evaluated 59 patients with only lower-extremity STS treated with preoperative image-guided IMRT. The primary end point was the incidence of major wound complications (defined as readmission for wound care, need for a secondary operation or invasive procedure, deep wound packing, graft revision surgery, or prolong dressing changes more than 6 weeks).[25] This trial involved a novel contouring method, where in addition to bone, "virtual skin flaps" anticipated to be used during closure were defined by the radiation oncologist and surgeon and entered into the optimization as avoidance structures. Although the reduction in wound complications was not significantly less than in the NCIC SR2 trial (30.5% compared with the 43% seen in the NCIC SR2 trial; $P = .2$), primary closure was possible more commonly in the IMRT-treated cohort ($P = .002$) and both reoperations and chronic morbidity seemed improved. In addition, the volume of "virtual surgical skin flaps" receiving the prescribed dose was higher for patients who experienced wound complications than those who did not have such complications (67.1 cm^3 vs 21.5 cm^3).

The prospective phase II RTOG 0630 trial evaluated the use of preoperative RT with image guidance (primarily with IMRT [75%]) and reduced margins.[26] The primary end point was late toxicity at 2 years. Of 79 patients, 10.5% experienced grade 2 or greater late toxicity (fibrosis, joint stiffness, or edema) compared with 37% in the NCIC trial. Furthermore, each of the five LRs was in the radiation field, despite the significantly decreased margins.

Taken together, the results of the NCIC IMRT trial and RTOG 0630[25,26] suggest the possibility of a reduction in late toxicity with the use of preoperative image-guided radiation, likely secondary to the reduced treatment volumes and optimal normal tissue sparing.

There may be a reduction in LR, although these recurrences are likely to occur in the radiation field, indicating that tumor biology, not RT, drives poorer outcomes in local control.

POSITIVE MARGIN AFTER NEOADJUVANT RADIATION AND SURGICAL RESECTION

Preoperative radiation has become an acceptable therapy sequence since publication of the trials discussed previously. However, the patient for whom resection does not achieve a wide negative margin is challenging to manage in light of the prior radiation.

Several retrospective cohorts have shown similar rates of local control despite marginal excision (defined as final surgical plane passes through pseudocapsule and/or reactive tissue surrounding the tumor but the inked margin is free of malignant cells). One analysis found no difference in local control at 5-years comparing wide/radical margins with marginal excision.[23] Additionally, univariate and multivariate analysis did not demonstrate difference in rates of distant metastases, cause-specific survival, or overall survival. The authors concluded that the lower dose of preoperative radiation may effectively sterilize the surrounding at-risk tissue and reactive zones, such that patients who have a marginal excision enjoy the same excellent local control as that of patients undergoing wide or radical excisions. However, a contaminated or intralesional (grossly positive) margin substantially reduces local control and these patients may benefit from a postoperative boost. A different analysis found that the postoperative boost (usually 16 Gy) in the setting of marginal excision did not provide improved local control.[27]

UNPLANNED EXCISION

Up to 40% of patients present with sarcoma having undergone nononcologic resection of a mass assumed to be benign and corresponding rates of LR are much higher because the tumor's pseudocapsule is not adequately removed.[28] The pseudocapsule is actually normal tissue compressed by centrifugal tumor growth, causing atrophy that gives the characteristic appearance.[29] Optimal treatment of these patients necessitates re-excision and adjuvant radiation to minimize the risk of LR. One institution reviewed 134 patients referred after excision of lesions presumed to be benign and retrospectively revealed microscopically or macroscopically involved margins for 90% of patients, most of whom underwent salvage surgery revealing close to half had residual pathologic disease.[28] A group of stage-matched patients treated with definitive surgery at the institution were compared with the referred patients, whom had more favorable stage 1 tumors but even after reresection, LR was higher (11% vs 23.8%; $P<.05$) with a shorter time to LR for stage 3 tumors (18 months vs 10.5 months). Among the referred patients with stage 3 tumors, the rate of distant metastases was higher (68.7% vs 38.7%; $P<.05$). Thus the unplanned excision, even with reresection and achievement of clear margins, increased the probability of LR (23.8% vs 11%; $P<.01$), and these recurrences were more likely to occur on multiple occasions, even after radiation (43.8% vs 17.4%), compared with the control group.[28]

In light of the poorer outcomes following unplanned excision, it is critical for medical professionals to consider the diagnosis of sarcoma and complete a thorough diagnostic work-up to include a thorough history and physical examination, limb and chest imaging, a biopsy, and evaluation by a multidisciplinary team.

RADIATION TREATMENT PLANNING

Once the decision is made to deliver external beam radiation, questions of radiation planning, including target delineation, margins, total dose and number of fractions, and sequence of therapy must be considered. Identification of the high-risk areas is the most critical component to consider in target delineation. For preoperative radiation, the radiation oncologist uses the physical examination and computed tomography and MRI imaging obtained in the treatment position, in collaboration with the surgeon, to optimally define to target. Particularly, the surgeon can identify areas for future drain sites and wound closure to allow the treatment plan to avoid high dose to these areas. More generally, target delineation attempts to avoid uninvolved compartments and joints, vital or reproductive organs, and treatment of the circumferential limb to spare lymphatic drainage. Consensus guidelines recommended a margin of 3 cm beyond the gross tumor in the proximal and distal directions and 1.5 cm radially, including any area not confined by an intact fascial barrier, bone, or skin surface. Suspicious edema seen on MRI T2 images can harbor malignant cells and so it should be covered, even if margins need to be extended, unless there is very low suspicion that edema harbors malignant cells or such an extension would lead to excessive toxicity.[29-31]

For postoperative radiation planning, additional data are obtained from the operative reports and postoperative imaging that includes clips, scars, and drains. Radiopaque clips placed at the time of resection indicate to the radiation oncologist areas identified intraoperatively that the surgeon believes are at increased risk. In general, given these contouring guidelines, postoperative volumes tend to be larger.[17]

RADIATION TOXICITY
Acute

In the early trials of LSS versus amputation, radiation was associated with decreased muscle strength and joint motion and increased limb edema, but overall quality of life and performance of activities of daily living were similar whether or not radiation was administered.[8] More modern trials report acute toxicity outcomes. The NCIC trial reported acute grade 2 or greater skin toxicity was observed in 64 of 94 (68%) of postoperatively treated patients, compared with 32 of 88 (36%) of preoperatively treated patients.[17] Limb function was superior 6 weeks after surgery for the postoperative group compared with the preoperative group. Quality of life indices were not different at 2 years.[18] The RTOG 0630 used image-guided preoperative radiation. Wound complications occurred in 36.6% of cases (all lower extremity), necessitating secondary debridement (25.4%), prolonged dressing changes (23.9%), and readmission for further wound care (21.1%).[26]

Late

Late toxicities of extremity radiation include fibrosis, limb edema, joint stiffness, and bone fracture. Based on the NCIC trial comparing preoperative with postoperative RT, at 2 years there was increased grade 2 or greater fibrosis in the postoperative group (48.2% compared with 31.5%) and joint stiffness and limb edema, which were more common but not significantly so, although the small same size prevented adequate power to detect these end points.[32] Only field size, not treatment sequence, was found to be a predictive risk factor.

A radiation-associated bone fracture (RABF) is defined as one that is associated with minimal or no trauma and occurs within the prior radiation field. RABF occurs more commonly in the lower extremity and treatment is complicated by delayed or incomplete bone union, often requiring multiple surgeries or in an extreme case, total prosthetic replacement or amputation. Risk factors for RABF include age greater than 50 years, female gender, and tumor location in the thigh. A dosimetry analysis of patients who experienced RABF demonstrated that for every one-unit increase in maximum or mean dose, there is an 8% to 10% increased risk of fracture. Additionally, mean field size for the fracture group was 37 ± 8 cm, compared with 32 ± 9 cm in the nonfracture group. There was no effect of preoperative versus postoperative radiation sequence.[21]

RADIATION-ASSOCIATED SARCOMA

More than 50% of patients with cancer receive radiation at some point during their course of therapy, either alone for tumors of the larynx, esophagus, cervix, or in combination with other modalities for breast, rectal, and musculoskeletal tumors, to name a few. The risk of radiation-associated malignancy is well less than 1%, but successful treatment of primary cancers and long-term survivorship necessitate consideration of this risk.[33,34] A proportion of radiation-associated tumors are sarcoma histology. A retrospective from Memorial Sloan Kettering Cancer Center of patients with radiation-associated sarcoma showed that 83% were high-grade, 87% were deep, and 61.5% were truncal. Median latency was 10 years (range, 1.3–74 years). Disease-specific survival was shown to be worse with radiation-associated sarcoma compared with sporadic sarcoma (hazard ratio, 1.7; confidence interval, 1.1–2.4; $P<.05$) despite adjustment for age, histologic type, tumor size, depth, site, and margin.[35] A small cohort found equivalent outcomes comparing radiation-associated bone sarcomas compared with sporadic osteosarcoma.[36]

RETROPERITONEAL SARCOMA

Retroperitoneal sarcomas (RPS) are challenging tumors to diagnose and treat. They are often quite large before diagnosis, and their large size and anatomic location near critical structures make complete surgical resection difficult. Most of the evidence regarding appropriate therapy available extrapolates from treatment of extremity sarcomas or small retrospective series of RPS cases.

Roughly 90% of recurrences are local and a positive gross margin predicts a fourfold increased risk of death (median survival, 103 months vs 18 months with R0 or R1 resection, respectively), thus local control is critical.[37] The French Federation Cancer Sarcoma Group published the largest retrospective cohort of RPS cases including 145 patients, of whom 60 had postoperative radiation (median, 50 Gy).[38] At 5-years, local control was 55% for patients who had radiation compared with 23% for patients who had surgery alone. A slightly smaller retrospective review from Memorial Sloan Kettering Cancer Center included 134 patients, of whom about one-quarter had radiation, which was shown on univariate analysis of long-term survivors to be the only significant factor.[39] This trial and others demonstrated that the risk of LR extends out to 10 years, because 40% of LRs were in the latter 5-year interval.

Similar to STS, the timing of RT for the treatment of RPS has been studied with respect to efficacy and toxicity. The benefits of postoperative radiation include immediate surgical resection and availability of full pathologic information. However, the challenges of delivery of postoperative radiation include an ill-defined and larger target volume, more bowel in the field, and the need to treat to a higher dose (typically 60–66 Gy). In contrast, preoperative RT (usually 50 Gy) is advantageous because bowel and other critical organs are displaced by the tumor, target volumes are more easily defined based on gross disease, there is improved tissue oxygenation allowing for radiation-induced free radical formation, and tumor shrinkage potentially improves resection and decreases intraoperative surgical seeding.

A small prospective study treated 16 patients with preoperative radiation using a dose painting integrated "boost" to the area of concern for potential positive margin, achieving negative margins in 14 patients of whom only two had an LR.[40] A prospective cohort from MDACC including 72 patients (25% with recurrent disease) demonstrated that preoperative radiation with intraoperative or postoperative BRT boost improved the rate of gross total resection and improved local control.[41] Despite the gains in local control, radiation has not been shown to impart an overall survival benefit.

In summary, intraoperative and postoperative radiation (50 Gy with boost to >60 Gy) seem to improve local control by 20% to 60%, with no improvement in overall survival. Surgical resection first is particularly helpful if a low-grade sarcoma is suspected. Preoperative radiation (45–50 Gy) has been shown to be well tolerated, with local control at 3 and 5 years to be about 90% and 70% to 80%, although the 2015 consensus guidelines recommend the use of this technique only at experienced centers. In the event of a positive margin after preoperative radiation, a boost with intraoperative or postoperative BRT or external beam radiation can be considered. Image-guided IMRT is preferred, with tracking of respiratory motion for tumors above the iliac crest to ensure accurate delivery of the radiation.[42] The EORTC 69092 trial is accruing patients with RPS to treatment with preoperative radiation and surgery versus surgery alone.

Toxicity of RT for RPS includes poor wound healing, enteritis, nausea and vomiting, gastric ulcers, and small bowel obstruction or strictures. Toxicity is reduced when preoperative RT is used. Specifically intraoperative radiation is associated with increased peripheral neuropathy.

SUMMARY

Radiation is an essential component of the limb-sparing approach to extremity STS. Managed correctly, the local control of extremity STS is expected to be extremely favorable. Although it is unclear how the sequencing of radiation and surgery influences outcomes, prospective data suggest that the use of IMRT/image-guided RT techniques can improve and limit treatment-related toxicity while maintaining excellent local control.

REFERENCES

1. Shieber W, Graham P. An experience with sarcomas of the soft tissues in adults. Surgery 1962;52:295–8.
2. Gerner RE, Moore GE, Pickren JW. Soft tissue sarcomas. Ann Surg 1975;181(6): 803–8.
3. Leibel SA, Tranbaugh RF, Wara WM, et al. Soft tissue sarcomas of the extremities: survival and patterns of failure with conservative surgery and postoperative irradiation compared to surgery alone. Cancer 1982;50(6):1076–83.
4. Markhede G, Angervall L, Stener B. A multivariate analysis of the prognosis after surgical treatment of malignant soft-tissue tumors. Cancer 1982;49(8): 1721–33.
5. Windeyer B, Dische S, Mansfield CM. The place of radiotherapy in the management of fibrosarcoma of the soft tissues. Clin Radiol 1966;17(1):32–40.
6. Rosenberg SA, Tepper J, Glatstein E, et al. The treatment of soft-tissue sarcomas of the extremities: prospective randomized evaluations of (1) limb-sparing surgery plus radiation therapy compared with amputation and (2) the role of adjuvant chemotherapy. Ann Surg 1982;196(3):305–15.

7. Lawrence W Jr, Donegan WL, Natarajan N, et al. Adult soft tissue sarcomas. A pattern of care survey of the American College of Surgeons. Ann Surg 1987; 205(4):349–59.

8. Yang JC, Chang AE, Baker AR, et al. Randomized prospective study of the benefit of adjuvant radiation therapy in the treatment of soft tissue sarcomas of the extremity. J Clin Oncol 1998;16(1):197–203.

9. Pisters PW, Harrison LB, Leung DH, et al. Long-term results of a prospective randomized trial of adjuvant brachytherapy in soft tissue sarcoma. J Clin Oncol 1996;14(3):859–68.

10. Gutierrez JC, Perez EA, Franceschi D, et al. Outcomes for soft-tissue sarcoma in 8249 cases from a large state cancer registry. J Surg Res 2007;141(1):105–14.

11. Hou CH, Lazarides AL, Speicher PJ, et al. The use of radiation therapy in localized high-grade soft tissue sarcoma and potential impact on survival. Ann Surg Oncol 2015;22(9):2831–8.

12. Lazarides AL, Eward WC, Speicher PJ, et al. The use of radiation therapy in well-differentiated soft tissue sarcoma of the extremities: an NCDB review. Sarcoma 2015;2015:186581.

13. Pisters PW, Pollock RE, Lewis VO, et al. Long-term results of prospective trial of surgery alone with selective use of radiation for patients with T1 extremity and trunk soft tissue sarcomas. Ann Surg 2007;246(4):675–81 [discussion: 681–2].

14. Cahlon O, Brennan MF, Jia X, et al. A postoperative nomogram for local recurrence risk in extremity soft tissue sarcomas after limb-sparing surgery without adjuvant radiation. Ann Surg 2012;255(2):343–7.

15. Pollack A, Zagars GK, Goswitz MS, et al. Preoperative vs. postoperative radiotherapy in the treatment of soft tissue sarcomas: a matter of presentation. Int J Radiat Oncol Biol Phys 1998;42(3):563–72.

16. Zagars GK, Ballo MT, Pisters PW, et al. Preoperative vs. postoperative radiation therapy for soft tissue sarcoma: a retrospective comparative evaluation of disease outcome. Int J Radiat Oncol Biol Phys 2003;56(2):482–8.

17. O'Sullivan B, Davis AM, Turcotte R, et al. Preoperative versus postoperative radiotherapy in soft-tissue sarcoma of the limbs: a randomised trial. Lancet 2002;359(9325):2235–41.

18. Davis AM, O'Sullivan B, Bell RS, et al. Function and health status outcomes in a randomized trial comparing preoperative and postoperative radiotherapy in extremity soft tissue sarcoma. J Clin Oncol 2002;20(22):4472–7.

19. Al-Absi E, Farrokhyar F, Sharma R, et al. A systematic review and meta-analysis of oncologic outcomes of pre- versus postoperative radiation in localized resectable soft-tissue sarcoma. Ann Surg Oncol 2010;17(5):1367–74.

20. Dickie CI, Griffin AM, Parent AL, et al. The relationship between local recurrence and radiotherapy treatment volume for soft tissue sarcomas treated with external beam radiotherapy and function preservation surgery. Int J Radiat Oncol Biol Phys 2012;82(4):1528–34.

21. Dickie CI, Parent AL, Griffin AM, et al. Bone fractures following external beam radiotherapy and limb-preservation surgery for lower extremity soft tissue sarcoma: relationship to irradiated bone length, volume, tumor location and dose. Int J Radiat Oncol Biol Phys 2009;75(4):1119–24.

22. Folkert MR, Singer S, Brennan MF, et al. Comparison of local recurrence with conventional and intensity-modulated radiation therapy for primary soft-tissue sarcomas of the extremity. J Clin Oncol 2014;32(29):3236–41.

23. Dagan R, Indelicato DJ, McGee L, et al. The significance of a marginal excision after preoperative radiation therapy for soft tissue sarcoma of the extremity. Cancer 2012;118(12):3199–207.

24. McGee L, Indelicato DJ, Dagan R, et al. Long-term results following postoperative radiotherapy for soft tissue sarcomas of the extremity. Int J Radiat Oncol Biol Phys 2012;84(4):1003–9.

25. O'Sullivan B, Griffin AM, Dickie CI, et al. Phase 2 study of preoperative image-guided intensity-modulated radiation therapy to reduce wound and combined modality morbidities in lower extremity soft tissue sarcoma. Cancer 2013; 119(10):1878–84.

26. Wang D, Zhang Q, Eisenberg BL, et al. Significant reduction of late toxicities in patients with extremity sarcoma treated with image-guided radiation therapy to a reduced target volume: results of radiation therapy oncology group RTOG-0630 Trial. J Clin Oncol 2015;33(20):2231–8.

27. Al Yami A, Griffin AM, Ferguson PC, et al. Positive surgical margins in soft tissue sarcoma treated with preoperative radiation: is a postoperative boost necessary? Int J Radiat Oncol Biol Phys 2010;77(4):1191–7.

28. Qureshi YA, Huddy JR, Miller JD, et al. Unplanned excision of soft tissue sarcoma results in increased rates of local recurrence despite full further oncological treatment. Ann Surg Oncol 2012;19(3):871–7.

29. Bahig H, Roberge D, Bosch W, et al. Agreement among RTOG sarcoma radiation oncologists in contouring suspicious peritumoral edema for preoperative radiation therapy of soft tissue sarcoma of the extremity. Int J Radiat Oncol Biol Phys 2013;86(2):298–303.

30. White LM, Wunder JS, Bell RS, et al. Histologic assessment of peritumoral edema in soft tissue sarcoma. Int J Radiat Oncol Biol Phys 2005;61(5): 1439–45.

31. Wang D, Bosch W, Roberge D, et al. RTOG sarcoma radiation oncologists reach consensus on gross tumor volume and clinical target volume on computed tomographic images for preoperative radiotherapy of primary soft tissue sarcoma of extremity in Radiation Therapy Oncology Group studies. Int J Radiat Oncol Biol Phys 2011;81(4):e525–8.

32. Davis AM, O'Sullivan B, Turcotte R, et al. Late radiation morbidity following randomization to preoperative versus postoperative radiotherapy in extremity soft tissue sarcoma. Radiother Oncol 2005;75(1):48–53.

33. Hall EJ, Wuu CS. Radiation-induced second cancers: the impact of 3D-CRT and IMRT. Int J Radiat Oncol Biol Phys 2003;56(1):83–8.

34. Mark RJ, Bailet JW, Poen J, et al. Postirradiation sarcoma of the head and neck. Cancer 1993;72(3):887–93.

35. Gladdy RA, Qin LX, Moraco N, et al. Do radiation-associated soft tissue sarcomas have the same prognosis as sporadic soft tissue sarcomas? J Clin Oncol 2010; 28(12):2064–9.

36. Shaheen M, Deheshi BM, Riad S, et al. Prognosis of radiation-induced bone sarcoma is similar to primary osteosarcoma. Clin Orthop Relat Res 2006;450:76–81.

37. Lewis JJ, Leung D, Woodruff JM, et al. Retroperitoneal soft-tissue sarcoma: analysis of 500 patients treated and followed at a single institution. Ann Surg 1998; 228(3):355–65.

38. Stoeckle E, Coindre JM, Bonvalot S, et al. Prognostic factors in retroperitoneal sarcoma: a multivariate analysis of a series of 165 patients of the French Cancer Center Federation Sarcoma Group. Cancer 2001;92(2):359–68.

39. Heslin MJ, Lewis JJ, Nadler E, et al. Prognostic factors associated with long-term survival for retroperitoneal sarcoma: implications for management. J Clin Oncol 1997;15(8):2832–9.
40. Tzeng CW, Fiveash JB, Popple RA, et al. Preoperative radiation therapy with selective dose escalation to the margin at risk for retroperitoneal sarcoma. Cancer 2006;107(2):371–9.
41. Pawlik TM, Pisters PW, Mikula L, et al. Long-term results of two prospective trials of preoperative external beam radiotherapy for localized intermediate- or high-grade retroperitoneal soft tissue sarcoma. Ann Surg Oncol 2006;13(4):508–17.
42. Baldini EH, Wang D, Haas RL, et al. Treatment guidelines for preoperative radiation therapy for retroperitoneal sarcoma: preliminary consensus of an international expert panel. Int J Radiat Oncol Biol Phys 2015;92(3):602–12.

Systemic Therapy for Advanced Soft Tissue Sarcoma

 CrossMark

Jennifer Y. Sheng, MD[a],*, Sujana Movva, MD[b]

KEYWORDS

- Advanced soft tissue sarcoma • Chemotherapy • Novel therapies

KEY POINTS

- Survival for advanced soft tissue sarcomas has improved significantly over the last 20 years because of advancements in histologic classification, improved treatment approaches, and novel agents.
- An important factor guiding choice of therapy is soft tissue sarcoma subtype, as drugs such as eribulin and trabectedin may have particular activity in leiomyosarcoma and liposarcoma.
- Focus on angiogenesis inhibition has led to the approval of pazopanib for soft tissue sarcoma, and the pathway continues to be investigated in this disease.
- Toxicity is an important area of investigation in soft tissue sarcoma, and new agents, such as aldoxorubicin, may be alternatives with better safety profiles.
- Future studies on treatment of advanced soft tissue sarcoma will continue to focus on identification of novel drug targets, personalization of therapy, and combination immunotherapies.

BACKGROUND

Sarcomas are rare tumors that arise from or are differentiated from tissues of mesodermal origin. They comprise less than 1% of all adult malignancies.[1] In 2015 there were approximately 14, 900 new cases diagnosed, with 6360 deaths in the United States. Sarcomas are grouped into 2 general categories: soft tissues sarcomas and primary bone sarcomas, which have different staging and treatment approaches.

This article includes a discussion of chemotherapy in advanced or refractory soft tissue sarcoma. Patients with metastatic disease are usually best managed with chemotherapy. Distant metastasis occurs in up to 10% of patients, with the lung being the most common site in 83% of cases.[2] Systemic therapy can involve cytotoxic

[a] Department of Oncology, Sidney Kimmel Comprehensive Cancer Center, Johns Hopkins University School of Medicine, Baltimore, MD, USA; [b] Department of Hematology/Oncology, Fox Chase Cancer Center, 333 Cottman Avenue, Philadelphia, PA 19111, USA
* Corresponding author.
E-mail address: jsheng7@jhmi.edu

Surg Clin N Am 96 (2016) 1141–1156
http://dx.doi.org/10.1016/j.suc.2016.06.006
0039-6109/16/$ – see front matter Published by Elsevier Inc.

surgical.theclinics.com

chemotherapy or targeted therapy with different toxicity profiles. In general, the response rates to doxorubicin and ifosfamide have ranged from 20% to 35%, while the response to other single-agent chemotherapy is low (10% or less).[3] In addition, combination and dose-intense regimens have largely failed to improve survival.[4] New therapies such as eribulin, olaratumab, and immunotherapy are promising and are under further investigation.

DOXORUBICIN

Doxorubicin is an anthracycline antibiotic isolated from *Streptomyces peucetius*, which intercalates in the DNA helix and prevents replication.[5] It has been used since the 1970s, with initial studies demonstrating a complete remission in 6.7% and partial remission in 20% of patients with metastatic soft tissue sarcoma.[6] More recent studies of doxorubicin 75 mg/m^2 administered every 3 weeks have demonstrated objective response rates (ORRs) ranging from 18.8% to 25.6%.[7,8]

A 2001 EORTC (European Organization for Research and Treatment of Cancer) phase II trial compared Doxil (pegylated liposomal doxorubicin) 50 mg/m^2 every 4 weeks with doxorubicin 75 mg/m^2 every 3 weeks (**Table 1**). Response rates in the cohort of patients with soft tissue sarcoma excluding gastrointestinal stromal tumor were 14% and 12% for Doxil and doxorubicin, respectively. Incidents of hematologic toxicity, febrile neutropenia, and alopecia were higher in the doxorubicin arm. However, more patients had palmar–plantar erythrodysesthesia in the Doxil arm.[9] Doxil has activity specifically in cutaneous angiosarcoma. A review of 8 cases in Germany demonstrated a complete response in 2 patients, partial response in 4 patients, and a response followed by progressive disease in 1 patient.[10] Another retrospective analysis of 119 patients with metastatic angiosarcoma showed that doxorubicin, Doxil, and taxanes resulted in similar response rates (30%) and median overall survival (OS) of 12.1 months.[11]

Response rates as high as 66% in patients receiving doxorubicin 75 to 90 mg/m^2 in combination with ifosfamide have been noted.[12] Combinations of Doxil and ifosfamide as first-line therapy for metastatic soft tissue sarcoma have demonstrated ORRs as high as 55.9%.[13] However, a meta-analysis of 2281 patients showed that although the response rate was marginally higher for patients receiving doxorubicin and ifosfamide versus single-agent doxorubicin, pooled analysis using random effects showed no statistically significant difference. Additionally, a significant difference was not achieved with 1-year year or 2-year mortality rate.[14] Some of these findings are supported by the multicenter phase III trial, EORTC 62012. Patients with locally advanced, unresectable, or metastatic high-grade soft tissue sarcomas were randomly assigned to receive doxorubicin (n = 228) or doxorubicin and ifosfamide (n = 227). Doxorubicin was given at 75 mg/m^2 on day 1 bolus or 72-hour infusion at 25 mg/m^2/d. In the combination arm, ifosfamide was given at 10 g/m^2 over 4 days with mesna and pegfilgastrim. There was no significant difference in OS between the 2 groups (hazard ratio [HR] 0.83, 95.5% confidence interval [CI], 0.67–1.03; P = .076), as OS was 12.8 months in doxorubicin group (95.5% CI, 10.5–14.3) and 14.3 months in the combination group (95.5% CI, 12.5–16.5). However, the median progression-free survival (PFS) was significantly higher for combination chemotherapy at 7.4 months (95% CI, 6.6–8.3) versus doxorubicin at 4.6 months (95% CI, 2.9–5.6); (HR 0.74, 95.5% CI, 0.60–0.90; P = .003).[15]

IFOSFAMIDE

Ifosfamide, a nitrogen mustard alkylating agent that crosslinks DNA, has demonstrated activity in soft tissue sarcoma at doses of 7.5 g/m^2 to 10 g/m^2. A phase III trial

Table 1
Select phase II/III trials of active drugs in soft tissue sarcoma

Author, Year	N	Subtype	Regimen	Previous Chemotherapy	Response Rate[a]	OS, median (months)[a] or PFS[b]
Judson et al,[9] 2001	95	Soft tissue sarcoma excluding gastrointestinal stromal tumor	Doxil 50 mg/m² every 4 wk vs doxorubicin 75 mg/m² every 3 wk	N	Doxil: 14% Doxorubicin: 12%	Doxil: 10.7 Doxorubicin: 8.2
Judson et al,[15] 2014	455	Locally advanced, unresectable or metastatic high-grade soft tissue sarcoma	Doxorubicin 75 mg/m² on day 1 bolus or 72-h infusion at 25 mg/m²/d vs Combination arm with ifosfamide 10 g/m² over 4 d every 3 wk	N	Doxorubicin: 14% Combination: 26% (P = .0006)	Doxorubicin: 12.8 Combination: 14.3
Lorigan et al,[16] 2007	326	Locally advanced or metastatic soft tissue sarcoma	Doxorubicin 75 mg/m² vs ifosfamide 9 g/m² over 3 d (continuous vs 3 h/d) every 3 wk	N	Doxorubicin: 11.8% Ifos 3h/d: 5.5% Ifos 9: 8.4%	Doxorubicin: 12.0 Ifos 3h/d: 10.9 Ifos 9: 10.9
Maki et al,[24] 2007	119	Soft tissue sarcoma excluding gastrointestinal stromal tumor and Kaposi sarcoma	Gemcitabine 1200 mg/m² on days 1 and 8 every 3 wk vs gemcitabine 900 mg/m² on days 1 and 8 with docetaxel 100 mg/m² on day 8 every 3 wk	Both treated and untreated	Gemcitabine: 8% Combination: 16%	Gemcitabine: 11.5 Combination: 17.9 Pr(β_GD > 0 | data) = .97
Pautier et al,[25] 2012	90	Uterine LMS and nonuterine LMS	Gemcitabine 1,000 mg/m² on days 1, 8, and 15 of a 28 d cycle vs combination gemcitabine 900 mg/m² on days 1 and 8 plus docetaxel at 100 mg/m² on day 8 of a 21 d cycle	Y	Uterine LMS: Gemcitabine: 19% Combination: 24% Non-uterine LMS: Gemcitabine: 14% Combination: 5%	Uterine LMS: Gemcitabine: 20 Combination: 23 Non-uterine LMS: Gemcitabine: 15 Combination: 13

(continued on next page)

Table 1
(continued)

Author, Year	N	Subtype	Regimen	Previous Chemotherapy	Response Rate[a]	OS, median (months)[a] or PFS[b]
Seddon,[28] 2015	257	Advanced soft tissue sarcoma	Doxorubicin 75 mg/m^2 every 3 wk vs gemcitabine 675 mg/m^2 days 1 and 8 and docetaxel 75 mg/m^2 day 8 every 3 wk	N	Includes Stable Disease: Doxorubicin: 65.9% Combination: 58.6%	Doxorubicin: 16.4 Combination: 14.5
Buesa et al,[29] 1991	44	Advanced soft tissue sarcoma	Dacarbazine 1.2 g/m^2 every 3 wk	Y	18%	NR
Penel et al,[36] 2008	30	Angiosarcoma	Paclitaxel 80 mg/m^2 on days 1, 8 and 15 of a 28 d cycle	Both treated and untreated	19% at 6 mo	8 mo
Sleijfer et al,[38] 2009	142	Advanced soft tissue sarcoma	Pazopanib 800 mg orally once daily	Y	6.3%	Adipocytic: 6.6 LMS: 11.8 Synovial: 10.3 Other: 10.0
van der Graaf et al,[39] 2012	369	Metastatic soft tissue sarcoma	Pazopanib 800 mg orally once daily vs placebo	Y	Pazopanib: 6% Placebo: 0	Pazopanib: 12.5 Placebo: 10.7
Yovine et al,[42] 2004	54	Soft tissue sarcoma	Trabectedin 1.5 mg/m^2 over 24 h every 3 wk	Y	3.7%	12.8 mo
Garcia-Carbonera et al,[43] 2004	36	Soft tissue sarcoma	Trabectedin 1.5 mg/m^2 over 24 h every 3 wk	Y	8%	12.1 mo
Le Cesne et al,[44] 2005	104	Soft tissue sarcoma	Trabectedin 1.5 mg/m^2 over 24 h every 3 wk	Y	8.1%	9.2 mo
Demetri et al,[45] 2009	270	Liposarcoma, LMS	Trabectedin 1.5 mg/m^2 over 24-h every 3 wk vs 0.58 mg/m^2 3-h infusion every week for 3 wk of a 4-wk cycle	Y	q3 wk 24-h: 5.6% qweek 3-h: 1.6%	q3 wk 24-h: 13.9 qweek 3-h: 11.8

Study	N	Population	Treatment	Statistically significant	Response rate	Median overall survival (mo)
Monk et al,[47] 2012	20	Uterine LMS	Trabectedin 1.5 mg/m² over 24-h every 3 wk	N	10%	>26.1 mo (median not reached)
Demetri et al,[50] 2015	518	Liposarcoma and LMS	Trabectedin 1.5 mg/m² over 24 h vs dacarbazine 1 g/m² every 3 wk	Y	Trabectedin: 9.9% Dacarbazine: 6.9%	Trabectedin: 12.4 Dacarbazine: 12.9
Schoffski et al,[56] 2011	128	LMS, synovial sarcoma, adipocytic sarcoma and other	Eribulin 1.4 mg/m² on days 1 and 8 of a 21 d cycle	Y	Adipocytic: 3% LMS: 5% Synovial: 5% Other: 5%	PFS: Adipocytic: 2.6 LMS: 2.9 Synovial: 2.6 Other: 2.1
Schoffski et al,[57] 2015	452	LMS, adipocytic sarcoma	Eribulin 1.4 mg/m² on days 1 and 8 of a 21 d cycle vs dacarbazine (850 or 1000 or 1200 mg/m²) every 3 wk	Y	Eribulin: 4% Dacarbazine: 5%	Eribulin: 13.5 Dacarbazine: 11.5 (P = .0169)
Chawla et al,[58] 2015	13	Soft tissue sarcoma	Aldoxorubicin 350 mg/m² every 3 wk (phase II portion of trial)	Y	38%	21.7
Chawla et al,[59] 2015	126	Advanced, unresectable or metastatic soft tissue sarcoma	Aldoxorubicin 350 mg/m² vs doxorubicin 75 mg/m² every 3 wk	N	Aldoxorubicin: 25% Doxorubicin: 0%	Aldoxorubicin: 15.8 Doxorubicin: 14.3
Tap,[8] 2015	133	Unresectable or metastatic soft tissue sarcoma	Doxorubicin (75 g/m²) with or without olaratumab (15 mg/kg on days 1 and 8) every 21 d	Both treated and untreated	Doxorubicin: 12.3% Combination: 18.8%	Doxorubicin: 14.7 Combination: 25.0
Dickson,[61] 2016	60	Liposarcoma	Palbociclib 125 mg orally daily for 21 d in 28 d cycles	Both treated and untreated	1.6%	PFS: 4.5

a Results are statistically nonsignificant unless otherwise specified.
b Where specified.
Data from Refs. [8,9,15,16,24,25,28,29,36,38,39,42–45,47,50,53–56,58]

of doxorubicin at 75 mg/m^2 versus ifosfamide at 9 g/m^2 showed no differences in PFS, OS, or response rates in a population of mostly leiomyosarcoma (LMS) and synovial sarcoma.[16] However, grade 4 hematologic toxicity and encephalopathy were higher in the ifosfamide arm. Despite increased toxicity, exposure to higher-dose ifosfamide (>10 g/m^2) per cycle has demonstrated higher rates of complete and partial responses, with overall response rates as high as 19% to 37.7%.[17,18] A retrospective analysis of 1319 patients by EORTC-STBSG (Soft Tissue and Bone Sarcoma Group) identified predictive factors of response to first-line ifosfamide-containing chemotherapy. Trending found that patients with liposarcoma and LMS benefited less from ifosfamide-containing therapy compared with doxorubicin alone. The response rate for synovial sarcoma patients was higher in the ifosfamide-containing regimen, but not statistically significant.[19] Other studies have demonstrated the sensitivity of synovial sarcoma to ifosfamide with a complete response rate of 30.7% in 13 patients.[20] The addition of ifosfamide to doxorubicin and dacarbazine in 340 patients improved response rates (32% vs 17%; P<.002) and time to progression (TTP 6 months vs 4 months; P<.02), with no significant advantage for OS.[21]

GEMCITABINE

Gemcitabine is a pyrimidine antimetabolite that inhibits DNA synthesis by inhibiting DNA polymerase and ribonucleotide reductase. In the United States, a phase II study of 56 patients with soft tissue sarcoma treated with gemcitabine at 2 different dose rates showed an ORR of 18% (95% CI, 7%–29%) and median duration of response of 3.5 months (range: 2–13 months). A pharmacology analysis demonstrated higher levels of gemcitabine triphosphate in peripheral blood mononuclear cells in patients receiving a fixed-dose rate infusion over 150 minutes compared with standard dosing over 30 minutes.[22]

Gemcitabine may also be synergistic with docetaxel.[23] A phase II trial (n = 119) conducted by Sarcoma Alliance for Research through Collaboration (SARC) compared fixed dose rate gemcitabine at 1200 mg/m^2 on days 1 and 8 every 21 days and fixed dose rate gemcitabine at 900 mg/m^2 over 90 minutes on days 1 and 8 in combination with docetaxel at 100 mg/m^2 over 1 hour on day 8 every 21 days. In the combination arm (n = 73), the ORR was 16% versus 8% in the single-agent arm (n = 49). The median PFS was 6.2 versus 3.0 months, and median OS was 17.9 versus 11.5 months in the combination versus single-agent arm, respectively. The posterior probability that combination therapy was superior to single-agent gemcitabine was 0.8 for PFS and 0.97 for OS. More than 40% of patients in the combination arm discontinued therapy within 6 months because of nonhematologic toxicity such as myalgia and fatigue, suggesting that cumulative toxicity with this regimen is prohibitive of long-term use. Grade 3 fatigue and myalgias or muscle weakness were observed in 25% of patients receiving combination therapy versus 10% of patients receiving gemcitabine only. Despite increase in toxicity of the combination as compared to gemcitabine alone, the authors concluded that the toxicity associated with gemcitabine and docetaxel compared favorably to the combination of doxorubicin and ifosfamide.[24] However, a separate phase II study of LMS in France, TAXOGEM, showed no difference in ORR in uterine LMS (n = 46) and nonuterine LMS (n = 44) groups receiving gemcitabine or the combination of gemcitabine and docetaxel. A total of 90 patients received either gemcitabine at 1,000 mg/m^2 on days 1, 8, and 15 of a 28-day cycle (n = 44) or combination gemcitabine at 900 mg/m^2 on days 1 and 8 plus docetaxel at 100 mg/m^2 on day 8 of a 21 day cycle (n = 46). ORR in uterine LMS was 19% in the gemcitabine arm (95% CI, 5%–42%) and 24% in the combination arm (95% CI, 8%–47%). For patients with nonuterine LMS, response rates were 14% (95% CI, 3%–35%) versus 5% (95%CI, 0%–26%). For uterine LMS, the median PFS was 5.5 months for gemcitabine and 4.7 months for the combination arm. For nonuterine LMS, the median PFS was 6.3 months for gemcitabine and 3.8 months for the combination arm.[25] The differences in these results as compared to the SARC trial may be due to inclusion of only patients with LMS who had failed first-line anthracycline regimen, whereas the SARC trial enrolled patients with all histologies who received none or a variety of regimens. Additionally, they had different designs (Bayesian vs classical randomization), schedules for drug intensity, and staging intervals.

Other studies have also demonstrated the activity of gemcitabine and docetaxel in LMS. In a phase II study of 34 patients with LMS who had not responded to up to 2 prior regimens, the ORR was 53%, with a median TTP of 5.6 months; 52.6% of patients had received no prior therapy.[26] Single-agent gemcitabine has also shown activity in angiosarcoma. In a retrospective case series of 25 patients with advanced angiosarcoma, there was an ORR of 68%, median OS of 17 months, and median PFS of 7 months (range: 1–40 months), suggesting that some patients may attain long-lasting responses.[27]

A phase III trial of gemcitabine and docetaxel with doxorubicin for soft tissue sarcomas (GeDDiS), compared gemcitabine and docetaxel with doxorubicin as first-line treatment in previously untreated advanced soft tissue sarcoma. Patients were randomized to receive 6 cycles of doxorubicin at 75 mg/m^2 day 1 every 3 weeks (n = 129) or gemcitabine 675 mg/m^2 intravenously on days 1 and 8 and docetaxel 75 mg/m^2 intravenously on day 8 every 3 weeks (n = 128). The primary endpoint of PFS at 24 weeks was achieved in 46.1% of the doxorubicin arm and 46.0% of the combination arm (HR 1.28, 95% CI, 0.98–1.67; P = .07). Median OS was 71 versus 63 weeks (HR 1.07; 95% CI, 0.77–1.49) for doxorubicin versus combination. Although PFS Kaplan-Meier curves did not violate the proportional hazards assumption (P = .53), they initially overlapped and then separated after 24 weeks in favor of doxorubicin. Patients receiving doxorubicin had higher grade 3 and 4 toxicities of febrile neutropenia and mucositis, while patients receiving combination had higher grade 3 and 4 rates of fatigue and diarrhea. The combination arm was also associated with greater dose delays of at least 1 day, patient withdrawal due to toxicity and lower mean dose intensity despite a lower starting dose of gemcitabine and docetaxel than previously published. Therefore, the investigators suggested that doxorubicin should be the preferred agent for first-line treatment in advanced soft tissue sarcoma.[28]

DACARBAZINE AND TEMOZOLOMIDE

Dacarbazine is an alkylating agent that breaks DNA strands. In a phase II EORTC study of 44 patients with advanced soft tissue sarcoma who had received previous chemotherapy, 1 complete remission and 7 partial remissions were seen with dacarbazine, for a response rate of 18%. Median duration of response was 8 weeks, with complete remission lasting 12 months.[29] Other investigators have suggested that second- or third-line dacarbazine may have comparable activity to other treatments but with a better profile toxicity.[30] The combination of doxorubicin and dacarbazine has yielded a response rate of 17%.[31]

Temozolomide is an oral agent and prodrug of the active metabolite of dacarbazine. An initial phase II study of temozolomide in soft tissue sarcoma (n = 41) suggested that it was well tolerated at a dose of 85 mg/m^2 orally for 21 days on a 28-day cycle. However, it had minimal efficacy (response rate of 5%) and a limited role in soft tissue sarcoma.[32] In a phase II study by the Spanish Group for Research on

Sarcomas, 49 patients with pretreated soft tissue sarcoma were given temozolomide 75 to 100 mg/m^2 continuously (doses were dependent on time of enrollment into the study due to an amendment). The response rate was 15.5%, most notable in patients with gynecologic LMS.[33]

The activity of temozolomide may be higher in patients with tumors lacking MGMT (O^6-methylguanine-DNA methyltransferase) gene expression. Retrospective analysis of 28 patients with metastatic LMS receiving temozolomide at 75 mg/m^2 daily for 21 days in 28-day cycles yielded an overall response rate of 17.8%. Median PFS was 126 days. MGMT was deficient in tumors from 6 of 20 patients with clinical benefit and in 1 of 8 without clinical benefit. Median PFS was 105 days for the MGMT-intact group and 203 days for the MGMT-deficient group.[34]

PACLITAXEL

Paclitaxel promotes microtubule assembly and interferes with cell replication by stabilizing existing microtubules. Paclitaxel is useful in treating several solid tumors and has demonstrated activity in angiosarcoma, especially of the scalp or face.

A phase II study of 28 patients with advanced soft tissue sarcoma treated with paclitaxel yielded only 2 partial responses. The responding patients included 1 patient with angiosarcoma and uterine LMS. Therefore, the activity of paclitaxel outside of angiosarcoma appears to be low. Two patients with angiosarcoma of the scalp who did not qualify for this study were treated with paclitaxel off protocol and experienced dramatic tumor regression. In another retrospective cohort of cutaneous angiosarcoma of the head and neck treated with single-agent paclitaxel at 250 mg/m^2 over 3 hours every 3 weeks, there was an ORR of 88.9% in 9 patients, with a clinical complete response in 4 patients. Median duration of response was 5 months (range: 2–13 months).[35] The phase II ANGIOTAX study of 30 patients with unresectable angiosarcoma formally evaluated the activity of paclitaxel in angiosarcoma. The agent was given at 80 mg/m^2, 3 weeks of 4. PFS at 2 and 4 months was 74% and 45%, respectively. With a median follow-up of 8 months, the median TTP was 4 months, and the median OS was 8 months.[36]

A retrospective study compared doxorubicin and paclitaxel in 117 patients with angiosarcoma treated in the first-line setting. The rates of complete response, partial response, and stable disease were 6%, 23.5%, and 29.5% in the doxorubicin group and 13%, 40%, and 29.5% in the paclitaxel group. Patients in the paclitaxel group were more likely to have a cutaneous angiosarcoma. Therefore, both agents appear to have similar activity in previously untreated angiosarcoma.[37]

PAZOPANIB

Pazopanib, a multitargeted tyrosine kinase inhibitor that limits tumor growth through inhibition of angiogenesis, has single-agent activity in advanced nonadipocytic STS. It is given as 800 mg orally once daily. In EORTC 62043, a phase II study, 142 patients with intermediate- or high-grade advanced STS who were ineligible for chemotherapy or who had received no more than 2 prior cytotoxic agents were given pazopanib. The primary endpoint was progression-free rate (PFR) at 12 weeks. The study met the predetermined cutoff for sufficient activity in 3 cohorts, with a PFR at 12 weeks of 44% for LMS (18 of 41 patients), 49% for synovial sarcoma (18 of 37 patients) and 39% in other STS types (16 of 41 patients). The study was closed in the adipocytic cohort of 19 patients after the first stage, given insufficient activity (primary endpoint achieved in only 26% of patients).[38] Another study, PALETTE (Pazopanib for metastatic soft-tissue sarcoma), an international, multicenter phase III study, randomized patients with angiogenesis inhibitor-naive, pretreated metastatic STS, to receive pazopanib (n = 246) or placebo (n = 123). Median PFS was significant at 4.6 months with pazopanib (95.5% CI, 3.7–4.8) versus 1.6 months with placebo (95.5% CI, 0.9–1.8; HR 0.31, 95.5% CI, 0.24–0.40; P<.0001). OS was not statistically different at 12.5 months with pazopanib (95.5% CI, 10.6–14.8) versus 10.7 months with placebo (95.5% CI, 8.7–12.8).[39]

In a pooled analysis of both the EORTC 62043 (n = 118) and PALETTE (n = 226), PFS was 4.4 months, and median OS was 11.7 months. One hundred twenty-four patients (36%) had a PFS greater than 6 months. One hundred sixteen patients (34%) survived more than 18 months. A total of 12 patients remained on pazopanib for over 2 years.[40] Additional studies are investigating the activity of pazopanib in liposarcoma and in combination with other therapies.

TRABECTEDIN

Trabectedin is a marine-derived compound that blocks the cell cycle by binding to the minor DNA groove, given at 1.5 mg/m^2 over 24 hours once every 3 weeks.[41] In a phase II European study, 54 patients with previously treated metastatic soft tissue sarcoma demonstrated an ORR of 3.7% by World Health Organization (WHO) criteria, with a median PFS of 1.9 months and median OS of 12.8 months. The PFR at 6 months was 24%.[42] In a phase II study in the United States, 36 patients with previously treated STS had an ORR of 8%, with TTP of 1.7 months and OS of 12.1 months. Notably, some responses were durable for up to 20 months.[43] The EORTC phase II study of trabectedin showed that the 6-month PFS (29%) compared favorably with other drugs tested as second-line chemotherapy. Of 104 patients with pretreated advanced STS, the progression arrest rate (sum of partial response and no change in disease) was 56% in LMS and 61% in synovial sarcoma. Toxicity involved reversible grade 3 to 4 asymptomatic elevation of transaminases (40%) and neutropenia (52%).[44] Another study evaluated different treatment regimens. It was a multicenter phase II study that randomized patients with pretreated liposarcomas and LMS to either trabectedin 1.5 mg/m^2 24-hour infusion once every 3 weeks (n = 136) or 0.58 mg/m^2 3-hour infusion every week for 3 weeks of a 4-week period (n = 134). The primary endpoint of median TTP was 3.7 months versus 2.3 months (HR 0.734; 95% CI, 0.554–0.974; P = .0302), favoring the every 3 weeks 24-hour arm. Median PFS was 3.3 months in the 24-hour arm versus 2.3 months in 3-hour arm (HR 0.755; 95% CI, 0.574–0.992; P = .0418).[45]

Trabectedin has also shown activity in the first-line setting. In 36 patients with previously untreated disease, the ORR was 17.1%, with an estimated 1-year PFS of 21% (95% CI, 11%–41%) and OS rate of 72% (95% CI, 59%–88%).[41] In the worldwide expanded access program of trabectedin, efficacy data on 807 patients with refractory disease were available. A stable disease rate of 43% was reported. Patients with LMS and liposarcoma demonstrated longer OS compared with other histologies, with OS of 16.2 months (95% CI, 14.1–19.5 months). They also had a higher ORR of 6.9% (95% CI, 4.8–9.6) versus 4.0% (95% CI, 2.1–6.8) for other histologies.[46] In a multicenter phase IIb study comparing single-agent doxorubicin (n = 43) with trabectedin (n = 47 for 3-hour infusion arm and n = 43 for 24-hour infusion arm), no significant improvement in PFS was observed in the trabectedin arm compared with the doxorubicin arm; therefore the study was terminated early.[7]

Liposarcomas and LMS are particularly sensitive to trabectedin. A phase II evaluation in 20 chemotherapy-naïve patients with advanced, persistent, or recurrent uterine LMS had a partial response noted in 10% of patients. Although there was a modest response rate, it is noteworthy that 50% of patients achieved stable disease with a PFS of 5.8 months. More than half the patients remained in the study for more than 10 cycles (>6 months).[47] Retrospective analysis of 5 phase II studies including 62 patients with pretreated advanced uterine LMS demonstrated a median PFS of 2.5 months (95% CI, 1.7–4.2). The primary endpoint of PFS at 6 months was achieved in 30.7% (95%CI, 19–43). Median OS was 12.1 months, with 52% alive at 12 months (95% CI, 39–64) and 20% alive at 24 months (95% CI, 10–30).[48] A retrospective analysis of 32 patients with myxoid liposarcoma receiving trabectedin demonstrated an ORR by RECIST of 50%, with a median PFS of 17 months (95% CI, 13.5–30.1) and a median OS that was not reached.[49]

In the multicenter phase III trial of previously treated patients with liposarcoma and LMS, trabectedin (n = 345) reduced risk of disease progression or death by 45% compared with dacarbazine (n = 173). Patients receiving trabectedin had a median PFS of 4.2 months versus 1.5 months with dacarbazine (HR 0.55, $P=<.001$). The ORR was 9.9% versus 6.9%, respectively, with trabectedin and dacarbazine ($P = .33$). The clinical benefit rates (partial response, complete response, or stable disease ≥18 weeks) were 34% and 19%, respectively ($P < .001$). Median OS was not significant, as it was similar across both arms at 12.4 months with trabectedin and 12.9 months with dacarbazine (HR 0.87, $P = .37$).[50] This study led to US Food and Drug Administration (FDA) approval of trabectedin in the United States for patients with LMS or liposarcoma previously treated with doxorubicin. Both the phase II and III studies demonstrated that the most common grade 3 to 4 adverse effects with trabectedin are related to myelosuppression and transient transaminitis.

NEOADJUVANT CHEMOTHERAPY FOR LOCALLY ADVANCED SOFT TISSUE SARCOMA

When managing patients with unresectable or borderline resectable localized soft tissue sarcoma, chemotherapy is often considered with the hope that sufficient cytoreduction will be achieved in order to convert the disease to resectable and/or to eradicate micrometastases. In a randomized study assessing the utility of neoadjuvant chemotherapy, patients with potentially radically resectable tumors were randomized to 3 cycles of preoperative chemotherapy with doxorubicin (50 mg/m^2) and ifosfamide (5 g/m^2) every 21 days or to no chemotherapy. Patients were required to have tumors that were at least 8 cm of any grade, or grade II/III tumors that were locally recurrent or required a second resection. Although there were no survival benefits, 29% of patients had a response (8% with a complete response), and none of the 18% of patients with progressive disease lost their surgical window or had a change in the scope of the procedure required.[51] Another randomized phase II study focused on differences in safety outcomes for 2 different chemotherapy regimens, doxorubicin and ifosfamide versus gemcitabine and docetaxel, given neoadjuvantly for resectable soft tissue sarcoma. The response rate with doxorubicin-based chemotherapy was 12.5%, and with gemcitabine-based chemotherapy, it was 3.4%.[52] Trabectedin has also been studied when given in the neoadjuvant fashion in 23 patients with myxoid liposarcoma, a histology known to be sensitive to this chemotherapy. Patients were required to have stage III disease for enrollment, and 17% had tumors greater than 10 cm. There was an ORR of 24%, with 13% of patients achieving a pathologic complete response. Importantly, no patients had progressive disease.[53] None of these studies specifically address whether patients whose tumors were unresectable could be rendered surgically resectable or if the scope of surgery could be down-staged with preoperative chemotherapy.

INVESTIGATIONAL AGENTS
Eribulin

Eribulin, a cytotoxic agent approved for advanced breast cancer, has demonstrated improvement in OS for patients with advanced STS. It is a nontaxane microtubule inhibitor dosed at 1.4 mg/m^2 on days 1 and 8 of a 21-day cycle.[54,55] A phase II study included 128 patients who had received no more than 1 previous combination chemotherapy or up to 2 single agents. Patients were stratified by histology: LMS (n = 40), synovial sarcoma (n = 19), adipocytic sarcoma (n = 37), and other sarcomas (n = 32). Only the LMS and liposarcoma cohorts met the primary endpoint of PFS at 12 weeks; 31.6% of patients with LMS and 46.9% with adipocytic sarcoma were progression free at 12 weeks. In the other groups, only 21.1% with synovial sarcoma and 19.2% with other sarcomas were progression free at 12 weeks.[56]

In a follow-up multicenter phase III trial, 452 patients with pretreated advanced LMS or adipocytic sarcoma were randomized to receive eribulin or dacarbazine. The primary endpoint was OS, which was significantly improved with eribulin. Median PFS was 2.6 months in both arms (HR 0.877, 95.5% CI, 0.710–1.085; P = .229). The median OS was 13.5 months with eribulin compared with 11.5 months with dacarbazine (HR 0.768, 95.5% CI, 0.618–0.954; P = .017). The 12-week PFS rate was 33% with eribulin and 29% with dacarbazine; however, this difference was not statistically significant. In the eribulin arm, 26% of patients required dose reductions, and 8% discontinued due to treatment-emergent adverse events (TEAEs) versus 14% and 5% in the dacarbazine arm, respectively. These TEAEs included neutropenia, pyrexia, peripheral sensory neuropathy, and alopecia.[57]

Aldoxorubicin

Aldoxorubicin is an albumin-binding prodrug of doxorubicin that has promising activity in advanced soft tissue sarcoma. A phase Ib/II study of aldoxorubicin included 17 patients (68%) with advanced soft tissue sarcoma, of whom 13 received aldoxrubicin at the maximum tolerated dose (MTD) of 350 mg/m^2. Among these patients, a partial response was achieved in 38% and stable disease in 46%.[58] In the subsequent international phase IIb study, 123 patients with previously untreated locally advanced, unresectable, or metastatic soft tissue sarcoma were randomized to aldoxorubicin at 350 mg/m^2 (n = 83) or doxorubicin 75 mg/m^2 (n = 40) once every 3 weeks for up to 6 cycles. Median PFS was significantly in favor of the aldoxorubicin arm: 5.6 months with aldoxorubicin (95.5% CI, 3.0–8.1) versus 2.7 months with doxorubicin (95.5% CI, 1.6–4.3) (P = .02). The rate of 6-month PFS was 46% versus 23% (P = .02). Median OS was not statistically different between the groups. Overall tumor response rate was higher with aldoxorubicin than with doxorubicin (25% vs 0%), as 20 patients achieved partial response with aldoxorubicin. No patient in either arm developed congestive heart failure or clinically significant abnormal cardiac function as measured by echocardiography or multigated acquisition scan. Three of 40 patients who received doxorubicin had a left ventricular ejection fraction (LVEF) that dropped below 50% while participating in the study. Twelve percent of patients in the aldoxorubicin group and 29% of patients in the doxorubicin group had at least a 10% decrease in LVEF at some point during treatment.[59] A phase III confirmatory trial comparing aldoxorubicin with physician choice chemotherapy recently completed enrollment, and results are awaited.

Olaratumab

Olaratumab (IMC-3G3) is a human antiplatelet-derived growth factor alpha (PDGFRα) monoclonal antibody that blocks ligand binding. A randomized phase Ib/II study evaluated the efficacy of doxorubicin (75 g/m^2 on day 1) with or without olaratumab (15 mg/kg on days 1 and 8 every 21 days) for up to 8 cycles in advanced STS. Patients randomized to the olaratumab arm were allowed to receive maintenance olaratumab until disease progression. Of 133 patients, median PFS was 6.6 months in the combination arm and 4.1 months in doxorubicin alone (HR 0.672; 95.5% CI, 0.442–1.021; $P = .0615$). Interim median OS was 25.0 months with combination therapy and 14.7 months with doxorubicin alone (HR 0.44, $P = .0005$). The study met its primary PFS endpoint and achieved an impressive 10.3 month improvement in median OS. Grade 3 or 4 adverse events occurred in over 5% of the population. Those in the olaratumab arm experienced neutropenia (51.5%), anemia (12.5%), fatigue (9.4%), and thrombocytopenia (9.4%), but had lower rates of febrile neutropenia (12.5%) and infections (6.3%). Overall, 64% of patients in the combination arm had a grade 3 or 4 adverse event, compared with 54% in the doxorubicin arm. Discontinuation of therapy was noted in 8 patients in the combination arm (including 4 with serious adverse events) versus 14 patients in the doxorubicin arm (including 8 with serious adverse events).[8] A phase III trial with a similar design is currently enrolling patients.

Palbociclib

In the mammalian cell cycle, G1 to S phase transition is tightly regulated by cyclin-dependent kinases 4 and 6 (CDK4/6). Palbociclib is a selective CDK4/CDK6 inhibitor. CDK4 is amplified in the majority of well-differentiated and dedifferentiated liposarcomas. In an open-label study of palbociclib 200 mg orally daily for 14 of 21 days, the PFS at 12 weeks was 66% (90% CI, 51–100) with a median PFS of 18 weeks. However, there was a high rate of hematologic toxicity, with 24% of patients requiring a dose reduction.[60] A subsequent study evaluated an alternate dosing regimen of palbociclib at 125 mg daily for 21 days in 28-day cycles. This dosing schedule was associated with less hematologic toxicity, as only 5% of patients required a dose reduction for this reason. The efficacy was comparable to the 200 mg dose.[61]

SUMMARY

The French Sarcoma Group has shown that on retrospective multivariate analysis, median OS for advanced STS has improved by 50% in the last 20 years. Contributing factors to this are the advancements in histologic and molecular classification of soft tissue sarcoma and improvements in treatment paradigms, as well as the development of new agents.[62] Specific soft tissue sarcoma subtype is one of the most important factors to guide choice of therapy, as drugs such as trabectedin and eribulin have shown particular activity in LMS and liposarcoma. Inhibition of signaling pathways related to angiogenesis has been effective therapeutically in soft tissue sarcoma with pazopanib, and is now under further investigation with olaratumab. Finally, mitigating toxicity has also been an important avenue of investigation in soft tissue sarcoma, with drugs such as aldoxorubicin. Unfortunately, investigation of prodrugs and/or metabolites of ifosfamide with potentially less toxicity has largely been unsuccessful thus far. In the future, studies will continue to focus on immunotherapy approaches for the management of, soft tissue sarcoma as well as personalization of therapy through identification of biomarkers of activity.

REFERENCES

1. Jo VY, Fletcher CD. WHO classification of soft tissue tumours: an update based on the 2013 (4th) edition. Pathology 2014;46(2):95–104.

2. Christie-Large M, James SL, Tiessen L, et al. Imaging strategy for detecting lung metastases at presentation in patients with soft tissue sarcomas. Eur J Cancer 2008;44(13):1841–5.

3. Ravi V, Patel S, Benjamin RS. Chemotherapy for soft-tissue sarcomas. Oncology (Williston Park) 2015;29(1):43–50.

4. Ray-Coquard I, Le Cesne A. A role for maintenance therapy in managing sarcoma. Cancer Treat Rev 2012;38(5):368–78.

5. Doxorubicin. 2016. Available at: https://pubchem.ncbi.nlm.nih.gov/compound/31703. Accessed December 20, 2015.

6. Benjamin RS, Wiernik PH, Bachur NR. Adriamycin: a new effective agent in the therapy of disseminated sarcomas. Med Pediatr Oncol 1975;1(1):63–76.

7. Bui-Nguyen B, Butrynski JE, Penel N, et al. A phase IIb multicentre study comparing the efficacy of trabectedin to doxorubicin in patients with advanced or metastatic untreated soft tissue sarcoma: The TRUSTS trial. Eur J Cancer 2015;51(10):1312–20.

8. Tap WD. A randomized phase ib/II study evaluating the safety and efficacy of olaratumab (IMC-3G3), a human anti-platelet-derived growth factor α (PDGFRα) monoclonal antibody, with or without doxorubicin (dox), in advanced soft tissue sarcoma (STS). J Clin Oncol 2015;33:10501.

9. Judson I, Radford JA, Harris M, et al. Randomised phase II trial of pegylated liposomal doxorubicin (DOXIL/CAELYX) versus doxorubicin in the treatment of advanced or metastatic soft tissue sarcoma: a study by the EORTC soft tissue and bone sarcoma group. Eur J Cancer 2001;37(7):870–7.

10. Wollina U, Hansel G, Schonlebe J, et al. Cutaneous angiosarcoma is a rare aggressive malignant vascular tumour of the skin. J Eur Acad Dermatol Venereol 2011;25(8):964–8.

11. D'Angelo SP, Munhoz RR, Kuk D, et al. Outcomes of systemic therapy for patients with metastatic angiosarcoma. Oncology 2015;89(4):205–14.

12. Patel SR, Vadhan-Raj S, Burgess MA, et al. Results of two consecutive trials of dose-intensive chemotherapy with doxorubicin and ifosfamide in patients with sarcomas. Am J Clin Oncol 1998;21(3):317–21.

13. De Sanctis R, Bertuzzi A, Basso U, et al. Non-pegylated liposomal doxorubicin plus ifosfamide in metastatic soft tissue sarcoma: results from a phase-II trial. Anticancer Res 2015;35(1):543–7.

14. Bramwell VH, Anderson D, Charette ML, Sarcoma Disease Site Group. Doxorubicin-based chemotherapy for the palliative treatment of adult patients with locally advanced or metastatic soft tissue sarcoma. Cochrane Database Syst Rev 2003;(3):CD003293.

15. Judson I, Verweij J, Gelderblom H, et al. Doxorubicin alone versus intensified doxorubicin plus ifosfamide for first-line treatment of advanced or metastatic soft-tissue sarcoma: a randomised controlled phase 3 trial. Lancet Oncol 2014; 15(4):415–23.

16. Lorigan P, Verweij J, Papai Z, et al. Phase III trial of two investigational schedules of ifosfamide compared with standard-dose doxorubicin in advanced or metastatic soft tissue sarcoma: a European organisation for research and treatment of cancer soft tissue and bone sarcoma group study. J Clin Oncol 2007;25(21): 3144–50.

17. Buesa JM, Lopez-Pousa A, Martin J, et al. Phase II trial of first-line high-dose ifosfamide in advanced soft tissue sarcomas of the adult: a study of the Spanish group for research on sarcomas (GEIS). Ann Oncol 1998;9(8):871–6.

18. Patel SR, Vadhan-Raj S, Papadopolous N, et al. High-dose ifosfamide in bone and soft tissue sarcomas: results of phase II and pilot studies–dose-response and schedule dependence. J Clin Oncol 1997;15(6):2378–84.
19. Sleijfer S, Ouali M, van Glabbeke M, et al. Prognostic and predictive factors for outcome to first-line ifosfamide-containing chemotherapy for adult patients with advanced soft tissue sarcomas: an exploratory, retrospective analysis on large series from the European organization for research and treatment of cancer-soft tissue and bone sarcoma group (EORTC-STBSG). Eur J Cancer 2010; 46(1):72–83.
20. Rosen G, Forscher C, Lowenbraun S, et al. Synovial sarcoma. uniform response of metastases to high dose ifosfamide. Cancer 1994;73(10):2506–11.
21. Antman K, Crowley J, Balcerzak SP, et al. An intergroup phase III randomized study of doxorubicin and dacarbazine with or without ifosfamide and mesna in advanced soft tissue and bone sarcomas. J Clin Oncol 1993;11(7):1276–85.
22. Patel SR, Gandhi V, Jenkins J, et al. Phase II clinical investigation of gemcitabine in advanced soft tissue sarcomas and window evaluation of dose rate on gemcitabine triphosphate accumulation. J Clin Oncol 2001;19(15):3483–9.
23. Maki RG. Gemcitabine and docetaxel in metastatic sarcoma: Past, present, and future. Oncologist 2007;12(8):999–1006.
24. Maki RG, Wathen JK, Patel SR, et al. Randomized phase II study of gemcitabine and docetaxel compared with gemcitabine alone in patients with metastatic soft tissue sarcomas: results of sarcoma alliance for research through collaboration study 002 [corrected]. J Clin Oncol 2007;25(19):2755–63.
25. Pautier P, Floquet A, Penel N, et al. Randomized multicenter and stratified phase II study of gemcitabine alone versus gemcitabine and docetaxel in patients with metastatic or relapsed leiomyosarcomas: a Federation Nationale des Centres de Lutte Contre le Cancer (FNCLCC) French Sarcoma Group study (TAXOGEM study). Oncologist 2012;17(9):1213–20.
26. Hensley ML, Maki R, Venkatraman E, et al. Gemcitabine and docetaxel in patients with unresectable leiomyosarcoma: results of a phase II trial. J Clin Oncol 2002; 20(12):2824–31.
27. Stacchiotti S, Palassini E, Sanfilippo R, et al. Gemcitabine in advanced angiosarcoma: a retrospective case series analysis from the italian rare cancer network. Ann Oncol 2012;23(2):501–8.
28. Seddon B. GeDDiS: a prospective randomised controlled phase III trial of gemcitabine and docetaxel compared with doxorubicin as first-line treatment in previously untreated advanced unresectable or metastatic soft tissue sarcomas (EudraCT 2009-014907-29). J Clin Oncol 2015;33:10500.
29. Buesa JM, Mouridsen HT, van Oosterom AT, et al. High-dose DTIC in advanced soft-tissue sarcomas in the adult. A phase II study of the E.O.R.T.C. soft tissue and bone sarcoma group. Ann Oncol 1991;2(4):307–9.
30. Zucali PA, Bertuzzi A, Parra HJ, et al. The "old drug" dacarbazine as a second/third line chemotherapy in advanced soft tissue sarcomas. Invest New Drugs 2008;26(2):175–81.
31. Gottlieb JA, Benjamin RS, Baker LH, et al. Role of DTIC (NSC-45388) in the chemotherapy of sarcomas. Cancer Treat Rep 1976;60(2):199–203.
32. Trent JC, Beach J, Burgess MA, et al. A two-arm phase II study of temozolomide in patients with advanced gastrointestinal stromal tumors and other soft tissue sarcomas. Cancer 2003;98(12):2693–9.
33. Garcia del Muro X, Lopez-Pousa A, Martin J, et al. A phase II trial of temozolomide as a 6-week, continuous, oral schedule in patients with advanced soft tissue

sarcoma: a study by the spanish group for research on sarcomas. Cancer 2005; 104(8):1706–12.

34. Marrari A. Expression of MGMT and response to treatment with temozolomide in patients with leiomyosarcoma. J Clin Oncol 2011;29:10074.

35. Fata F, O'Reilly E, Ilson D, et al. Paclitaxel in the treatment of patients with angiosarcoma of the scalp or face. Cancer 1999;86(10):2034–7.

36. Penel N, Bui BN, Bay JO, et al. Phase II trial of weekly paclitaxel for unresectable angiosarcoma: The ANGIOTAX study. J Clin Oncol 2008;26(32):5269–74.

37. Italiano A, Cioffi A, Penel N, et al. Comparison of doxorubicin and weekly paclitaxel efficacy in metastatic angiosarcomas. Cancer 2012;118(13):3330–6.

38. Sleijfer S, Ray-Coquard I, Papai Z, et al. Pazopanib, a multikinase angiogenesis inhibitor, in patients with relapsed or refractory advanced soft tissue sarcoma: a phase II study from the European Organisation for Research and Treatment of Cancer–Soft Tissue and Bone Sarcoma Group (EORTC study 62043). J Clin Oncol 2009;27(19):3126–32.

39. van der Graaf WT, Blay JY, Chawla SP, et al. Pazopanib for metastatic soft-tissue sarcoma (PALETTE): A randomised, double-blind, placebo-controlled phase 3 trial. Lancet 2012;379(9829):1879–86.

40. Kasper B, Sleijfer S, Litiere S, et al. Long-term responders and survivors on pazopanib for advanced soft tissue sarcomas: subanalysis of two European Organisation for Research and Treatment of Cancer (EORTC) clinical trials 62043 and 62072. Ann Oncol 2014;25(3):719–24.

41. Garcia-Carbonero R, Supko JG, Maki RG, et al. Ecteinascidin-743 (ET-743) for chemotherapy-naive patients with advanced soft tissue sarcomas: multicenter phase II and pharmacokinetic study. J Clin Oncol 2005;23(24):5484–92.

42. Yovine A, Riofrio M, Blay JY, et al. Phase II study of ecteinascidin-743 in advanced pretreated soft tissue sarcoma patients. J Clin Oncol 2004;22(5): 890–9.

43. Garcia-Carbonero R, Supko JG, Manola J, et al. Phase II and pharmacokinetic study of ecteinascidin 743 in patients with progressive sarcomas of soft tissues refractory to chemotherapy. J Clin Oncol 2004;22(8):1480–90.

44. Le Cesne A, Blay JY, Judson I, et al. Phase II study of ET-743 in advanced soft tissue sarcomas: a European Organisation for the Research and Treatment of Cancer (EORTC) Soft Tissue and Bone Sarcoma Group trial. J Clin Oncol 2005;23(3):576–84.

45. Demetri GD, Chawla SP, von Mehren M, et al. Efficacy and safety of trabectedin in patients with advanced or metastatic liposarcoma or leiomyosarcoma after failure of prior anthracyclines and ifosfamide: results of a randomized phase II study of two different schedules. J Clin Oncol 2009;27(25):4188–96.

46. Samuels BL, Chawla S, Patel S, et al. Clinical outcomes and safety with trabectedin therapy in patients with advanced soft tissue sarcomas following failure of prior chemotherapy: results of a worldwide expanded access program study. Ann Oncol 2013;24(6):1703–9.

47. Monk BJ, Blessing JA, Street DG, et al. A phase II evaluation of trabectedin in the treatment of advanced, persistent, or recurrent uterine leiomyosarcoma: a gynecologic oncology group study. Gynecol Oncol 2012;124(1):48–52.

48. Judson IR. Trabectedin (tr) in the treatment of advanced uterine leiomyosarcomas (U-LMS): Results of a pooled analysis of five single-agent phase II studies using the recommended dose. J Clin Oncol 2010;28:10028.

49. Grosso F, Sanfilippo R, Virdis E, et al. Trabectedin in myxoid liposarcomas (MLS): a long-term analysis of a single-institution series. Ann Oncol 2009;20(8):1439–44.

50. Demetri GD, von Mehren M, Jones RL, et al. Efficacy and safety of trabectedin or dacarbazine for metastatic liposarcoma or leiomyosarcoma after failure of conventional chemotherapy: results of a phase III randomized multicenter clinical trial. J Clin Oncol 2015;34(8):786–93.

51. Gortzak E, Azzarelli A, Buesa J, et al. A randomised phase II study on neoadjuvant chemotherapy for 'high-risk' adult soft-tissue sarcoma. Eur J Cancer 2001;37(9):1096–103.

52. Davis EJ, Chugh R, Zhao L, et al. A randomised, open-label, phase II study of neo/adjuvant doxorubicin and ifosfamide versus gemcitabine and docetaxel in patients with localised, high-risk, soft tissue sarcoma. Eur J Cancer 2015; 51(13):1794–802.

53. Gronchi A, Bui BN, Bonvalot S, et al. Phase II clinical trial of neoadjuvant trabectedin in patients with advanced localized myxoid liposarcoma. Ann Oncol 2012; 23(3):771–6.

54. Cortes J, O'Shaughnessy J, Loesch D, et al. Eribulin monotherapy versus treatment of physician's choice in patients with metastatic breast cancer (EMBRACE): a phase 3 open-label randomised study. Lancet 2011;377(9769):914–23.

55. Swami U, Shah U, Goel S. Eribulin in cancer treatment. Mar Drugs 2015;13(8): 5016–58.

56. Schoffski P, Ray-Coquard IL, Cioffi A, et al. Activity of eribulin mesylate in patients with soft-tissue sarcoma: A phase 2 study in four independent histological subtypes. Lancet Oncol 2011;12(11):1045–52.

57. Schoffski P. Randomized, open-label, multicenter, phase III study of eribulin versus dacarbazine in patients (pts) with leiomyosarcoma (LMS) and adipocytic sarcoma (ADI). J Clin Oncol 2015;33:10502.

58. Chawla SP, Chua VS, Hendifar AF, et al. A phase 1B/2 study of aldoxorubicin in patients with soft tissue sarcoma. Cancer 2015;121(4):570–9.

59. Chawla SP, Papai Z, Mukhametshina G, et al. First-line aldoxorubicin vs doxorubicin in metastatic or locally advanced unresectable soft-tissue sarcoma: a phase 2b randomized clinical trial. JAMA Oncol 2015;1(9):1272–80.

60. Dickson MA, Tap WD, Keohan ML, et al. Phase II trial of the CDK4 inhibitor PD0332991 in patients with advanced CDK4-amplified well-differentiated or dedifferentiated liposarcoma. J Clin Oncol 2013;31(16):2024–8.

61. Dickson MA, Schwartz GK, Keohan ML, et al. Progression-free survival among patients with well-differentiated or dedifferentiated liposarcoma treated with CDK4 inhibitor palbociclib: a phase 2 clinical trial. JAMA Oncol 2016. http://dx.doi.org/10.1001/jamaoncol.2016.0264.

62. Italiano A, Le Cesne A, Mendiboure J, et al. Prognostic factors and impact of adjuvant treatments on local and metastatic relapse of soft-tissue sarcoma patients in the competing risks setting. Cancer 2014;120(21):3361–9.

Local Recurrence of Extremity Soft Tissue Sarcoma

Whitney M. Guerrero, MD[a], Jeremiah L. Deneve, DO[a,b,*]

KEYWORDS

- Sarcoma • Recurrence • Metastasis • Radiation • Amputation • Limb salvage
- Isolated limb infusion • Hyperthermic isolated limb perfusion

KEY POINTS

- Multimodality management of recurrent extremity soft tissue sarcoma is dependent upon prior therapy and includes surgery, irradiation, brachytherapy and systemic chemotherapy.
- Amputation may provide local control and palliation of symptoms for recurrent extremity soft tissue sarcoma.
- Regional therapy in the form of hyperthermic isolated limb perfusion or isolated limb infusion has a role in the management of recurrent extremity soft tissue sarcoma to provide local control as a limb-salvage therapy treatment option.

INTRODUCTION

Soft tissue sarcomas (STSs) are a heterogeneous group of malignancies with distinct clinical and pathologic features, all characterized by mesodermal differentiation.[1] STS is relatively rare, accounting for only 1% of adult malignancies with an estimated 11,900 people diagnosed annually and approximately 4870 deaths in the United States.[2] More than 50 different subtypes have been identified with undifferentiated pleomorphic sarcoma, gastrointestinal stromal tumors, liposarcoma, leiomyosarcoma, synovial sarcoma, and malignant peripheral nerve sheath tumors being the most common.[3] These tumors may arise from the extremity, head or neck, truncal region, retroperitoneum or chest wall, as well as, other locations. The anatomic location of these tumors is important because it influences treatment and outcome. Several prognostic factors, such as tumor stage, size, grade, and anatomic location, have

[a] Department of Surgery, University of Tennessee Health Science Center, 910 Madison Ave, Suite 300, Memphis, TN 38163, USA; [b] Division of Surgical Oncology, University of Tennessee Health Science Center, 910 Madison Avenue, Suite 300, Memphis, TN 38163, USA
* Corresponding author. Division of Surgical Oncology, University of Tennessee Health Science Center, 910 Madison Avenue, Suite 300, Memphis, TN 38163.
E-mail address: jdeneve@uthsc.edu

Surg Clin N Am 96 (2016) 1157–1174
http://dx.doi.org/10.1016/j.suc.2016.05.002
0039-6109/16/$ – see front matter © 2016 Elsevier Inc. All rights reserved.
surgical.theclinics.com

been demonstrated to have an impact on overall survival in the management of primary extremity STS.[4–6] Similarly, margin of resection, low-grade histology, and the use of radiotherapy are important factors in achieving local disease control.[7–9]

Treatment involves a multidisciplinary effort by those specializing in the management of sarcoma. Surgery is the standard treatment of primary extremity STS. The objective of surgical resection is to obtain negative margins but this may be difficult in situations of abutment or involvement of critical neurovascular structures. In these situations, radiation therapy (RT) may be administered as either neoadjuvant therapy or in the adjuvant setting. Neoadjuvant RT is recommended in situations in which a microscopic positive margin is anticipated. The disadvantage of neoadjuvant RT is that it does result in an increased risk of wound healing complications. Positive margins after surgical resection are associated with an increased risk of local recurrence.[10,11] Re-resection to negative margins is preferred but may not be possible, especially in situations of critical nerve or vascular involvement, or when resection may result in loss of function or significant impairment of the involved extremity. Postoperative RT is recommended and has been demonstrated to improve the local control of patients with positive surgical margins.[12,13] Postoperative RT, although associated with a lower risk of short-term wound complications, is associated with higher rates of long-term treatment-related effects, possibly related to the higher dosages of radiation.[14]

The role of systemic chemotherapy in the management of primary extremity STS varies among institutions. The relative indications of systemic chemotherapy include high-grade tumors larger than 5 cm or intermediate-grade tumors larger than 10 cm, especially in younger patients. The use of chemotherapy in the treatment of primary extremity STS is controversial and has yielded inconsistent results. In a randomized controlled trial of preoperative chemotherapy followed by surgery compared with surgical resection alone of subjects with high-risk tumors, there was no difference in 5-year disease-free survival or overall survival.[15] In smaller tumors in a retrospective cohort of subjects receiving neoadjuvant chemotherapy in high-grade extremity sarcomas, Grobmyer and colleagues[16] demonstrated an improvement in disease-specific survival for tumors larger than 10 cm receiving neoadjuvant chemotherapy but not in smaller tumors. Generally accepted indications for adjuvant chemotherapy include synovial sarcoma and pediatric rhabdomyosarcoma, as well as situations of local recurrence and metastatic disease. Single-agent and anthracycline-based regimens are generally accepted and frequently used in situations of locally advanced, unresectable, or metastatic STS.[17–20]

Despite appropriate aggressive multimodality therapy, local recurrence is not uncommon, affecting up to 7% to 24%.[11,21,22] Management of recurrent STS is a challenge because often patients have undergone neoadjuvant therapy before surgical resection. Local recurrence for those who may not have undergone preoperative therapy may be associated with a better prognosis than for those treated with a combined multimodality initial approach.[23] Little is known about the effect of local recurrence on overall outcome. It is generally thought that local recurrence of STS is associated with a poor prognosis and has a negative impact on distant metastasis and survival.[24]

Historically, local recurrences of extremity sarcomas were managed with amputation.[25] Amputation offers definitive local control but often at the expense of patient function, with potential for significant morbidity and a negative impact on overall quality of life. Furthermore, amputation does not have an impact on distant metastasis or overall outcome.[26–28] For this reason many suggest that attempts to surgically manage local recurrence a second time should be more aggressive than the initial treatment approach. Re-resection of extremity STS recurrence is a treatment option, as well as the repeated use of irradiation for those receiving radiation during initial management. Both of these treatment approaches are associated with a high risk of treatment-related morbidity and may negatively affect extremity function. Selecting an appropriate therapy that allows patients to maintain function and quality of life without negatively affecting long-term outcome is important. The regional delivery of chemotherapy, in the form of hyperthermic isolated limb perfusion (HILP) or isolated limb infusion (ILI), as a potential adjunct to surgical resection with RT, may be an additional treatment option for these complex patients.

How to most appropriately manage local recurrence remains an active area of debate among clinicians who devote their practices to the management of STS. This article focuses on the management of locally recurrent STS of the extremity.

MANAGEMENT OF RECURRENCE
Surgical Resection and Irradiation of Sarcoma Recurrence

Local recurrence after previous resection with or without previous radiation can be a devastating development for patients. Management of the local recurrence is complicated by previous therapies and development of the recurrence within a previously irradiated field. There is a growing trend toward limb-salvage therapy, even in the setting of recurrent disease, with an emphasis on the maintenance of extremity function and preservation of quality of life. Wide resection is important when treating local recurrence to prevent further local relapse from sarcoma. Unfortunately, positive margins are common after repeated resection for recurrence, as high as 30%.[21,29,30] In addition, the risk of a second relapse after undergoing limb salvage for local recurrence is also high, up to 21%.[22,31] Because many patients have undergone multimodality treatment before the development of recurrence, management of the recurrence is, therefore, associated with higher morbidity. This may limit repeated use of potential therapeutic modalities for the management of recurrent disease. These factors in the initial treatment of the primary sarcoma tumor, as well as others such as anatomic constraints, synchronous distant metastasis, and aggressive tumor biology, are present and must be considered in the management of the local recurrence.

Salvage treatment options after local recurrence include limited re-excision; radical surgical resection, often necessitating plastic surgery reconstruction; amputation; additional RT; and, in selected cases, systemic chemotherapy. Although many investigators report on the management of recurrence using combined modality therapies, one series in particular highlights the role of surgical management alone in managing these complex patients. A retrospective review was performed on 62 patients at MD Anderson Cancer Center who were treated for an isolated first recurrence of STS within a previously irradiated field.[32] All subjects underwent previous resection and external beam radiation (EBRT) with a median time to development to recurrence of 25 months. The investigators attempted a conservative, limb-sparing approach to the management of the local recurrence and attempted to obtain a 1 to 3 cm negative surgical margin when possible. Twenty-five subjects underwent wide local excision (WLE) alone, 33 underwent WLE with brachytherapy (BCT), 3 had WLE with preoperative EBRT (45, 46, 50 Gy), and 1 had WLE with postoperative EBRT (64 Gy). When EBRT was used, a 5 to 7 cm treatment margin was administered to the tumor bed. There were 39 relapses (69%), 29 were local (12, WLE group and 17, RT group) resulting in a 5-year actuarial local control (LC) rate of 51%. The use of additional RT was associated with a higher rate of complication compared with WLE alone (80% vs 17%, P<.001) and was the only factor significant for late complication on multivariate analysis (P<.001). With respect to tumor biology and outcome, 71% of subjects had high-grade tumors but only 27% developed distant metastasis and 50% developed local recurrence within 5 years. The investigators go on to suggest that consideration should be given to a surgery-alone approach when possible, primarily because of the toxicity associated with additional RT and lack of a local control benefit.

Others investigators, however, have identified that limb salvage after initial conservative treatment is possible and that additional radiation in the management of recurrence results in improved local control with acceptable toxicity. Catton and colleagues[29] reported on 25 subjects treated with surgery alone or surgery and re-irradiation for locally recurrent STS. Two subjects with synchronous metastasis were treated palliatively, whereas 7 subjects were managed with early amputation. Eleven subjects underwent conservative resection without irradiation, 7 of which relapsed, and 5 underwent subsequent conservative surgery and irradiation. A total of 10 subjects were treated with combined surgery and irradiation (Brachy-6, Brachy/EBRT-3, EBRT-1). The investigators reported a local control of 91% with 36% local control for conservative excision alone (4/11) and 100% for excision with reirradiation (10/10). Sixty percent of the reirradiation group did develop significant postirradiation complications but 3 eventually recovered function. Although the numbers are small, the investigators suggest that inappropriate initial management is a risk factor for relapse and the use of combined conservative surgery with re-irradiation provides superior local control and a better functional outcome to amputation.

The initial treatment of primary extremity STS has an impact on the subsequent management of recurrence. Additional cumulative radiation is associated with potential increased morbidity. Furthermore, obtaining negative margins may be difficult and incomplete resection of isolated recurrences is associated with a high rate of relapse. Moureau and colleagues[22] reported on 83 adult subjects with isolated local recurrence of STS sarcoma (74 located on the extremity). The recurrences were managed with wide excision (number [N] = 29), marginal resection (N = 43) and 5 required amputation. The margin of resection (R) was R0 (N = 33), R1 (N = 47), or R2 (N = 3). Twenty-three subjects received EBRT and 26 underwent BCT (22, BCT alone; 4, BCT plus EBRT). Thirty-seven subjects (45%) developed further local recurrence within a mean of 23 months, giving an actuarial local control rate of 42% at 5 years. The investigators note that when conservative treatment is feasible, it should combine surgery and radiotherapy with BCT being best used in previously irradiated patients. The use of BCT may decrease the high complication rates associated with reirradiation but recognize that the cumulative dose of radiation is high and late complications may develop.

One of the difficulties in managing patients with isolated local recurrence after previous surgical resection and radiation is the high morbidity associated with subsequent treatment. Repeated irradiation carries the potential for significant complication and many of these complications may require subsequent reconstructive surgery or even amputation.[33,34] One study reported that 34% of patients previously irradiated required re-intervention for wound healing complications.[35] The University of Florida reported on 14 patients treated over a 30-year period with isolated recurrence after initial primary conservative resection and irradiation.[36] Thirteen of the 14 received EBRT with or without BCT and 1 received BCT alone. The incidence of serious complication requiring either reoperation or leading to permanent functional impairment was 50%.

To reduce the effect of compounded toxicity with repeat irradiation in the recurrent setting, advanced techniques such as intraoperative RT (IORT) and BCT have been used to deliver high-dose irradiation while minimizing normal tissue toxicity. IORT has been well studied when combined with salvage limb-sparing surgery for recurrent disease with favorable local control, limb salvage, and overall survival results.[37,38] Investigators from the University of California, San Francisco reported a 23% acute treatment-related toxicity and grade 3 late toxicity developing in 31% of subjects when using IORT for recurrence.[37] No grade 4 or 5 toxicity was observed and no subject required amputation for complication when treated with IORT for recurrence. Pearlstone and colleagues[33] reported on 26 subjects who developed sarcoma recurrence within a previously irradiated field treated with re-resection and BCT. Re-resection was performed with BCT with a mean dose of 47.2 Gy delivered at the implant procedure. Half of the subjects underwent tissue flap transfer over the resection bed. Complications, primarily wound breakdown, occurred in 5 subjects, 4 of whom required operative intervention. Each of the 4 had initially undergone primary closure without tissue transfer. The 5-year recurrence-free survival was good at 52%, suggesting that local control can be achieved with re-irradiation of recurrent STS by BCT with acceptable complication rates, potentially sparing the need for more radical surgery or even amputation.

Amputation for Sarcoma Recurrence

Although limb-salvage therapies offer local control in up to 85% to 90% of patients, the development of local recurrence may make conservative management difficult. Tumors involving proximal nerves or vessels may compromise local control if limited resection is attempted and limb-salvage, therefore, may not be possible. Furthermore, the development of treatment-related toxicities, such as wound healing complications or nonhealing wounds, may represent a source of significant pain and render the involved extremity functionless. Fungating, foul-smelling tumors, bleeding, or intractable pain may further complicate patient quality of life and management of recurrent STS tumors.[39] Amputation in this setting may offer palliation of tumor or treatment-related symptoms. Investigators from the University of California, Los Angeles (UCLA), found the development of local recurrence to be extremely morbid with 38% of subjects eventually requiring amputation.[8] Some subjects, unfortunately, are not amenable to resection at presentation and require early amputation for management of recurrent disease.[29]

Distal extremity amputations range from resection of individual digits to above-elbow or above-knee amputations. In situations of proximal vascular or neural involvement, forequarter or hindquarter amputation may be required. Forequarter amputation, or interscapulothoracic disarticulation, involves the removal of the whole upper limb girdle, including the humerus, scapula, distal clavicle, and chest wall musculature. Hindquarter amputation, or hemipelvectomy, involves removal of the femur and the bony pelvis, typically through the sacroiliac joint.

Morbidity after radical amputations, especially hindquarter, may be significant occurring in up to 60% or more of patients.[40,41] Most commonly, wound healing complications and flap necrosis have been described. Hernia formation may also develop long term.[41] Complications after forequarter amputation are generally fewer. Mortality is also high for those undergoing hindquarter amputation but a more recent report of 40 subjects undergoing radical amputation demonstrated a 2.5% mortality with only one subject succumbing to postoperative sepsis.[42] Phantom pain may be a problem after amputation, especially in those who present with significant pain preamputation.[43] However, for those who present with symptomatic, disabling disease, radical amputation may offer palliation of symptoms with improvement in pain in up to 78%.[42] Advances in limb prostheses allow restoration of limited function, cosmesis, and maintenance of independence for motivated patients.

Although there is no effect on overall survival for patients who undergo amputation for recurrence, for those who have exhausted all other treatment options, amputation remains a treatment option. Local and distant recurrences are high after amputation and likely reflect aggressive tumor biology.[42] The palliation of complex wounds, improvement of pain, and potential impact on improved quality of life renders amputation a reasonable treatment option for the symptomatic patient.

Chemotherapy for Sarcoma Recurrence

The routine use of adjuvant chemotherapy in the treatment of recurrent extremity sarcoma continues to be an area of active debate. In general, the regimens commonly used in the management of primary extremity STS are highly toxic and have failed to demonstrate a sustained long-term survival benefit. Although individual center results vary widely, a meta-analysis of 1568 subjects demonstrated a benefit to local recurrence (6%) and distant recurrence (10%) at 10 years when doxorubicin-based chemotherapy regimens were combined with surgery for local control.[44] There was no benefit when overall survival was analyzed at 10 years. A retrospective review from Memorial Sloan-Kettering and MD Anderson Cancer center demonstrated a statistically significant benefit when chemotherapy was used for stage III extremity STS with respect to local control, distant metastases, overall disease-free survival, and disease-specific survival at 1 year.[45] The benefits were not maintained overtime, however, and were not observed at 5 years.

One of the difficulties in interpreting and broadly generalizing these results is that various histologic subtypes are frequently treated in these series, hence confounding results. Certain histologic subtypes have demonstrated more chemosensitive behavior, notably pediatric rhabdomyosarcoma and synovial sarcoma. Synovial sarcoma has been found to respond favorably to adjuvant chemotherapy and metastatic lesions are also sensitive to chemotherapy.[46,47] Pediatric rhabdomyosarcoma also responds favorably and when treated with chemotherapy has a 5-year overall survival of 71%.[48] Broadly accepted indications for systemic chemotherapy include pediatric rhabdomyosarcoma, synovial sarcoma, local recurrence, and distant metastasis.

In the setting of recurrent disease, recommendations are less clear. The National Comprehensive Cancer Network (NCCN) guidelines for limited metastasis confined to a single organ or disseminated metastases are similar to those of stage IV disease at presentation; that is, doxorubicin based regimens.[49] There are limited data on the use of systemic chemotherapy in patients who undergo metastasectomy and results suggest minimal impact on survival of patients with metastatic extremity STS who undergo metastasectomy.[50] NCCN guidelines describe the use of systemic chemotherapy in the recurrent setting as a category 2B recommendation, suggesting that the intervention may be appropriate based on lower-level evidence. Despite a lack of consensus, several centers have suggested a potential benefit to the use of systemic chemotherapy for the management of local recurrence. Investigators from McGill University demonstrated that local recurrence occurred at or before the development of distant metastasis in 34% of patients.[31] Eilber and colleagues[8] from the UCLA Sarcoma Research Group noted that local recurrence was the most significant factor for decreased survival and, therefore, patients should be strongly considered for adjuvant systemic chemotherapy. Patients who develop recurrence should undergo referral to a multidisciplinary team that specializes in the management of these complex patients with consideration for clinical trial enrollment.

Regional Lymphadenectomy for Sarcoma Recurrence

Regional lymph node metastasis (RLNM) is a rare event in the natural history of STS with an estimated incidence of less than 5% of all patients.[51] For this reason, elective lymphadenectomy is generally not indicated in the initial management of STS.[52,53] Certain subtypes, however, are more commonly associated with regional nodal metastasis. Lymph node metastasis as regional recurrence is more common for epithelioid sarcoma, synovial sarcoma, and rhabdomyosarcomas, particularly in the pediatric population.[53–55] The predilection for regional metastasis has led some investigators to suggest the routine use of sentinel lymph node biopsy (SLNB) in the management of these particular histologies.[56–58] Results have been inconclusive, however, and limited to single-institution, small-volume, retrospective series. Most likely, a multicenter trial will be required to demonstrate any effect of routine SLNB on overall STS outcome for at-risk pathologic conditions.

Although lymph node metastasis is rare, in the absence of distant disease, formal lymphadenectomy may offer potential for cure and is recommended. In one of the larger series reported, Fong and colleagues[51] reported on 1772 sarcoma subjects treated at Memorial Sloan-Kettering Cancer Center with lymph node metastasis from STS. Forty-six subjects (2.6%) were identified with lymph node metastasis over a 10-year treatment period. The most common histologies included angiosarcoma, embryonal rhabdomyosarcoma, and epithelioid sarcoma. Leiomyosarcoma and malignant fibrous histiocytoma were also common but, because of a higher prevalence of these tumors, represented a smaller percentage overall. Forty-five of the 46 subjects had high-grade tumors. Thirty-one subjects went onto radical lymphadenectomy with the remainder undergoing either simple excision or noncurative procedures. Those who underwent radical lymphadenectomy had an improved outcomes compared with those with noncurative procedures (16.3 months survival vs 5.9 months survival, $P = .027$). Although the 5-year survival for nodal metastasis was poor (34%), radical lymphadenectomy did offer the potential for long-term survival in a select few with isolated lymph node metastasis.

Results from the United Kingdom give additional insight on the impact of RLNM and the outcome of STS in adults. Seventy-three subjects who developed RLNM of 2127 patients with STS were reported.[59] The most common histology was similar to that of the Memorial Sloan-Kettering series and also included angiosarcoma. Fifty-seven subjects (78%) had lymph node metastasis alone as the site of initial spread, whereas 16 subjects (22%) had regional and distant metastasis. Forty-two subjects presented with synchronous RLNM with the primary tumor. The remainder presented with RLNM a median of 13.5 months from diagnosis of the primary tumor. Most interesting, the 1-year survival for RLNM alone was 77.5% compared with 36% for those with regional and distant metastasis at initial diagnosis ($P = .005$) suggesting that those with RLNM only fare better. The investigators also identified that those who presented with RLNM at the time of initial diagnosis had a poorer outcome than those who presented with metachronous RLNM metastasis.

Regional Therapy for Sarcoma Recurrence

For patients with STS who present with bulky recurrent tumors involving critical neurovascular structures, or with concomitant distant disease, selecting an appropriate therapy that provides local control without compromising quality of life, limb function, or long-term outcome is a challenge. Amputation, as previously mentioned, may provide local control at the expense of loss of function but does nothing to address distant disease and has no impact on overall outcome.[26,60] There has been a growing trend over the last several decades toward limb-preservation therapies when treating these complicated patients with recurrent or unresectable STS. Regional delivery of chemotherapy can be used as an adjunct to surgical resection with RT for advanced STS of the extremity. Furthermore, regional therapy offers the potential for local control, especially in situations of unresectable, isolated recurrent disease or recurrent disease in the presence of distant metastasis.

Two techniques, HILP and ILI, allow the regional administration of chemotherapy, delivering drug concentrations 15 to 25 times higher than systemic dosages without the systemic side effects.[61] There are numerous potential indications for regional therapy for STS, most notably: multifocal primary tumors,[62] recurrent disease,[63] those undergoing previous resection with irradiation,[64] bulky primary tumors,[65,66] or high-grade tumors.[65] Elderly patients[67] and those with distant metastasis treated in a palliative setting[68] have been shown to gain a benefit in local control and limb-salvage rates using regional therapy.

HILP, first reported in the 1950s for treating melanoma patients with regional in-transit disease, was the first regional chemoperfusion therapy to demonstrate improved salvage rates in patients with extremity STS.[61] The technique is invasive and requires an extracorporeal bypass circuit.[69] HILP requires surgical exposure and cannulation of the iliac or femoral vessels for lower extremity disease or subclavian or axillary vessels for upper extremity tumors. The cannulae are connected to an extracorporeal circuit that contains a membrane oxygenator and a heat exchanger. To ensure vascular isolation and target tumor perfusion, a pneumatic cuff or esmarch tourniquet is applied proximally on the affected extremity. Systemic leakage is measured continuously throughout the procedure by a precordial Geiger counter that monitors ^{99}Tc radiolabeled human serum albumin or red blood cells previously injected into the perfusate. Flow rates are set as high as possible, generally 35 to 40 mL/L of limb volume per minute. The procedure is performed under hyperthermic conditions (38.5–40°C). Melphalan is the drug of choice for HILP and dosage is calculated according to the liter-volume method.[70] In many European centers, a combination of melphalan (10 mg/L for lower limb and 13 mg/L for upper limb), as well as TNF-α (2–4 mg) is commonly used.[63,65,66] Actinomycin-D is frequently used with melphalan in most centers in the United States.[71] Chemoperfusion is performed for a total of 90 minutes. At the completion of HILP, the limb is flushed with 2 to 4 L of isotonic saline solution, tourniquets are released, and vascular anatomy is reconstructed. Patients are observed in an intensive care setting for monitoring of systemic toxicity and reperfusion injury. Average postoperative length of stay ranges from 8 to 10 days.

ILI is a less invasive approach for administering regional chemotherapy and was first reported on by the Sydney Melanoma Unit.[72] ILI, first described for the treatment of in-transit metastases in melanoma patients, is a less complex procedure with overall response rates close to those observed with conventional HILP. ILI is essentially a low-flow HILP performed under hyperthermic, nonoxygenated conditions by percutaneously placed catheters. High-flow 5Fr to 6Fr arterial and 6Fr to 8Fr venous catheters are inserted by way of the uninvolved lower extremity and advanced fluoroscopically into the involved extremity. This may be done preoperatively by interventional radiology or by vascular surgery after the induction of general anesthesia. Heparin is administered to achieve full systemic anticoagulation with a target activated clotting time (ACT) greater than or equal to 350 seconds. The catheters are connected to an infusion circuit that consists of a heat exchanger and bubble excluder. Once subcutaneous temperatures of greater than 37°C are achieved, a pneumatic tourniquet or an Esmark wrap is placed on the proximal aspect of the limb to be infused, isolating the limb from the systemic circulation. Papaverine (60 mg) is injected into the arterial catheter and chemoperfusion is initiated. The cytotoxic agents, often melphalan and actinomycin D, are circulated for 30 minutes. After infusion is complete, the limb is manually flushed with 1 L of isotonic crystalloid solution, heparinization is reversed with protamine, and the catheters are removed when the ACT is at or near baseline. Patients are monitored daily for regional toxicity with serial creatine phosphokinase (CPK) measurements and discharged home when CPK levels peak and decrease back towards baseline, generally within 4 to 6 days.[73]

There are treatment-related toxicities to HILP and ILI that are worth discussion. In general, the toxicity of HILP is more severe than that experienced by patients who undergo ILI procedures. Systemic toxicities are more commonly observed with HILP procedures and are related to the type of chemotherapy used and the amount of leakage of the chemotherapeutic into the systemic circulation. Leakage rates less than 3% to 4% are generally well tolerated. Continuous precordial monitoring for systemic leakage is mandatory for patients undergoing HILP procedures. TNF-α, commonly used in many European centers, is thought to be responsible for many of the systemic toxicities experienced with HILP. Systemic leakage of TNF-α can induce a severe systemic inflammatory response syndrome with hypotension and shock-like symptoms, which necessitates aggressive hydration and vasopressor resuscitation. Systemic toxicity related to ILI is much less common than HILP. Rhabdomyolysis, as measured by serum CPK, may be encountered in patients undergoing this form of regional therapy. CPK levels often increase greater than 1000 IU/L and require daily blood urea nitrogen and creatinine level monitoring to avoid myoglobin-induced renal failure. Aggressive hydration with isotonic saline and maintaining urine output greater than 0.5 mL/kg/h may reduce the risk of renal failure caused by myoglobinuria.[74] Patients with CPK levels greater than 1000 IU/L are hydrated and given corticosteroids to decrease muscle edema or inflammation and monitored until CPK levels decrease towards baseline. Regional toxicity after HILP or ILI is more common than systemic toxicity. A commonly used classification system characterizing acute tissue reactions was first reported by Wieberdink and colleagues[70] and has standardized regional toxicity reporting for patients undergoing HILP or ILI therapy (**Table 1**). Acute regional toxicity-related symptoms are seen within the first 48 hours after HILP, or 72 to 96 hours after ILI.[72,75] Typical reactions to either therapy include mild erythema, edema, and pain (Wieberdink II-III). Mild to moderate blistering is frequently seen up to several days post-therapy. The development of compartment syndrome progressing to the need for amputation has been reported but is generally uncommon.

Table 1 Wieberdink toxicity	
Grade	**Clinical Characteristics**
I	No subjective or objective evidence of reaction
II	Slight erythema or edema
III	Considerable erythema or edema with some blistering; slightly disturbed motility permissible
IV	Extensive epidermolysis or obvious damage to the deep tissues causing definite functional disturbances; threatened or manifest compartmental syndromes
V	Reaction that may necessitate amputation

From Wieberdink J, Benckhuysen C, Braat RP et al. Dosimetry in isolation perfusion of the limbs by assessment of perfused tissue volume and grading of toxic tissue reactions. Eur J Cancer. 1982;18:906; with permission.

Table 2
Treatment and outcome data for regional therapy for advanced extremity soft tissue sarcoma

Author, Year	Number of Subjects	Modality	Chemotherapy	Follow-up (mo)	ORR (%)	CR/PR/SD (%)	Limb Preservation (%)
Eggermont et al,[65] 1996	186	HILP	TNF-α INF-γ (N = 55) Melphalan	22	82	29/53/18	82
Eggermont et al,[87] 1996	55	HILP	TNF-α INF-γ Melphalan	26	87	36/51/13	84
Gutman et al,[66] 1997	35	HILP	TNF-α Melphalan	14	91	37/54/9	85
Olieman et al,[68] 1998	34	HILP	TNF-α INF-γ Melphalan	34	94	35/59/6	85
Lejeune et al,[80] 2000	22	HILP	TNF-α INF-γ (N = 4) Melphalan	19	82	18/64/18	86
Noorda et al,[77] 2003	49	HILP	TNF-α INF-γ (N = 4) Melphalan	26	63	8/55/35	57
Rossi et al,[88] 2005	21	HILP	TNF-α Doxorubicin	30	62	5/57/38	71

	N	Procedure	Drugs			CR/PR/SD	ORR
Grunhagen et al,[64] 2005	53	HILP	TNF-α / Melphalan	22	88	42/45/13	82
Bonvalot et al,[89] 2005	100	HILP	TNF-α / Melphalan	24	65	36/29/35	87
Lans et al,[90] 2005	26	HILP	TNF-α / Melphalan	22	70	20/50/30	65
Grunhagen et al,[76] 2006	197	HILP	TNF-α / Melphalan	22	75	26/49/25	87
Hegazy et al,[62] 2007	40	ILI	Doxorubicin	15	85	—/85/—	83
Moncrieff et al,[78] 2008	21	ILI	Melphalan / Actin D	28	90	57/33/10	76
Turaga et al,[73] 2011	12	ILI	Melphalan / Actin D	8.6	78	14/64/—	78
Vohra et al,[79] 2013	26	ILI	Melphalan / Actin D	11	42	24/18/18	71
Rastrelli et al,[91] 2016	117	HILP	Doxorubicin (N = 47) / TNF/Doxorubicin (N = 30) / TNF/Melphalan (N = 40)	36	—	47/30/—	78

Abbreviations: Actin D, actinomycin D; CR, complete response; ORR, overall response rate; PR, partial response; SD, stable disease.

Long-term toxicity is infrequently reported and may include paresthesias or permanent nerve dysfunction.

The treatment and outcome data for patients undergoing regional therapy for extremity STS are listed in **Table 2**. Tumor response rates range from 68% to 91% for patients with advanced extremity STS previously only considered for patients with amputation who undergo HILP.[65,66,76,77] Early results for ILI therapy for limb-threatening STS have also produced encouraging results comparable with those for HILP. Tumor response rates range from 79% to 90% for patients treated with ILI.[62,73,78] In general, despite similar overall response rates, HILP is thought to produce more complete responders than ILI.

In addition to tumor response, both HILP and ILI spare these complex patients the potential morbidity and need for amputation with well-documented limb-salvage rates. HILP limb preservation rates have been consistently reported to range from 57% to 87% when treating advanced extremity STS.[65,68,76] ILI also is an attractive limb-sparing alternative to amputation for extremity STS recurrence with equal salvage rates to HILP and without the potential toxicity. Four of the larger ILI series for STS sarcoma document limb-preservation rates of 71% to 83%.[62,72,73,79] Local or regional recurrence after HILP and ILI treatment have been reported and can occur as high as up to 42% to 48%, respectively.[62,65,78,80] Additional regional therapy remains an option for patients who may recur or progress after previous HILP or ILI. Repeat HILP or ILI, for instance, offers the potential for local control, even in the presence of distant metastases. Furthermore, both procedures can be used either as definitive treatment or neoadjuvant therapy combined with surgery and radiation for advanced, unresectable or metastatic STS.

OVERALL SURVIVAL AFTER LOCAL RECURRENCE

The impact of local recurrence on overall outcome remains an area of active debate. Randomized clinical trials have not demonstrated an impact on overall survival whereas others have demonstrated conflicting results ranging from no impact to decreased survival.[11,81–84] Although no consensus exists, the long-term prognosis after development of local recurrence is guarded. Determinants of survival, such as grade, size, location, and histologic type, have all been well described for primary extremity STS.[11,27,28,85] Many of these primary tumor factors are also at play in the management of recurrent disease. Recurrence is a marker of high-grade tumor biology is associated with the development of additional recurrence and is associated with distant metastasis. Indirectly, therefore, these factors do potentially have a negative impact on survival. The UCLA Sarcoma Research Group demonstrated that local recurrence in subjects with high-grade extremity STS is associated with the development of subsequent local recurrences.[8] When reporting on 753 subjects treated over a 20-year period, subjects who developed local recurrence were 3 times more likely to eventually die of disease compared with those who had not developed a local recurrence. Local recurrence was the most significant factor associated with decreased survival.

Local recurrence may also present with concomitant distant disease in up to 30% of patients.[30,31,86] The management of local recurrence in the setting of distant metastasis is a challenging problem. The synchronous development of local recurrence in the setting of distant failure represents a grave prognosis. Furthermore, although many subjects in the aforementioned studies represent those who undergo additional treatment, these studies may not capture patients with recurrence that rapidly progress locally or systemically, or fail to complete treatment, and are thus excluded. In the setting of local recurrence, referral to a multidisciplinary regional sarcoma center is strongly recommended with consideration for clinical trial enrollment.

SUMMARY

Local recurrence of extremity STS is a difficult clinical entity to treat. Treatment should aim for limb-salvage therapies when possible. Resection and irradiation of recurrence are associated with potentially significant morbidity that may negatively affect function. Amputation may be required for management of the recurrence or of complications related to treatment of the recurrence; however, it has no impact on survival and a potentially negative impact on patient function and quality of life. Regional therapies in the form of HILP and ILI are attractive treatment options as either definitive or adjuvant therapy, especially in the presence of distant disease. Local recurrence has a guarded prognosis and early referral to a center specializing in the management of these complex patients is warranted.

REFERENCES

1. Cormier JN, Pollock RE. Soft tissue sarcomas. CA Cancer J Clin 2004;54:94–109.
2. Siegel RL, Miller KD, Jemal A. Cancer statistics, 2015. CA Cancer J Clin 2015;65: 5–29.
3. Coindre JM, Terrier P, Guillou L, et al. Predictive value of grade for metastasis development in the main histologic types of adult soft tissue sarcomas: a study of 1240 patients from the French Federation of Cancer Centers Sarcoma Group. Cancer 2001;91:1914–26.
4. Collin C, Hajdu SI, Godbold J, et al. Localized operable soft tissue sarcoma of the upper extremity. Presentation, management, and factors affecting local recurrence in 108 patients. Ann Surg 1987;205:331–9.
5. Sim FH, Pritchard DJ, Reiman HM, et al. Soft-tissue sarcoma: Mayo Clinic experience. Semin Surg Oncol 1988;4:38–44.
6. Pisters PW, Pollock RE. Staging and prognostic factors in soft tissue sarcoma. Semin Radiat Oncol 1999;9:307–14.
7. Davis AM, Kandel RA, Wunder JS, et al. The impact of residual disease on local recurrence in patients treated by initial unplanned resection for soft tissue sarcoma of the extremity. J Surg Oncol 1997;66:81–7.
8. Eilber FC, Rosen G, Nelson SD, et al. High-grade extremity soft tissue sarcomas: factors predictive of local recurrence and its effect on morbidity and mortality. Ann Surg 2003;237:218–26.
9. Trovik CS, Bauer HC, Alvegard TA, et al. Surgical margins, local recurrence and metastasis in soft tissue sarcomas: 559 surgically-treated patients from the Scandinavian Sarcoma Group Register. Eur J Cancer 2000;36:710–6.
10. Wilson AN, Davis A, Bell RS, et al. Local control of soft tissue sarcoma of the extremity: the experience of a multidisciplinary sarcoma group with definitive surgery and radiotherapy. Eur J Cancer 1994;30A:746–51.
11. Singer S, Corson JM, Gonin R, et al. Prognostic factors predictive of survival and local recurrence for extremity soft tissue sarcoma. Ann Surg 1994;219:165–73.
12. Delaney TF, Kepka L, Goldberg SI, et al. Radiation therapy for control of soft-tissue sarcomas resected with positive margins. Int J Radiat Oncol Biol Phys 2007;67:1460–9.
13. Sadoski C, Suit HD, Rosenberg A, et al. Preoperative radiation, surgical margins, and local control of extremity sarcomas of soft tissues. J Surg Oncol 1993;52: 223–30.

14. Zagars GK, Ballo MT, Pisters PW, et al. Preoperative vs. postoperative radiation therapy for soft tissue sarcoma: a retrospective comparative evaluation of disease outcome. Int J Radiat Oncol Biol Phys 2003;56:482–8.

15. Gortzak E, Azzarelli A, Buesa J, et al. A randomised phase II study on neo-adjuvant chemotherapy for 'high-risk' adult soft-tissue sarcoma. Eur J Cancer 2001;37:1096–103.

16. Grobmyer SR, Maki RG, Demetri GD, et al. Neo-adjuvant chemotherapy for primary high-grade extremity soft tissue sarcoma. Ann Oncol 2004;15:1667–72.

17. Mouridsen HT, Bastholt L, Somers R, et al. Adriamycin versus epirubicin in advanced soft tissue sarcomas. A randomized phase II/phase III study of the EORTC Soft Tissue and Bone Sarcoma Group. Eur J Cancer 1987;23:1477–83.

18. Buesa JM, Mouridsen HT, van Oosterom AT, et al. High-dose DTIC in advanced soft-tissue sarcomas in the adult. A phase II study of the E.O.R.T.C. Soft Tissue and Bone Sarcoma Group. Ann Oncol 1991;2:307–9.

19. Zalupski M, Metch B, Balcerzak S, et al. Phase III comparison of doxorubicin and dacarbazine given by bolus versus infusion in patients with soft-tissue sarcomas: a Southwest Oncology Group study. J Natl Cancer Inst 1991;83:926–32.

20. Reichardt P, Tilgner J, Hohenberger P, et al. Dose-intensive chemotherapy with ifosfamide, epirubicin, and filgrastim for adult patients with metastatic or locally advanced soft tissue sarcoma: a phase II study. J Clin Oncol 1998;16:1438–43.

21. Eilber FC, Brennan MF, Riedel E, et al. Prognostic factors for survival in patients with locally recurrent extremity soft tissue sarcomas. Ann Surg Oncol 2005;12: 228–36.

22. Moureau-Zabotto L, Thomas L, Bui BN, et al. Management of soft tissue sarcomas (STS) in first isolated local recurrence: a retrospective study of 83 cases. Radiother Oncol 2004;73:313–9.

23. Robinson M, Barr L, Fisher C, et al. Treatment of extremity soft tissue sarcomas with surgery and radiotherapy. Radiother Oncol 1990;18:221–33.

24. Novais EN, Demiralp B, Alderete J, et al. Do surgical margin and local recurrence influence survival in soft tissue sarcomas? Clin Orthop Relat Res 2010;468: 3003–11.

25. Shiu MH, Castro EB, Hajdu SI, et al. Surgical treatment of 297 soft tissue sarcomas of the lower extremity. Ann Surg 1975;182:597–602.

26. Williard WC, Collin C, Casper ES, et al. The changing role of amputation for soft tissue sarcoma of the extremity in adults. Surg Gynecol Obstet 1992;175:389–96.

27. Collin CF, Friedrich C, Godbold J, et al. Prognostic factors for local recurrence and survival in patients with localized extremity soft-tissue sarcoma. Semin Surg Oncol 1988;4:30–7.

28. Collin C, Godbold J, Hajdu S, et al. Localized extremity soft tissue sarcoma: an analysis of factors affecting survival. J Clin Oncol 1987;5:601–12.

29. Catton C, Davis A, Bell R, et al. Soft tissue sarcoma of the extremity. Limb salvage after failure of combined conservative therapy. Radiother Oncol 1996;41:209–14.

30. Trovik CS, Gustafson P, Bauer HC, et al. Consequences of local recurrence of soft tissue sarcoma: 205 patients from the Scandinavian Sarcoma Group Register. Acta Orthop Scand 2000;71:488–95.

31. Abatzoglou S, Turcotte RE, Adoubali A, et al. Local recurrence after initial multidisciplinary management of soft tissue sarcoma: is there a way out? Clin Orthop Relat Res 2010;468:3012–8.

32. Torres MA, Ballo MT, Butler CE, et al. Management of locally recurrent soft-tissue sarcoma after prior surgery and radiation therapy. Int J Radiat Oncol Biol Phys 2007;67:1124–9.

33. Pearlstone DB, Janjan NA, Feig BW, et al. Re-resection with brachytherapy for locally recurrent soft tissue sarcoma arising in a previously radiated field. Cancer J Sci Am 1999;5:26–33.

34. Fontanesi J, Mott MP, Lucas DR, et al. The role of irradiation in the management of locally recurrent non-metastatic soft tissue sarcoma of extremity/trunkal locations. Sarcoma 2004;8:57–61.

35. Cambeiro M, Aristu JJ, Moreno Jimenez M, et al. Salvage wide resection with intraoperative electron beam therapy or HDR brachytherapy in the management of isolated local recurrences of soft tissue sarcomas of the extremities and the superficial trunk. Brachytherapy 2015;14:62–70.

36. Indelicato DJ, Meadows K, Gibbs CP Jr, et al. Effectiveness and morbidity associated with reirradiation in conservative salvage management of recurrent soft-tissue sarcoma. Int J Radiat Oncol Biol Phys 2009;73:267–72.

37. Tinkle CL, Weinberg V, Braunstein SE, et al. Intraoperative Radiotherapy in the Management of Locally Recurrent Extremity Soft Tissue Sarcoma. Sarcoma 2015;2015:913565.

38. Oertel S, Treiber M, Zahlten-Hinguranage A, et al. Intraoperative electron boost radiation followed by moderate doses of external beam radiotherapy in limb-sparing treatment of patients with extremity soft-tissue sarcoma. Int J Radiat Oncol Biol Phys 2006;64:1416–23.

39. Merimsky O, Kollender Y, Inbar M, et al. Palliative major amputation and quality of life in cancer patients. Acta Oncol 1997;36:151–7.

40. Douglass HO Jr, Razack M, Holyoke ED. Hemipelvectomy. Arch Surg 1975;110: 82–5.

41. Kraybill WG, Standiford SB, Johnson FE. Posthemipelvectomy hernia. J Surg Oncol 1992;51:38–41.

42. Parsons CM, Pimiento JM, Cheong D, et al. The role of radical amputations for extremity tumors: a single institution experience and review of the literature. J Surg Oncol 2012;105:149–55.

43. Nikolajsen L, Jensen TS. Phantom limb pain. Br J Anaesth 2001;87:107–16.

44. Tierney JF, Mosseri V, Stewart LA, et al. Adjuvant chemotherapy for soft-tissue sarcoma: review and meta-analysis of the published results of randomised clinical trials. Br J Cancer 1995;72:469–75.

45. Cormier JN, Huang X, Xing Y, et al. Cohort analysis of patients with localized, high-risk, extremity soft tissue sarcoma treated at two cancer centers: chemotherapy-associated outcomes. J Clin Oncol 2004;22:4567–74.

46. Ferrari A, Gronchi A, Casanova M, et al. Synovial sarcoma: a retrospective analysis of 271 patients of all ages treated at a single institution. Cancer 2004;101: 627–34.

47. Rosen G, Forscher C, Lowenbraun S, et al. Synovial sarcoma. Uniform response of metastases to high dose ifosfamide. Cancer 1994;73:2506–11.

48. Stevens MC, Rey A, Bouvet N, et al. Treatment of nonmetastatic rhabdomyosarcoma in childhood and adolescence: third study of the International Society of Paediatric Oncology–SIOP Malignant Mesenchymal Tumor 89. J Clin Oncol 2005;23:2618–28.

49. von Mehren M, Randall RL, Benjamin RS, et al. Soft tissue sarcoma, version 2.2014. J Natl Compr Canc Netw 2014;12:473–83.

50. Canter RJ, Qin LX, Downey RJ, et al. Perioperative chemotherapy in patients undergoing pulmonary resection for metastatic soft-tissue sarcoma of the extremity: a retrospective analysis. Cancer 2007;110:2050–60.

51. Fong Y, Coit DG, Woodruff JM, et al. Lymph node metastasis from soft tissue sarcoma in adults. Analysis of data from a prospective database of 1772 sarcoma patients. Ann Surg 1993;217:72–7.
52. Gerner RE, Moore GE, Pickren JW. Soft tissue sarcomas. Ann Surg 1975;181: 803–8.
53. Weingrad DN, Rosenberg SA. Early lymphatic spread of osteogenic and soft-tissue sarcomas. Surgery 1978;84:231–40.
54. Mazeron JJ, Suit HD. Lymph nodes as sites of metastases from sarcomas of soft tissue. Cancer 1987;60:1800–8.
55. Lawrence W Jr, Hays DM, Moon TE. Lymphatic metastasis with childhood rhabdomyosarcoma. Cancer 1977;39:556–9.
56. Maduekwe UN, Hornicek FJ, Springfield DS, et al. Role of sentinel lymph node biopsy in the staging of synovial, epithelioid, and clear cell sarcomas. Ann Surg Oncol 2009;16:1356–63.
57. Andreou D, Boldt H, Werner M, et al. Sentinel node biopsy in soft tissue sarcoma subtypes with a high propensity for regional lymphatic spread–results of a large prospective trial. Ann Oncol 2013;24:1400–5.
58. Alcorn KM, Deans KJ, Congeni A, et al. Sentinel lymph node biopsy in pediatric soft tissue sarcoma patients: utility and concordance with imaging. J Pediatr Surg 2013;48:1903–6.
59. Behranwala KA, A'Hern R, Omar AM, et al. Prognosis of lymph node metastasis in soft tissue sarcoma. Ann Surg Oncol 2004;11:714–9.
60. Pisters PW, Leung DH, Woodruff J, et al. Analysis of prognostic factors in 1,041 patients with localized soft tissue sarcomas of the extremities. J Clin Oncol 1996;14:1679–89.
61. Creech O Jr, Krementz ET, Ryan RF, et al. Chemotherapy of cancer: regional perfusion utilizing an extracorporeal circuit. Ann Surg 1958;148:616–32.
62. Hegazy MA, Kotb SZ, Sakr H, et al. Preoperative isolated limb infusion of Doxorubicin and external irradiation for limb-threatening soft tissue sarcomas. Ann Surg Oncol 2007;14:568–76.
63. Lienard D, Ewalenko P, Delmotte JJ, et al. High-dose recombinant tumor necrosis factor alpha in combination with interferon gamma and melphalan in isolation perfusion of the limbs for melanoma and sarcoma. J Clin Oncol 1992;10:52–60.
64. Grunhagen DJ, Brunstein F, Graveland WJ, et al. Isolated limb perfusion with tumor necrosis factor and melphalan prevents amputation in patients with multiple sarcomas in arm or leg. Ann Surg Oncol 2005;12:473–9.
65. Eggermont AM, Schraffordt Koops H, Klausner JM, et al. Isolated limb perfusion with tumor necrosis factor and melphalan for limb salvage in 186 patients with locally advanced soft tissue extremity sarcomas. The cumulative multicenter European experience. Ann Surg 1996;224:756–64 [discussion: 764–5].
66. Gutman M, Inbar M, Lev-Shlush D, et al. High dose tumor necrosis factor-alpha and melphalan administered via isolated limb perfusion for advanced limb soft tissue sarcoma results in a >90% response rate and limb preservation. Cancer 1997;79:1129–37.
67. van Etten B, van Geel AN, de Wilt JH, et al. Fifty tumor necrosis factor-based isolated limb perfusions for limb salvage in patients older than 75 years with limb-threatening soft tissue sarcomas and other extremity tumors. Ann Surg Oncol 2003;10:32–7.
68. Olieman AF, Pras E, van Ginkel RJ, et al. Feasibility and efficacy of external beam radiotherapy after hyperthermic isolated limb perfusion with TNF-alpha and

melphalan for limb-saving treatment in locally advanced extremity soft-tissue sarcoma. Int J Radiat Oncol Biol Phys 1998;40:807–14.

69. Lejeune FJ, Ghanem GE. A simple and accurate new method for cytostatics dosimetry in isolation perfusion of the limbs based on exchangeable blood volume determination. Cancer Res 1987;47:639–43.

70. Wieberdink J, Benckhuysen C, Braat RP, et al. Dosimetry in isolation perfusion of the limbs by assessment of perfused tissue volume and grading of toxic tissue reactions. Eur J Cancer 1982;18:905–10.

71. Wong J, Chen YA, Fisher KJ, et al. Isolated limb infusion in a series of over 100 infusions: a single-center experience. Ann Surg Oncol 2013;20:1121–7.

72. Thompson JF, Kam PC, Waugh RC, et al. Isolated limb infusion with cytotoxic agents: a simple alternative to isolated limb perfusion. Semin Surg Oncol 1998; 14:238–47.

73. Turaga KK, Beasley GM, Kane JM 3rd, et al. Limb preservation with isolated limb infusion for locally advanced nonmelanoma cutaneous and soft-tissue malignant neoplasms. Arch Surg 2011;146:870–5.

74. Santillan AA, Delman KA, Beasley GM, et al. Predictive factors of regional toxicity and serum creatine phosphokinase levels after isolated limb infusion for melanoma: a multi-institutional analysis. Ann Surg Oncol 2009;16:2570–8.

75. Vrouenraets BC, Klaase JM, Kroon BB, et al. Long-term morbidity after regional isolated perfusion with melphalan for melanoma of the limbs. The influence of acute regional toxic reactions. Arch Surg 1995;130:43–7.

76. Grunhagen DJ, de Wilt JH, Graveland WJ, et al. Outcome and prognostic factor analysis of 217 consecutive isolated limb perfusions with tumor necrosis factor-alpha and melphalan for limb-threatening soft tissue sarcoma. Cancer 2006; 106:1776–84.

77. Noorda EM, Vrouenraets BC, Nieweg OE, et al. Isolated limb perfusion with tumor necrosis factor-alpha and melphalan for patients with unresectable soft tissue sarcoma of the extremities. Cancer 2003;98:1483–90.

78. Moncrieff MD, Kroon HM, Kam PC, et al. Isolated limb infusion for advanced soft tissue sarcoma of the extremity. Ann Surg Oncol 2008;15:2749–56.

79. Vohra NA, Turaga KK, Gonzalez RJ, et al. The use of isolated limb infusion in limb threatening extremity sarcomas. Int J Hyperthermia 2013;29:1–7.

80. Lejeune FJ, Pujol N, Lienard D, et al. Limb salvage by neoadjuvant isolated perfusion with TNFalpha and melphalan for non-resectable soft tissue sarcoma of the extremities. Eur J Surg Oncol 2000;26:669–78.

81. Rosenberg SA, Tepper J, Glatstein E, et al. The treatment of soft-tissue sarcomas of the extremities: prospective randomized evaluations of (1) limb-sparing surgery plus radiation therapy compared with amputation and (2) the role of adjuvant chemotherapy. Ann Surg 1982;196:305–15.

82. Brennan MF, Hilaris B, Shiu MH, et al. Local recurrence in adult soft-tissue sarcoma. A randomized trial of brachytherapy. Arch Surg 1987;122:1289–93.

83. Potter DA, Kinsella T, Glatstein E, et al. High-grade soft tissue sarcomas of the extremities. Cancer 1986;58:190–205.

84. Lewis JJ, Leung D, Heslin M, et al. Association of local recurrence with subsequent survival in extremity soft tissue sarcoma. J Clin Oncol 1997;15:646–52.

85. Berlin O, Stener B, Angervall L, et al. Surgery for soft tissue sarcoma in the extremities. A multivariate analysis of the 6-26-year prognosis in 137 patients. Acta Orthop Scand 1990;61:475–86.

86. Ramanathan RC, A'Hern R, Fisher C, et al. Prognostic index for extremity soft tissue sarcomas with isolated local recurrence. Ann Surg Oncol 2001;8:278–89.

87. Eggermont AM, Schraffordt Koops H, Lienard D, et al. Isolated limb perfusion with high-dose tumor necrosis factor-alpha in combination with interferon-gamma and melphalan for nonresectable extremity soft tissue sarcomas: a multicenter trial. J Clin Oncol 1996;14:2653–65.
88. Rossi CR, Mocellin S, Pilati P, et al. Hyperthermic isolated perfusion with low-dose tumor necrosis factor alpha and doxorubicin for the treatment of limb-threatening soft tissue sarcomas. Ann Surg Oncol 2005;12:398–405.
89. Bonvalot S, Laplanche A, Lejeune F, et al. Limb salvage with isolated perfusion for soft tissue sarcoma: could less TNF-alpha be better? Ann Oncol 2005;16:1061–8.
90. Lans TE, Grunhagen DJ, de Wilt JH, et al. Isolated limb perfusions with tumor necrosis factor and melphalan for locally recurrent soft tissue sarcoma in previously irradiated limbs. Ann Surg Oncol 2005;12:406–11.
91. Rastrelli M, Campana LG, Valpione S, et al. Hyperthermic isolated limb perfusion in locally advanced limb soft tissue sarcoma: A 24-year single-centre experience. Int J Hyperthermia 2016;32:165–72.

Surgical Management of Metastatic Disease

Emily Z. Keung, MD[a], Mark Fairweather, MD[a], Chandrajit P. Raut, MD, MSc[a,b],*

KEYWORDS

- Soft tissue sarcoma • Metastatic sarcoma • Liver metastasis
- Pulmonary metastasis • Metastasectomy

KEY POINTS

- The lung and liver are the most common sites of metastasis in sarcoma.
- First-line treatment of metastatic sarcoma is chemotherapy. In appropriate patients, sarcoma metastasectomy may be considered and may prolong survival in those with good performance status, longer disease-free interval between resection of primary tumor and appearance of metastatic disease, and oligometastasis, and when complete resection can be achieved.
- There is an extensive body of retrospective data on the surgical management of pulmonary sarcoma metastases. There are sparse retrospective data on the surgical management of hepatic sarcoma metastases and there is no consensus on the role of surgery.
- Additional local treatment modalities include radiation therapy and ablative techniques.
- Patients with soft tissue and bone sarcomas should be referred to specialty sarcoma centers and treatment decisions made in conjunction with a multidisciplinary team of medical, radiation, and surgical oncologists who specialize in the care of such patients.

INTRODUCTION

Sarcomas, including soft tissue sarcomas (STSs) and bone sarcomas, are rare cancers of mesenchymal cell origin that include more than 50 histologic subtypes and many more molecularly distinct entities.[1–3] After gastrointestinal stromal tumors (GISTs), (the management and survival outcomes of which have improved greatly following the introduction of targeted tyrosine kinase inhibitor [TKI] therapies), the next most common subtypes of STS are liposarcoma and leiomyosarcoma. The annual incidence of STS ranges from 2.4 to 3.6 new cases per 100,000 in population-based studies.[4] The American Cancer Society estimates that 12,310

a Department of Surgery, Brigham and Women's Hospital, 75 Francis Street, Boston, MA 02115, USA; b Center for Sarcoma and Bone Oncology, Dana-Farber Cancer Institute, 450 Brookline Avenue, Boston, MA 02115, USA
* Corresponding author. Center for Sarcoma and Bone Oncology, Dana-Farber Cancer Institute, 450 Brookline Avenue, Boston, MA 02115.
E-mail address: craut@bwh.harvard.edu

Surg Clin N Am 96 (2016) 1175–1192
http://dx.doi.org/10.1016/j.suc.2016.05.010
0039-6109/16/$ – see front matter © 2016 Elsevier Inc. All rights reserved.

surgical.theclinics.com

new cases of STS will be diagnosed and 4990 patients will die in 2016 in the United States alone.[5] Despite treatment, approximately 50% of patients with STS are diagnosed with or develop distant metastatic STS (mSTS), reducing their 5-year overall survival (OS) to less than 10% and their median OS to approximately 8 to 15 months.[2,6]

For primary resectable STS, surgery is the mainstay of treatment. However, for patients with mSTS, systemic therapy with conventional chemotherapy remains the primary treatment modality. Increased OS has been achieved in some patients who receive multimodality therapy, including surgery, for their metastatic disease. Thus, patients with mSTS should be evaluated and managed by a multidisciplinary team of medical, radiation, surgical, thoracic, and orthopedic oncologists specializing in the treatment of STS.

This article provides an overview of the multimodality therapies for metastatic sarcoma, including chemotherapy, radiation therapy, and ablative techniques, with an emphasis on surgical metastasectomy for mSTS.

DIAGNOSIS AND PATTERN OF METASTATIC SOFT TISSUE SARCOMA

The probability of distant metastases from STS depends on primary tumor grade, size, depth of location, and whether it is recurrent disease or not. High-grade STS tends to metastasize more frequently than low-grade tumors and earlier in the clinical course.[2]

The lungs and liver are by far the most common sites of distant mSTS, with primary STS site influencing the pattern of metastasis.[7] Jaques and colleagues[7] reported that the proportion of lung/liver as a site of distant spread from a primary extremity sarcoma is 75:1, in contrast to primary retroperitoneal sarcoma, in which the ratio is 1:1.5, and visceral sarcomas in which the ratio is 1:10.

Leiomyosarcomas tend to show a higher rate of metastasis to the lungs, liver, and soft tissues. Metastases to bone are more often detected in myxoid round cell and metastatic dedifferentiated liposarcoma. Lymph node metastases are rare events, present in only 2.6% to 16% of all patients with STS.[6] Clear cell sarcoma, epithelioid sarcoma, and synovial sarcoma metastasize to lymph nodes in up to 10% of cases. Soft tissue metastasis usually presents as a late event associated with widely disseminated disease.[6] Brain metastases are uncommon in adult STS (1%); however, children with Ewing sarcoma or osteosarcoma are more often affected.[2]

Thus, distant staging of STS should include high-resolution contrast-enhanced chest computed tomography (CT) for moderate and high-grade tumors to evaluate for pulmonary metastases, and abdominal CT to evaluate for intra-abdominal metastases. Paraspinal MRI may be necessary in cases of myxoid liposarcoma because of its tendency to develop extrapulmonary metastases in this area.[8] PET imaging may be considered to identify additional sites of metastasis outside the lung in specific circumstances.

THE ROLE OF METASTASECTOMY FOR SARCOMA

In select patients with limited metastatic disease, multimodality treatment including surgical metastasectomy has been shown in some retrospective series to offer longer median OS after diagnosis of mSTS (33–39 months) and 5-year OS (30%–50%) compared with historical controls.[1,3,4,9–12] However, there are no randomized trials or prospective data available to establish standards of care for treatment sequencing in patients with potentially resectable mSTS.[13] Most studies evaluating the role of metastasectomy in patients with mSTS have focused on pulmonary metastasectomies with limited studies on hepatic resection.

Patient Selection for Metastasectomy

When evaluating patients for potential metastasectomy, several criteria should be met including[3]:

1. The presence of a controlled or controllable primary tumor
2. The presence of completely resectable metastatic disease
3. The absence of multivisceral metastatic disease
4. A medically fit surgical candidate

Across studies, the most consistent prognostic factor in patients undergoing pulmonary metastasectomy is the ability to achieve a complete (R0) resection. In these patients, median OS is 19 to 33 months compared with 6 to 16 months following incomplete (R1/R2) resection.[3,14–18] In addition, the decision to perform metastasectomy should factor in the disease-free interval (DFI) between resection of primary tumor and appearance of metastatic recurrence. Longer DFI has been shown to be a positive prognostic factor following metastasectomy for lung resection for metastatic sarcoma.[6,12,13,19] Other studies have identified additional prognostic factors associated with improved survival in patients undergoing metastasectomy for STS, albeit inconsistently across studies and institutions. These factors include histologic subtype, tumor size, and number of metastatic lesions.[3,12,20]

Pulmonary Metastasectomy for Sarcoma

Sarcomas show a predilection for metastasis to the lungs. Approximately 20% to 25% of all patients with STS develop pulmonary metastases, and this is the only site of recurrence in more than half of patients with both soft tissue and bone sarcomas who develop distant metastases.[2] Most patients with sarcoma pulmonary metastases are asymptomatic. Typically, patients initially develop a limited number of pulmonary metastases that are detected during follow-up staging. Most lung metastases are found within the first 2 years following diagnosis.[15,18,21–23]

The reported median OS for pulmonary metastatic disease with current multidisciplinary treatment of STS is 12 to 14 months.[16] For a small subset of patients with resectable disease and favorable tumor biology, pulmonary metastasectomy has become accepted standard therapy based on an abundance of retrospective and nonrandomized studies showing improved survival with complete resection compared with historical controls without resection (**Table 1**).[16] In an important landmark publication from the International Registry of Lung Metastasectomy, Pastorino and colleagues[24] reported a wide difference in 5-year survival among 5206 patients from Europe and North America following pulmonary metastasectomy depending on the type of cancer: 68% for germ cell, 37% for epithelial cancer, 31% for sarcoma, and 21% for melanoma. In more recent studies, 5-year OS following pulmonary metastasectomy for sarcoma have been reported to be as high as 50% (typically ~30%).[15–17,25,26]

Although pulmonary metastasectomy is now routinely considered for patients with STS, it is important to remember that the published evidence to support this practice consists almost entirely of retrospective studies,[10–12,14,15,17,18,22–24,27–46] which are inevitably subject to biases, including selection bias. Longer OS rates observed among patient cohorts undergoing pulmonary metastasectomy may be a reflection of patient selection bias rather than a true survival benefit afforded by resection.[16,21,47–49] Because only 2% to 3% of patients with pulmonary metastases ultimately undergo metastasectomy,[49] those selected for resection are likely to have more favorable features (including solitary or low number of metastases and long

Table 1
Results of sarcoma pulmonary metastasectomy series

Reference	Institution	Patients Undergoing Metastasectomy (N)	5-y OS (%)	Median OS	Factors Associated with Longer Survival
Soft Tissue Sarcoma: Mixed Histologies					
Van Geel et al,[46] 1996	Multi-institutional	255	38	NR	DFI >2.5 y, complete resection, lower tumor grade, age <40 y
Pastorino et al,[24] 1997	Multi-institutional	1917	31	NR	DFI >36 mo, fewer metastases
Billingsley[18] 1999	Memorial Sloan-Kettering	161	46 (3-y OS)	33 mo	DFI >1 y, complete resection, lower tumor grade, age <50 y
Weiser et al,[11] 2000	Memorial Sloan-Kettering	86 (all underwent multiple pulmonary metastasectomies)	36	42.8 mo	DFI >1 y, complete resection, ≤2 nodules
Canter et al,[30] 2007	Memorial Sloan-Kettering	138	29 (DSS)	30 mo	DFI >1 y, complete resection
Rehders et al,[14] 2007	Hamburg, Germany	61	25	33 mo	—
Smith et al,[15] 2009	Roswell Park	94	15	16 mo	DFI >25 mo, complete resection
Stephens et al,[44] 2011	MD Anderson	81 (metastasectomy after chemotherapy)	32 vs 0[a]	35.5 vs 17.2 mo[a]	DFI <2 y, ≤2 nodules, no progression after neoadjuvant chemotherapy
Schur et al,[43] 2014	Vienna, Austria	46	32	45.3 mo	—
Dossett et al,[39] 2015	Moffitt	120	NR	48 mo	—
Lin et al,[40] 2015	UCLA	155	34.8	35.4 mo	DFI >1 y, complete resection

Leiomyosarcoma					
Burt et al,[35] 2011	Brigham and Women's Hospital	31	52	69.9 mo	DFI >1 y, age <45 y
Lin et al,[40] 2015	UCLA	26	61	NR	Longer DFI
STS/Bone Sarcoma: Mixed Histologies					
Burt et al,[35] 2011	Brigham and Women's Hospital	51	32	23.9 mo	Longer DFI
Kim et al,[12] 2011	Massachusetts General Hospital	97	50	60.2 mo	DFI ≥1 y, complete resection, unilateral metastatic disease
Mizuno et al,[41] 2013	Nagoya, Japan	52	50.9	NR	Complete resection, ≤2 nodules
Osteogenic Sarcoma					
Briccoli et al,[32] 2005	Bologna, Italy	127	38	NR	Longer DFI
García Franco et al,[17] 2009	Pamplona, Spain	52	31	36 mo	Longer DFI
Lin et al,[40] 2015	UCLA	21	57	57%	—

Abbreviations: DSS, disease-specific survival; NR, not recorded; UCLA, University of California, Los Angeles.
[a] Nonprogressors versus progressors after neoadjuvant chemotherapy.

interoperative interval) associated with longer survival regardless of treatment. Thus, it is difficult to discern how much benefit pulmonary metastasectomy provides.

That the improved survival seen in most reported cohorts of patients undergoing pulmonary metastasectomy may be caused by underlying favorable tumor biology and patient selection bias rather than by surgical resection itself is also suggested by reports from Treasure and colleagues[45] and Stephens and colleagues.[44] In 2012, Treasure and colleagues[45] performed a systematic review of published reports that included survival rates following pulmonary metastasectomy for metastatic sarcoma. Among 1196 patients included in 18 studies, 5-year OS following first pulmonary metastasectomy for osteogenic sarcoma and STS were 34% and 25%, respectively. Compared with 5-year OS among all patients with metastatic sarcoma in the Thames Cancer Registry for 1985 to 1994 and 1995 to 2004 (20% and 25% for bone sarcoma, 13% and 15% for STS), these survival rates were better (P values not reported). However, the investigators commented that, "Given that pulmonary metastasectomy is used in a highly selected favorable minority, this suggests that the benefit from metastasectomy cannot be large. Although it is a standard component of sarcoma care, the evidence for benefit is weak."[45] In 2001, Stephens and colleagues[44] examined 81 patients with bone and soft tissue sarcoma who underwent pulmonary metastasectomy following neoadjuvant chemotherapy. Patients whose pulmonary metastatic disease progressed as determined by CT imaging following systemic therapy had markedly worse median OS (35.5 vs 17.2 months; $P > .001$) and 5-year survival (0% vs 32%; P value not reported) following pulmonary metastasectomy. The survival rates among nonprogressors in this study are comparable with pulmonary metastatic cohorts in other studies despite patients in this study having a higher average number of pulmonary nodules (progressors 5.1, nonprogressors 5.9; P value not significant). Clearly, there is a need for randomized trials to determine the true, rather than the perceived, effect of pulmonary metastasectomy in STS and bone sarcoma.

Pulmonary metastasectomy can be performed either via thoracoscopy or thoracotomy for unilateral disease. For bilateral pulmonary metastases, bilateral thoracoscopy/thoracotomy, median sternotomy, or clamshell thoracotomy can be performed. The main principle of pulmonary metastasectomy is complete resection and limiting resection to preserve pulmonary function.[21]

Preoperative planning should include pulmonary function tests (PFTs) and evaluation of the patient's ability to tolerate an operation. Special consideration should be given to patients who received chemotherapeutic agents associated with drug-induced lung disease. Patients should also cease smoking for at least 3 weeks before surgery to decrease the risk of postoperative pneumonia and other complications.[21]

Postoperative follow-up for those with metastatic STS to the lungs (as described by Jaklitsch and colleagues[36]) includes physical examination and CT scan of the chest every 4 months for 2 years then every 6 months for 6 years. Postoperative follow-up for those with metastatic bone sarcoma to the lungs (as described by Briccoli and colleagues[32]) includes physical examination and CT scan of the chest and imaging of primary tumor site every 3 months for 4 years and then every 6 months for 10 years and total-body bone scintigraphy every year.[33]

Outcomes following pulmonary metastasectomy for soft tissue sarcoma

Although there are numerous retrospective series reporting outcomes following pulmonary metastasectomy for sarcoma,[10–12,14,15,17,18,22–24,27–29,31–46] patient cohorts in these studies are highly heterogenous. These studies not only include patients with primary tumors of mixed STS histologies and primary tumor sites (extremity, trunk, visceral, retroperitoneal), but often also include patients with osteogenic sarcoma.[40,41] These studies inconsistently also include patients with synchronous pulmonary metastases, those who received chemotherapy, and/or those who underwent repeated pulmonary resections. Nevertheless, reported 5-year OS rates generally range from 15% to 43% and median OS range from 30 to 48 months in the literature.

The most consistently reported prognostic factor for survival following pulmonary metastasectomy is completeness of resection.[12,15,18,23,38,41,42,46] Reported median survival ranges from 19 to 33 months for patients who underwent complete resection compared with 6 to 16 months with incomplete resection.[15,18,22,24,25] Billingsley and colleagues[18] examined 3149 adult patients with STS treated at Memorial Sloan-Kettering Cancer Center from July 1982 and February 1997. Of these, 719 patients either presented with or developed pulmonary metastases. Median OS for all patients from time of diagnosis of pulmonary metastasis was 15 months. Patients who underwent complete resection of pulmonary metastatic disease had a median OS of 33 months, those who underwent incomplete resection had a median OS of 16 months, whereas those treated nonoperatively had a median OS of 11 months ($P<.001$).[18] In a study of 94 patients with mSTS of mixed primary sites, Smith and colleagues[15] reported median OS for R0 resection was 22 months, 11.5 months for R1 resection, and 9.5 months for R2 resection ($P<.0001$). Pogrebniak and colleagues[38] similarly reported longer median OS in patients undergoing complete resection of pulmonary metastases compared with those undergoing incomplete resection (25 vs 10 months; $P = .0007$).

Other reported prognostic factors for survival following pulmonary metastasectomy are DFI between resection of primary tumor and appearance of metastatic disease,[12,15,18,23,24,35,37,39,45,46] number of metastatic pulmonary nodules,[11,12,24,39,41,45] tumor grade,[11,18,46] tumor size,[11,12] and patient age.[18,23,46] Kim and colleagues[12] reported that DFI greater than or equal to 1 year was associated with improved 5-year OS compared with DFI less than 1 year (65% vs 21%; $P<.0001$).

Several investigators have noted improved survival among patients undergoing pulmonary metastasectomy for leiomyosarcoma.[35,40] Burt and colleagues[35] in 2011 reported longer median OS for patients undergoing repeated pulmonary metastasectomy for leiomyosarcoma compared with other histologies (69.9 vs 23.9 months; $P = .049$) and better 5-year OS (52% vs 32%; $P = .049$). More recently, Lin and colleagues[40] reported that patients with metastatic leiomyosarcoma (n = 26) undergoing pulmonary metastasectomy experienced longer 5-year OS compared with other histologies (61% vs 37%; $P = .02$).

Outcomes following pulmonary metastasectomy for bone sarcoma

Patients with STS are distinct from those with osteogenic sarcoma. Compared with STS, patients with osteogenic sarcoma tend to be younger at diagnosis.[17,28,29,31–34] Although there are few prospective studies and no randomized trials evaluating pulmonary metastasectomy in patients with osteogenic sarcoma, chemotherapy and pulmonary metastasectomy have transformed metastatic osteosarcoma from a uniformly fatal condition to one with reasonable expectation of survival, with 5-year OS up to 47% with complete resection of pulmonary metastases.[28] García-Franco and colleagues[17] examined 52 patients with pulmonary metastases from bone sarcomas, all treated with neoadjuvant chemotherapy before pulmonary metastasectomy. Five-year OS was 31%. In their study of 94 patients with metastatic, Briccoli and colleagues[32] reported a 5-year OS from first metastasectomy for osteosarcoma of 38%.[50]

Multiple groups have reported improved survival compared with patients with mSTS to the lungs.[28,40] Lin and colleagues[40] reported that patients with osteogenic sarcoma (n = 21) undergoing pulmonary metastasectomy experienced longer 5-year OS compared with those with STS (53% vs 37%; P = .03). Similar to mSTS, longer DFI, completeness of resection, and number of pulmonary metastases have been shown to be associated with improved survival following pulmonary metastasectomy for osteogenic sarcoma metastasis.[17,32]

As with mSTS, patients who present with synchronous pulmonary metastasis at the time of the initial sarcoma diagnosis have reported worse OS.[29,33] Kager and colleagues[29] reported outcomes of 202 patients with high-grade osteosarcoma with clinically detectable metastases at initial presentation registered in the neoadjuvant Cooperative Osteosarcoma Study Group before 1999. The most frequent metastatic site was the lung (164 patients, 81.2%). Five-year OS was 29%; in the 124 patients with lung-only metastasis, 5-year OS was 33%.

Long-term pulmonary function has been studied among patients who undergo recurrent pulmonary metastasectomy for osteogenic sarcoma during childhood.[31] Denbo and colleagues[31] examined 21 patients who had PFTs after pulmonary metastasectomy for osteosarcoma. Mean age at diagnosis of osteosarcoma was 13.2 years; mean age at PFTs was 34.9 years. Patients who underwent pulmonary metastasectomy for osteosarcoma as children often had abnormal PFTs on long-term follow-up but reductions in lung volumes and diffusing capacity for carbon monoxide were mild except in those who underwent multiple pulmonary metastasectomies.

Approach to recurrent metastases

Despite aggressive surgical management, recurrence rates are greater than 50% following pulmonary metastasectomy for STS.[2,16,22,51] Some series have shown that repeated resection of recurrent metastasis can be associated with improved survival,[3,11,12,25,35–38,52] although less invasive approaches may be associated with fewer morbidities and shorter hospital stay.[2,3,25] Jaklitsch and colleagues[36] reported that 5-year OS remained greater than 33% for up to 4 procedures. With 5 or more procedures, the ability to maintain control of intrathoracic metastases became very low and median survival decreased to 8 months. The investigators concluded that repeating pulmonary metastasectomy may be indicated as long as removal of all clinically apparent disease is practical.[36] More recently, Kim and colleagues[12] reported that patients who underwent multiple pulmonary metastasectomies had longer 5-year OS compared with those who had undergone a single operation (69% vs 41%; P = .017). To be able to undergo repeated metastasectomy likely identifies a subset of patients with good physiologic condition and favorable tumor biology.[16,48] Whether repeated pulmonary metastasectomy extends survival is unclear because it is unclear what the survival of these patients would have been without surgery.

Patients presenting with synchronous metastases

Approximately 10% of patients with STS have synchronous pulmonary metastases at initial presentation.[16,53] It is known that patients with STS and synchronous metastases at presentation generally have poor prognosis. One study based on the American Joint Committee on Cancer staging system for sarcoma reported that patients who presented with metastatic disease (stage IV) had a 6% 5-year disease-specific survival.[53] Several groups have examined whether pulmonary metastasectomy for synchronous metastases offers any benefit.[6,53]

In 2002, Kane and colleagues[6] reported that, among 48 patients with synchronous metastases, 30 had pulmonary metastases. Thirteen patients underwent pulmonary metastasectomy with no difference in median OS between those who underwent resection and those who did not (16 vs 14 months; $P = .3$). More recently, Ferguson and colleagues[53] examined 112 patients with bone sarcoma and STS who presented with synchronous metastases. Eighty-eight patients (79%) had pulmonary metastases at the time of presentation with STS. Of these, 18 patients underwent pulmonary metastasectomy. Median OS was 9 months for all patients with synchronous pulmonary metastases with no difference in OS between those who underwent pulmonary metastasectomy and those who did not.[53] Other investigators have reported pulmonary metastasis synchronous to the primary tumor to be a significant predictor of worse survival following pulmonary metastasectomy.[39,40,42]

Thus, patients with pulmonary metastases at the time of STS diagnosis do not benefit from metastasectomy. Chemotherapy should be the initial treatment of those who have short DFI or a large number of metastatic lesions.[53] Subsequent surgery could be considered if the patient benefits from chemotherapy.

Hepatic Resection for Metastatic Sarcoma

Isolated liver metastases of STS are uncommon compared with pulmonary metastases. Patients with retroperitoneal and intra-abdominal/visceral STS are more likely to develop liver-only metastatic disease compared with patients with extra-abdominal primary STS.[13,22] Although hepatic resection is increasingly being performed for colorectal and neuroendocrine liver metastases, surgical resection of hepatic metastases from STS remains controversial and hepatic metastases from STS are most often treated nonsurgically.[13]

There is currently no consensus on the role of resection for STS metastases to the liver and no prospective data available to guide surgical treatment.[13,54,55] The available data regarding resection of hepatic STS metastases are limited to retrospective series reporting on resection of noncolorectal nonneuroendocrine liver metastases,[20,56–59] case reports,[60] and case series reporting specifically on the treatment of STS liver metastases.[7,26,50,61–64] In addition to limitations and biases inherent in retrospective studies, the available data also represent heterogeneous patient groups with mixed primary sarcoma histologies. Such studies often include patients with GIST, which is inappropriate because these tumors have significantly better outcomes and different management following the introduction of targeted TKI therapies.[54] In these studies, median OS ranged between 34 and 37 months and 5-year OS ranged between 20% and 39% for patients undergoing hepatic resection for sarcoma metastases.[54,56,61,63,64] Survival outcomes are highly dependent on histologic subtypes, with leiomyosarcoma associated with worse outcomes and GIST associated with better outcomes in the postimatinib era, so hepatic resection may be considered with careful patient selection and may prolong survival in those with good performance status, longer DFI, oligometastasis, and when all gross hepatic disease is resectable.[13,54]

As in sarcoma pulmonary metastasis, consistently reported prognostic factors in patients undergoing hepatic metastasectomy for liver metastases include ability to achieve a complete (R0) resection and longer DFI between resection of primary tumor and appearance of metastatic recurrence (**Table 2**).[3,6,7,19,26,57,59,62]

Postoperative follow-up (described by Rehders and colleagues[50]) includes physical examination and CT scan of the chest/abdomen/pelvis every 3 months for 2 years, then every 6 months until the end of the fifth postoperative year, then annually.

Outcomes following hepatic resection for metastatic soft tissue sarcoma

There are several large retrospective studies of patients undergoing liver resection for noncolorectal nonneuroendocrine metastases. In general, these patient cohorts are highly heterogeneous and the data difficult to apply.[56,58] They do show the highly

Table 2
Results of sarcoma hepatic metastasectomy series

Reference	Institution	Patients Undergoing Metastasectomy (N)	Perioperative Mortality (%)	5-y OS (%)	Median OS (mo)	Factors Associated with Longer Survival
Leiomyosarcoma						
Chen et al,[26] 1998	Johns Hopkins	11	0	NR	39	Complete resection
Ercolani et al,[57] 2005	Bologna, Italy	10	NR	36	44	—
Lang et al,[62] 2000	Hannover, Germany	26	6	20	NR	None found
Yedibela et al,[59] 2005	Erlangen, Germany	15	NR	NR	NR	Complete resection
Mixed Histologies						
Adam et al,[56] 2006	Multi-institutional	125 (excluding GIST)	NR	31	32	—
DeMatteo et al,[61] 2001	Memorial Sloan-Kettering	56 (34 with GIST)	0	30	39	DFI >2 y, complete resection
Marudanayagam et al,[63] 2011	Birmingham, UK	36 (5 with GIST)	0	31.8	24	Histologies other than leiomyosarcoma
Pawlik et al,[64] 2006	MD Anderson	53 (of 66 patients, 36 with GIST)	0	27	47	No adjuvant therapy
Rehders et al,[50] 2009	Dusseldorf, Germany	27 (of 45 patients, 6 with GIST)	7	49	44	DFI >2 y, no RFA treatment

Abbreviation: RFA, radiofrequency ablation.

variable survival outcomes between sarcoma histologies. In a study of 1452 patients who underwent hepatic resection for noncolorectal nonneuroendocrine liver metastases, Adam and colleagues[56] reported the highest 5-year OS among patients with GIST (70%, median survival not reached), whereas patients with all other sarcoma histologies had 5-year OS of 30% (median survival, 32 months; P value not reported).

DeMatteo and colleagues[61] examined 331 patients with liver metastases from sarcoma admitted to Memorial Sloan-Kettering Cancer Center from 1982 to 2000. Fifty-six patients underwent resection of all gross hepatic disease. Of these, 34 (61%) had GIST or leiomyosarcoma. The sites of primary tumor in the resected patients were predominantly intra-abdominal (38 patients, 68%) or retroperitoneal (8 patients, 14%) and less commonly extremity/trunk (5, 9%) or head/neck (5, 9%). Five-year OS for patients who underwent R0 surgery was 30% compared with 4% among those who did not undergo complete resection (P<.0001). On multivariate analysis, only DFI from diagnosis of the primary tumor to the development of liver metastasis greater than 2 years was associated with longer OS after hepatic resection. Repeated liver resection for recurrent tumor was performed in 17 patients.

More recently, Rehders and colleagues[50] reported their series of 45 patients with liver metastases from sarcoma of whom 27 underwent surgery. Again, a significant proportion of these patients had leiomyosarcoma (30%) or GIST (22%). In this cohort, median OS was 44 months and 5-year OS was 49%. Longer DFI (>2 years) was associated with improved survival. Repeated liver resection for recurrent tumor was performed in 8 patients; median survival in this subset of patients was 76 months.

Both DeMatteo and colleagues[61] and Rehders and colleagues[50] found that longer DFI (before development of liver metastatic disease) was associated with improved survival following hepatic resection for mSTS. However, the investigators of the former study emphasized that patients who underwent hepatectomy were highly selected and tended to have favorable characteristics, including longer DFI, fewer liver metastases (1–2), and smaller lesions (<10 cm). The observation that the DFI between resection of a primary cancer and subsequent tumor recurrence affects survival has been made across malignancies, including malignant melanoma, breast, and renal carcinoma, as well as in a large study of 2123 patients with completely resected primary STS.[19] Thus, whether hepatic resection of sarcoma metastatic disease itself provides a survival benefit is unclear. It may be that patients selected for hepatic resection of metastatic disease tend to have longer DFI reflecting better/more indolent tumor biology, which may also result in these patients having metastatic disease that is more amenable to complete resection.

Outcomes following hepatic resection for metastatic leiomyosarcoma

Leiomyosarcoma is among the most commonly resected metastatic tumors to the liver, along with colorectal, neuroendocrine, and GIST hepatic metastases. Patients who undergo hepatic resection for leiomyosarcoma metastasis have worse survival outcomes compared with patients who undergo hepatic resection for GIST.[26,57,59,62,63] Marudanayagam and colleagues[63] reported that, among their series of 36 patients who underwent hepatic resection for mSTS, factors associated with poor survival on univariate analysis included positive resection margin of liver metastasis, tumor grade, and primary leiomyosarcoma; only primary leiomyosarcoma remained prognostic as a risk factor for poor survival on multivariate analysis (P = .01).

Across studies, incomplete gross resection was associated with worse OS following liver resection for metastatic leiomyosarcoma. Median OS ranged between 20.5 and 44.4 months and 5-year OS ranged between 13% and 36% for those patients able to undergo resection of leiomyosarcoma liver metastases, depending on whether R0 or R1/R2 resection was achieved.[7,26,57,59,62]

Jaques and colleagues[7] reported that, among 981 adult patients with STS admitted to Memorial Sloan-Kettering Cancer Center between July 1982 and July 1987, 65 patients had hepatic metastases. The primary sarcoma in most patients was leiomyosarcoma (n = 55, 85%); the remainder were angiosarcomas, rhabdomyosarcomas, liposarcomas, and malignant fibrous histiocytomas. Thirteen patients (20%) had liver metastases on initial presentation. In the remaining patients, the median time from primary diagnosis to development of hepatic metastases was 12 months. Hepatic metastases were predominantly seen among patients with primary intra-abdominal (visceral or retroperitoneal) rather than extremity/trunk sarcomas. Hepatic resection was performed in 14 patients (22%) with median OS of 30 months in the resected group (vs 12 months in patients with unresectable disease; P value not significant). There were no 5-year survivors in this study.

In 1998, Chen and colleagues[26] examined outcomes of hepatic resection specifically for metastatic leiomyosarcoma. Of 11 patients in this series, 5 had retroperitoneal leiomyosarcoma and 6 had visceral primary leiomyosarcoma (3 gastric, 2 small bowel, 1 uterine/adnexal). Patients underwent hepatic lobectomies/extended lobectomies (n = 4), segmentectomies/wedge resections (n = 5), and complex liver resections (n = 2) with complete resection (R0) achieved in 6 patients. Average disease-free survival (DFS) was 16 months and median OS was 39 months. Only resection margin status was associated with OS (P = .03). The median survival time for the 6 patients who underwent R0 resection was not reached at 56-month follow-up; all 5 patients with incomplete (R1/R2) resection died by 39 months (median 25 months). In this small series, there was no association between OS and number or size of liver lesions, extent of hepatic resection, or tumor grade.

Lang and colleagues[62] reported their series of 26 patients who underwent a total of 34 liver resections for leiomyosarcoma metastases. Of 23 first hepatic resections, R0 resection was achieved in 15 patients, R1 in 3 patients, and incomplete gross resection (R2) in 5 patients. Median OS after R0 resection was 32 months compared with 20.5 months after R1/R2 resection (P = .31). Five-year OS was 13% for all patients and 20% after R0 resection.

More recently, Ercolani and colleagues[57] and Yedibela and colleagues[59] studied the role of liver resection for noncolorectal metastases and reported outcomes for subsets of patients with metastatic leiomyosarcoma. Although the heterogeneity of these two patient cohorts makes interpretation of their data challenging, 5-year OS among patients who underwent liver resection for metastatic leiomyosarcoma were 36.4%[57] and 26%, respectively.[59] Yedibela and colleagues[59] reported that, among 9 patients who underwent hepatic resection for leiomyosarcoma metastases, those who underwent R0 resection experienced longer 5-year OS (42 vs 26 months) and median survival (41 vs 21 months; P value not reported). Ercolani and colleagues[57] reported a median survival of 44.4 months among 10 patients who underwent hepatic resection for metastatic leiomyosarcoma.

OTHER TREATMENT MODALITIES FOR METASTATIC SARCOMA
Chemotherapy

The first-line treatment of mSTS is chemotherapy.[3,8,16] Doxorubicin and ifosfamide are the most active drugs and constitute the standard treatment of advanced STS. The recommended first-line treatment is doxorubicin at a dose of 75 mg/m^2. Ifosfamide is an alternative in patients with contraindication to doxorubicin or as second-line treatment after doxorubicin failure. Ifosfamide in monotherapy is used at doses of 5 to 9 g/m^2. Doxorubicin and ifosfamide may be used in combination when obtaining an objective response to improve symptoms or before surgical resection.[1,4,8]

Second-line therapy for unresectable mSTS is palliative. For most STS, there is no evidence that a particular drug sequence is superior to another. Some tumor types may be more sensitive to certain drugs and this may aid in selection of second-line therapy: high-dose ifosfamide for synovial sarcoma, trabectedin for myxoid liposarcoma and leiomyosarcoma, or gemcitabine with docetaxel or with dacarbazine (dimethyl triazeno imidazole carboxamide [DTIC]) in leiomyosarcoma. Symptomatic patients with good performance status are candidates for clinical trials. For symptomatic patients with poor performance status, radiation therapy or supportive care alone are appropriate options.

Gemcitabine and DTIC alone have limited activity in STS; however, the combination of gemcitabine (1800 mg/m^2 at 10 mg/m^2/min) with DTIC (500 mg/m^2) every 14 days seems to provide benefit, particularly in leiomyosarcoma. Gemcitabine in combination with docetaxel has also been reported in uterine leiomyosarcoma and undifferentiated pleomorphic sarcoma.[8]

Trabectedin has been explored in phase I to II trials with modest objective response rates and higher progression arrest rates in myxoid liposarcoma, synovial sarcoma, and leiomyosarcoma. In a phase III trial, trabectedin improved disease control compared with standard second-line DTIC in advanced metastatic liposarcoma and leiomyosarcoma.[8] Trabectedin is now approved in Europe and the United States for patients with STS after failure on doxorubicin and ifosfamide or in patients unable to receive these first-line treatments.

Patients previously treated with ifosfamide may be treated with high-dose ifosfamide (>10 g/m^2), which has shown activity in synovial sarcoma. Pazopanib, a multitargeted TKI, now constitutes a second-line option after first-line failure for nonadipocytic sarcoma.

Two recent retrospective analyses examined treatment patterns in patients with metastatic/relapsed STS. The earlier study, from 2012, was a multicenter, multicountry retrospective review,[4] whereas the later study, from 2015, was performed in the United States.[1] In the former study, the most common first-line regimens were doxorubicin (34%) or anthracycline plus ifosfamide (30%) with median progression-free survival (PFS) and OS of 8.3 and 23.5 months from first favorable response to chemotherapy.[4] In the latter study, the most common first-line regimens were anthracycline based (44%) or gemcitabine based (28%) with median PFS from initiation of second-line treatment of 5.4 months and median OS from first diagnosis of mSTS of 39 months.[1] Most patients receive multiple lines of chemotherapy with higher likelihood of favorable response to first-line therapy compared with second or later lines of therapy. Both studies highlight that PFS and OS in patients with metastatic STS with favorable response to chemotherapy are short and that there remains a significant unmet need in the treatment of patients with metastatic STS.[1,4]

Radiation Therapy

For patients who are not candidates for surgical metastasectomy, radiation therapy can be used for control of limited metastatic disease.[3] Stereotactic body radiation therapy (SBRT) delivers high doses of radiation with precise localization and limited exposure of adjacent tissue. Good local control rates have been noted in studies of SBRT for patients with liver and lung metastases from various primary tumors.[65–67] In STS specifically, local control rates for patients with pulmonary metastases have been reported to be as high as 80% to 88%.[68,69] Further data on long-term toxicity and outcomes, particularly compared with metastasectomy, are needed.

Ablative Techniques

As thermoablative techniques continue to evolve, these techniques have been increasingly used as adjuncts in combination with surgical metastasectomy or as primary therapy in nonsurgical candidates for some disease processes.[2,3,16] Thermal ablative methods include radiofrequency ablation (RFA) and microwave ablation. To date, there have been no studies to compare thermoablative techniques with surgical metastasectomy in patients with mSTS.[3]

Liver ablation

One retrospective study by Pawlik and colleagues[64] examined 66 patients who underwent hepatic resection, RFA, or both for mSTS liver lesions. Although most patients had GIST, patients with leiomyosarcoma and other sarcoma histologies were included. Compared with patients who underwent surgery alone, those who received RFA (either alone or combined with surgery) had shorter DFS ($P = .002$) with no difference in OS. RFA alone was used in patients who were deemed poor surgical candidates or who had lesions in unfavorable locations, whereas RFA plus surgery was used in those with large lesions not amenable to surgery alone.

Lung ablation

For patients with limited pulmonary metastatic disease but whose performance status or comorbidities prohibit surgery, minimally invasive procedures such as RFA may be of benefit. Palussiere and colleagues[70] published a series of 100 patients with mSTS of whom 47 had lung metastasis. Twenty-nine patients (with 47 lesions) were treated with RFA, and the remainder received chemotherapy. In 4 of 47 lesions ablated, there was progression on follow-up scans consistent with incomplete response. DFS was 7 months with 1-year and 3-year survival of 92.2% and 65.2%, similar to surgical series. Complications of ablation included pneumothorax (68.7% of cases). Similar results were reported by Nakamura and colleagues,[71] with 1-year and 3-year survival of 88.9% and 59.2% and with pneumothorax occurring in 54% of procedures, with chest tube drainage required in 9%. In contrast, failure to eradicate all pulmonary metastases resulted in significantly worse 1-year and 3-year survival rates (29.6% and 0%).

SUMMARY

Half of all patients with sarcoma are diagnosed with or develop distant metastases during their disease course. The presence of distant metastatic disease significantly affects patient survival, reducing 5-year OS to less than 10% and median overall survival to 8 to 15 months. The most common sites of distant metastatic disease in STS are the lungs and liver. Those with limited metastatic disease may benefit from surgical metastasectomy or minimally invasive ablative approaches for disease control. In retrospective series, 5-year survival rates up to 30% to 50% have been reported. Given the absence of randomized controlled trials and other prospective data and the diversity of STS behavior, treatment decisions should be made in a specialty sarcoma center and with a multidisciplinary team of medical, radiation, and surgical oncologists who specialize in the care of such patients.

REFERENCES

1. Wagner MJ, Amodu LI, Duh MS, et al. A retrospective chart review of drug treatment patterns and clinical outcomes among patients with metastatic or recurrent soft tissue sarcoma refractory to one or more prior chemotherapy treatments. BMC Cancer 2015;15:175.
2. Hohenberger P, Kasper B, Ahrar K. Surgical management and minimally invasive approaches for the treatment of metastatic sarcoma. Am Soc Clin Oncol Educ Book 2013;457–64. http://dx.doi.org/10.1200/EdBook_AM.2013.33.457.
3. Cardona K, Williams R, Movva S. Multimodality therapy for advanced or metastatic sarcoma. Curr Probl Cancer 2013;37:74–86.
4. Leahy M, Garcia Del Muro X, Reichardt P, et al. Chemotherapy treatment patterns and clinical outcomes in patients with metastatic soft tissue sarcoma. The SArcoma treatment and Burden of illness in North America and Europe (SABINE) study. Ann Oncol 2012;23:2763–70.
5. Siegel R, Naishadham D, Jemal A. Cancer statistics, 2012. CA Cancer J Clin 2012;62(1):10–29.
6. Kane JM, Finley JW, Driscoll D, et al. The treatment and outcome of patients with soft tissue sarcomas and synchronous metastases. Sarcoma 2002;6:69–73.
7. Jaques DP, Coit DG, Casper ES, et al. Hepatic metastases from soft-tissue sarcoma. Ann Surg 1995;221:392–7.
8. Garcia Del Muro X, de Alava E, Artigas V, et al. Clinical practice guidelines for the diagnosis and treatment of patients with soft tissue sarcoma by the Spanish Group for Research in Sarcomas (GEIS). Cancer Chemother Pharmacol 2016; 77(1):133–46.
9. Gossot D, Radu C, Girard P, et al. Resection of pulmonary metastases from sarcoma: can some patients benefit from a less invasive approach? Ann Thorac Surg 2009;87:238–43.
10. Predina JD, Puc MM, Bergey MR, et al. Improved survival after pulmonary metastasectomy for soft tissue sarcoma. J Thorac Oncol 2011;6:913–9.
11. Weiser MR, Downey RJ, Leung DH, et al. Repeat resection of pulmonary metastases in patients with soft-tissue sarcoma. J Am Coll Surg 2000;191(2):184–90 [discussion: 190–1].
12. Kim S, Ott HC, Wright CD, et al. Pulmonary resection of metastatic sarcoma: prognostic factors associated with improved outcomes. Ann Thorac Surg 2011; 92:1780–7.
13. Abdalla EK, Pisters PW. Metastasectomy for limited metastases from soft tissue sarcoma. Curr Treat Options Oncol 2002;3(6):497–505.
14. Rehders A, Hosch SB, Scheunemann P, et al. Benefit of surgical treatment of lung metastasis in soft tissue sarcoma. Arch Surg 2007;142:70–5.
15. Smith R, Pak Y, Kraybill W, et al. Factors associated with actual long-term survival following soft tissue sarcoma pulmonary metastasectomy. Eur J Surg Oncol 2009; 35(4):356–61.
16. Smith R, Demmy TL. Pulmonary metastasectomy for soft tissue sarcoma. Surg Oncol Clin N Am 2012;21:269–86.
17. García Franco CE, Algarra SM, Ezcurra AT, et al. Long-term results after resection for soft tissue sarcoma pulmonary metastases. Interact Cardiovasc Thorac Surg 2009;9:223–6.
18. Billingsley K, Burt ME, Jara EG, et al. Pulmonary metastases from soft tissue sarcoma: analysis of patterns of diseases and postmetastasis survival. Ann Surg 1999;229:602–10 [discussion: 610–2].

19. Stojadinovic A, Leung DH, Allen P, et al. Primary adult soft tissue sarcoma: time-dependent influence of prognostic variables. J Clin Oncol 2002;20:4344–52.

20. Groeschl RT, Nachmany I, Steel JL, et al. Hepatectomy for noncolorectal non-neuroendocrine metastatic cancer: a multi-institutional analysis. J Am Coll Surg 2012;214:769–77.

21. Ceppa DP. Results of pulmonary resection sarcoma and germ cell tumors pulmonary metastasis lung resection sarcoma germ cell tumor outcomes. Thorac Surg Clin 2016;26:49–54.

22. Gadd MA, Casper ES, Woodruff JM, et al. Development and treatment of pulmonary metastases in adult patients with extremity soft tissue sarcoma. Ann Surg 1993;218:705–12.

23. Billingsley KG, Lewis JJ, Leung DH, et al. Multifactorial analysis of the survival of patients with distant metastasis arising from primary extremity sarcoma. Cancer 1999;85(2):389–95.

24. Pastorino U, Buyse M, Friedel G, et al. Long-term results of lung metastasectomy: prognostic analyses based on 5206 cases. J Thorac Cardiovasc Surg 1997;113:37–49.

25. Casson AG, Putnam JB, Natarajan G, et al. Efficacy of pulmonary metastasectomy for recurrent soft tissue sarcoma. J Surg Oncol 1991;47:1–4.

26. Chen H, Pruitt A, Nicol TL, et al. Complete hepatic resection of metastases from leiohyosarcoma prolongs survival. J Gastrointest Surg 1998;2(2):151–5.

27. Paik ES, Yoon A, Lee YY, et al. Pulmonary metastasectomy in uterine malignancy: outcomes and prognostic factors. J Gynecol Oncol 2015;26(4):270–6.

28. Skinner KA, Eilber FR, Holmes EC, et al. Surgical treatment and chemotherapy for pulmonary metastases from osteosarcoma. Arch Surg 1992;127:1061–5.

29. Kager L, Zoubek A, Pötschger U, et al. Primary metastatic osteosarcoma: presentation and outcome of patients treated on neoadjuvant cooperative osteosarcoma study group protocols. J Clin Oncol 2003;21:2011–8.

30. Canter RJ, Qin LX, Downey RJ, et al. Perioperative chemotherapy in patients undergoing pulmonary resection for metastatic soft-tissue sarcoma of the extremity: a retrospective analysis. Cancer 2007;110:2050–60.

31. Denbo JW, Zhu L, Srivastava D, et al. Long-term pulmonary function after metastasectomy for childhood osteosarcoma: a report from the St Jude Lifetime Cohort Study. J Am Coll Surg 2014;219:265–71.

32. Briccoli A, Rocca M, Salone M, et al. Resection of recurrent pulmonary metastases in patients with osteosarcoma. Cancer 2005;104:1721–5.

33. Briccoli A, Rocca M, Salone M, et al. High grade osteosarcoma of the extremities metastatic to the lung: long-term results in 323 patients treated combining surgery and chemotherapy, 1985-2005. Surg Oncol 2010;19:193–9.

34. Gelderblom H, Jinks RC, Sydes M, et al. Survival after recurrent osteosarcoma: data from 3 European Osteosarcoma Intergroup (EOI) randomized controlled trials. Eur J Cancer 2011;47:895–902.

35. Burt BM, Ocejo S, Mery CM, et al. Repeated and aggressive pulmonary resections for leiomyosarcoma metastases extends survival. Ann Thorac Surg 2011;92:1202–7.

36. Jaklitsch MT, Mery CM, Lukanich JM, et al. Sequential thoracic metastasectomy prolongs survival by re-establishing local control within the chest. J Thorac Cardiovasc Surg 2001;121:657–67.

37. Kandioler D, Krömer E, Tüchler H, et al. Long-term results after repeated surgical removal of pulmonary metastases. Ann Thorac Surg 1998;65:909–12.

38. Pogrebniak HW, Roth JA, Steinberg SM, et al. Reoperative pulmonary resection in patients with metastatic soft tissue sarcoma. Ann Thorac Surg 1991;52:197–203.
39. Dossett LA, Toloza EM, Fontaine J, et al. Outcomes and clinical predictors of improved survival in a patients undergoing pulmonary metastasectomy for sarcoma. J Surg Oncol 2015;112:103–6.
40. Lin AY, Kotova S, Yanagawa J, et al. Risk stratification of patients undergoing pulmonary metastasectomy for soft tissue and bone sarcomas. J Thorac Cardiovasc Surg 2015;149:85–92.
41. Mizuno T, Taniguchi T, Ishikawa Y, et al. Pulmonary metastasectomy for osteogenic and soft tissue sarcoma: who really benefits from surgical treatment? Eur J Cardiothorac Surg 2013;43(4):795–9.
42. Reza J, Sammann A, Jin C, et al. Aggressive and minimally invasive surgery for pulmonary metastasis of sarcoma. J Thorac Cardiovasc Surg 2014;147: 1193–200 [discussion: 1200–1].
43. Schur S, Hoetzenecker K, Lamm W, et al. Pulmonary metastasectomy for soft tissue sarcoma–report from a dual institution experience at the Medical University of Vienna. Eur J Cancer 2014;50:2289–97.
44. Stephens EH, Blackmon SH, Correa AM, et al. Progression after chemotherapy is a novel predictor of poor outcomes after pulmonary metastasectomy in sarcoma patients. J Am Coll Surg 2011;212:821–6.
45. Treasure T, Fiorentino F, Scarci M, et al. Pulmonary metastasectomy for sarcoma: a systematic review of reported outcomes in the context of Thames Cancer Registry data. BMJ Open 2012;2:e001736.
46. van Geel AN, Pastorino U, Jauch KW, et al. Surgical treatment of lung metastases: The European Organization for Research and Treatment of Cancer-Soft Tissue and Bone Sarcoma Group study of 255 patients. Cancer 1996;77:675–82.
47. Åberg T. Selection mechanisms as major determinants of survival after pulmonary metastasectomy. Ann Thorac Surg 1997;63(3):611–2.
48. Treasure T, Moller H, Fiorentino F, et al. Editorial comment: forty years on: pulmonary metastasectomy for sarcoma. Eur J Cardiothorac Surg 2013;43:799–800.
49. Treasure T, Milosevic M, Fiorentino F, et al. Pulmonary metastasectomy: what is the practice and where is the evidence for effectiveness? Thorax 2014;69(10): 946–9.
50. Rehders A, Peiper M, Stoecklein NH, et al. Hepatic metastasectomy for soft-tissue sarcomas: is it justified? World J Surg 2009;33(1):111–7.
51. Sonett JR. Pulmonary metastases: biologic and historical justification for VATS. Video assisted thoracic surgery. Eur J Cardiothorac Surg 1999;16:13–5 [discussion: S15–6].
52. Blackmon SH, Shah N, Roth JA, et al. Resection of pulmonary and extrapulmonary sarcomatous metastases is associated with long-term survival. Ann Thorac Surg 2009;88:877–84 [discussion: 884–5].
53. Ferguson PC, Deheshi BM, Chung P, et al. Soft tissue sarcoma presenting with metastatic disease: outcome with primary surgical resection. Cancer 2011;117: 372–9.
54. Neri F, Ercolani G, Di Gioia P, et al. Liver metastases from non-gastrointestinal non-neuroendocrine tumours: review of the literature. Updates Surg 2015;67(3): 223–33.
55. Page AJ, Weiss MJ, Pawlik TM. Surgical management of noncolorectal cancer liver metastases. Cancer 2014;120(20):3111–21.
56. Adam R, Chiche L, Aloia T, et al. Hepatic resection for noncolorectal nonendocrine liver metastases. Ann Surg 2006;244:524–35.

57. Ercolani G, Grazi GL, Ravaioli M, et al. The role of liver resections for noncolorectal, nonneuroendocrine metastases: experience with 142 observed cases. Ann Surg Oncol 2005;12:459–66.

58. Lendoire J, Moro M, Andriani O, et al. Liver resection for non-colorectal, non-neuroendocrine metastases: analysis of a multicenter study from Argentina. HPB (Oxford) 2007;9:435–9.

59. Yedibela S, Gohl J, Graz V, et al. Changes in indication and results after resection of hepatic metastases from noncolorectal primary tumors: a single-institutional review. Ann Surg Oncol 2005;12:778–85.

60. Vij M, Perumalla R, Srivastava M, et al. Liver metastasis of extremity pleomorphic liposarcoma treated with hepatic resection. J Gastrointest Cancer 2014;45(Suppl 1):51–4.

61. Dematteo RP, Shah A, Fong Y, et al. Results of hepatic resection for sarcoma metastatic to liver. Ann Surg 2001;234(4):540–7 [discussion: 547–8].

62. Lang H, Nussbaum KT, Kaudel P, et al. Hepatic metastases from leiomyosarcoma a single-center experience with 34 liver resections during a 15-year period. Ann Surg 2000;231(4):500–5.

63. Marudanayagam R, Sandhu B, Perera MT, et al. Liver resection for metastatic soft tissue sarcoma: an analysis of prognostic factors. Eur J Surg Oncol 2011;37: 87–92.

64. Pawlik TM, Vauthey JN, Abdalla EK, et al. Results of a single-center experience with resection and ablation for sarcoma metastatic to the liver. Arch Surg 2006; 141(6):537–43 [discussion: 543–4].

65. Rusthoven KE, Kavanagh BD, Cardenes H, et al. Multi-institutional phase I/II trial of stereotactic body radiation therapy for liver metastases. J Clin Oncol 2009;27: 1572–8.

66. Rusthoven KE, Kavanagh BD, Burri SH, et al. Multi-institutional phase I/II trial of stereotactic body radiation therapy for lung metastases. J Clin Oncol 2009; 27(10):1579–84.

67. Fumagalli I, Bibault JE, Dewas S, et al. A single-institution study of stereotactic body radiotherapy for patients with unresectable visceral pulmonary or hepatic oligometastases. Radiat Oncol 2012;7:164.

68. Dhakal S, Corbin KS, Milano MT, et al. Stereotactic body radiotherapy for pulmonary metastases from soft-tissue sarcomas: excellent local lesion control and improved patient survival. Int J Radiat Oncol Biol Phys 2012;82:940–5.

69. Stragliotto CL, Karlsson K, Lax I, et al. A retrospective study of SBRT of metastases in patients with primary sarcoma. Med Oncol 2012;29:3431–9.

70. Palussière J, Italiano A, Descat E, et al. Sarcoma lung metastases treated with percutaneous radiofrequency ablation: results from 29 patients. Ann Surg Oncol 2011;18:3771–7.

71. Nakamura T, Matsumine A, Yamakado K, et al. Lung radiofrequency ablation in patients with pulmonary metastases from musculoskeletal sarcomas [corrected]. Cancer 2009;115:3774–81.

Index

Note: Page numbers of article titles are in **boldface** type.

UNITED STATES POSTAL SERVICE® Statement of Ownership, Management, and Circulation (All Periodicals Publications Except Requester Publications)

1. Publication Title	2. Publication Number	3. Filing Date
SURGICAL CLINICS OF NORTH AMERICA	529 – 800	9/18/2016

4. Issue Frequency	5. Number of Issues Published Annually	6. Annual Subscription Price
FEB, APR, JUN, AUG, OCT, DEC	6	$370.00

7. Complete Mailing Address of Known Office of Publication (Not printer) (Street, city, county, state, and ZIP+4®)

ELSEVIER INC.
360 PARK AVENUE SOUTH
NEW YORK, NY 10010-1710

Contact Person
STEPHEN R. BUSHING

Telephone (Include area code)
215-239-3688

8. Complete Mailing Address of Headquarters or General Business Office of Publisher (Not printer)

ELSEVIER INC.
360 PARK AVENUE SOUTH
NEW YORK, NY 10010-1710

9. Full Names and Complete Mailing Addresses of Publisher, Editor, and Managing Editor (Do not leave blank)

Publisher (Name and complete mailing address)

LINDA BELFUS, ELSEVIER INC.
1600 JOHN F KENNEDY BLVD. SUITE 1800
PHILADELPHIA, PA 19103-2899

Editor (Name and complete mailing address)

JOHN VASSALLO, ELSEVIER INC.
1600 JOHN F KENNEDY BLVD. SUITE 1800
PHILADELPHIA, PA 19103-2899

Managing Editor (Name and complete mailing address)

ADRIANNE BRIGIDO, ELSEVIER INC.
1600 JOHN F KENNEDY BLVD. SUITE 1800
PHILADELPHIA, PA 19103-2899

10. Owner (Do not leave blank. If the publication is owned by a corporation, give the name and address of the corporation immediately followed by the names and addresses of all stockholders owning or holding 1 percent or more of the total amount of stock. If not owned by a corporation, give the names and addresses of the individual owners. If owned by a partnership or other unincorporated firm, give its name and address as well as those of each individual owner. If the publication is published by a nonprofit organization, give its name and address.)

Full Name	Complete Mailing Address
WHOLLY OWNED SUBSIDIARY OF REED/ELSEVIER, US HOLDINGS	1600 JOHN F KENNEDY BLVD. SUITE 1800 PHILADELPHIA, PA 19103-2899

11. Known Bondholders, Mortgagees, and Other Security Holders Owning or Holding 1 Percent or More of Total Amount of Bonds, Mortgages, or Other Securities. If none, check box ► ☐ None

Full Name	Complete Mailing Address
N/A	

12. Tax Status (For completion by nonprofit organizations authorized to mail at nonprofit rates) (Check one)
The purpose, function, and nonprofit status of this organization and the exempt status for federal income tax purposes:
☐ Has Not Changed During Preceding 12 Months
☐ Has Changed During Preceding 12 Months (Publisher must submit explanation of change with this statement)

13. Publication Title	14. Issue Date for Circulation Data Below
SURGICAL CLINICS OF NORTH AMERICA	JUNE 2016

15. Extent and Nature of Circulation			Average No. Copies Each Issue During Preceding 12 Months	No. Copies of Single Issue Published Nearest to Filing Date
a. Total Number of Copies (Net press run)			861	852
b. Paid Circulation (By Mail and Outside the Mail)	(1)	Mailed Outside-County Paid Subscriptions Stated on PS Form 3541 (Include paid distribution above nominal rate, advertiser's proof copies, and exchange copies)	284	351
	(2)	Mailed In-County Paid Subscriptions Stated on PS Form 3541 (Include paid distribution above nominal rate, advertiser's proof copies, and exchange copies)	0	0
	(3)	Paid Distribution Outside the Mails Including Sales Through Dealers and Carriers, Street Vendors, Counter Sales, and Other Paid Distribution Outside USPS®	271	371
	(4)	Paid Distribution by Other Classes of Mail Through the USPS (e.g., First-Class Mail®)	0	0
c. Total Paid Distribution (Sum of 15b (1), (2), (3), and (4))		►	555	722
d. Free or Nominal Rate Distribution (By Mail and Outside the Mail)	(1)	Free or Nominal Rate Outside-County Copies Included on PS Form 3541	30	110
	(2)	Free or Nominal Rate In-County Copies Included on PS Form 3541	0	0
	(3)	Free or Nominal Rate Copies Mailed at Other Classes Through the USPS (e.g., First-Class Mail)	0	0
	(4)	Free or Nominal Rate Distribution Outside the Mail (Carriers or other means)	0	0
e. Total Free or Nominal Rate Distribution (Sum of 15d (1), (2), (3) and (4))		►	30	110
f. Total Distribution (Sum of 15c and 15e)		►	585	832
g. Copies not Distributed (See Instructions to Publishers #4 (page #3))		►	276	20
h. Total (Sum of 15f and g)		►	861	852
i. Percent Paid (15c divided by 15f times 100)			95%	87%

* If you are claiming electronic copies, go to line 16 on page 3. If you are not claiming electronic copies, skip to line 17 on page 3.

16. Electronic Copy Circulation	Average No. Copies Each Issue During Preceding 12 Months	No. Copies of Single Issue Published Nearest to Filing Date
a. Paid Electronic Copies ►	0	0
b. Total Paid Print Copies (Line 15c) + Paid Electronic Copies (Line 16a) ►	555	722
c. Total Print Distribution (Line 15f) + Paid Electronic Copies (Line 16a) ►	585	832
d. Percent Paid (Both Print & Electronic Copies) (16b divided by 16c × 100) ►	95%	87%

☒ I certify that 50% of all my distributed copies (electronic and print) are paid above a nominal price.

17. Publication of Statement of Ownership

☒ If the publication is a general publication, publication of this statement is required. Will be printed ☐ Publication not required.
in the OCTOBER 2016 issue of this publication.

18. Signature and Title of Editor, Publisher, Business Manager, or Owner

STEPHEN R. BUSHING - INVENTORY DISTRIBUTION CONTROL MANAGER

Date 9/18/2016

I certify that all information furnished on this form is true and complete. I understand that anyone who furnishes false or misleading information on this form or who omits material or information requested on the form may be subject to criminal sanctions (including fines and imprisonment) and/or civil sanctions (including civil penalties).

PS Form 3526, July 2014 (Page 3 of 4)

PRIVACY NOTICE: See our privacy policy on www.usps.com.

PS Form 3526, July 2014 [Page 1 of 4 (see instructions page 4)] PSN 7530-01-000-9631   PRIVACY NOTICE: See our privacy policy on www.usps.com.

Moving?

Make sure your subscription moves with you!

To notify us of your new address, find your **Clinics Account Number** (located on your mailing label above your name), and contact customer service at:

Email: journalscustomerservice-usa@elsevier.com

800-654-2452 (subscribers in the U.S. & Canada)
314-447-8871 (subscribers outside of the U.S. & Canada)

Fax number: 314-447-8029

Elsevier Health Sciences Division
Subscription Customer Service
3251 Riverport Lane
Maryland Heights, MO 63043

*To ensure uninterrupted delivery of your subscription, please notify us at least 4 weeks in advance of move.

Printed and bound by CPI Group (UK) Ltd, Croydon, CR0 4YY

07/10/2024

01040500-0008